AF776368

Current Cancer Treatment

Edited by Mirjana Rajer and Eva Segelov

Published in London, United Kingdom

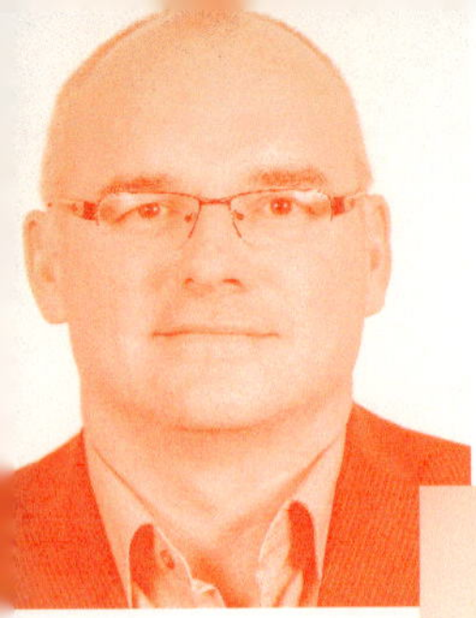
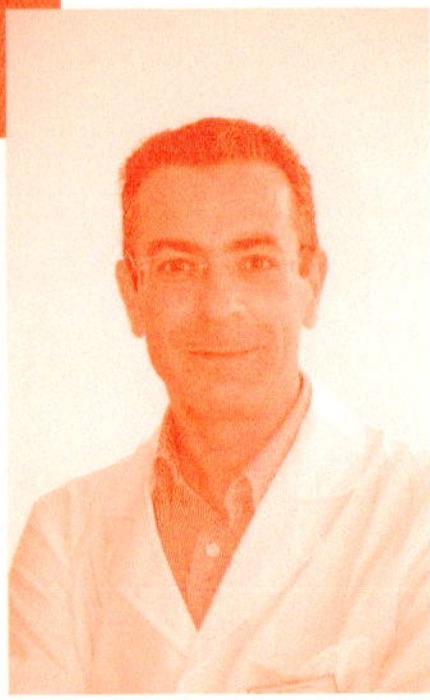
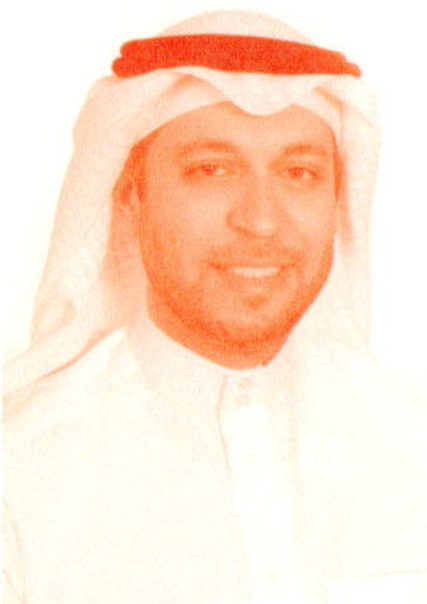
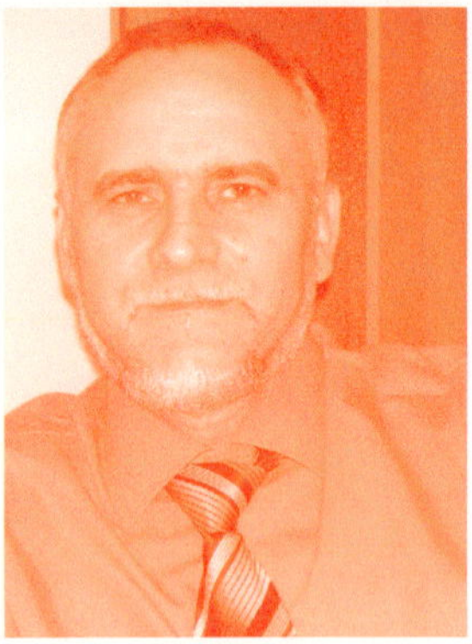
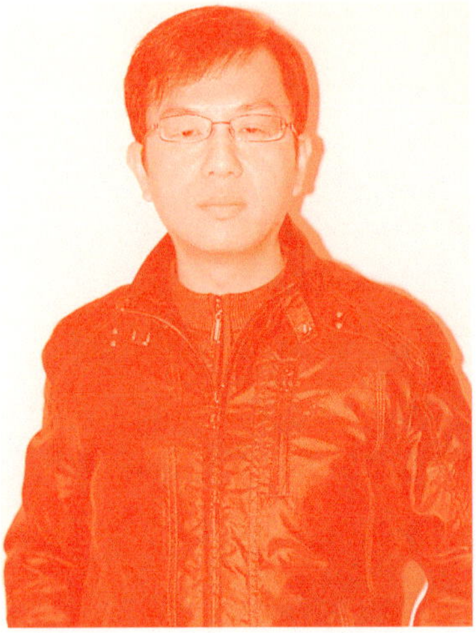
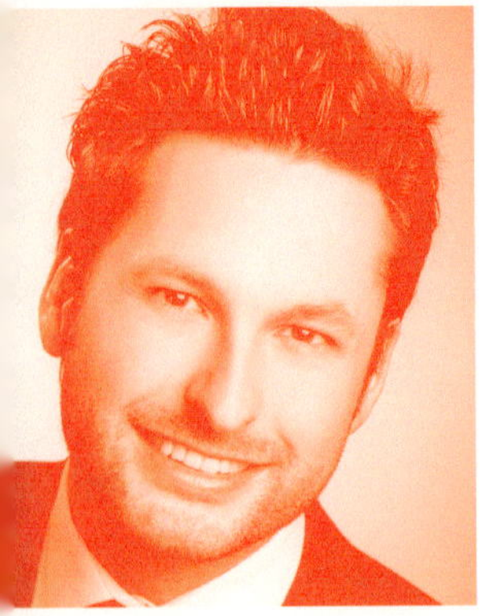
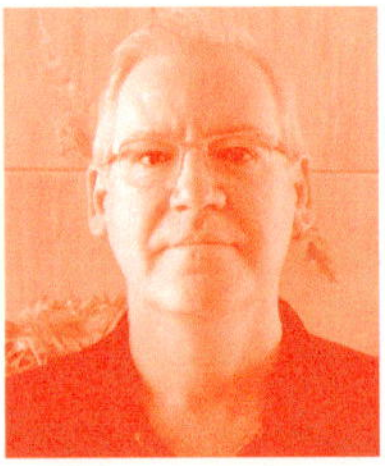

IntechOpen

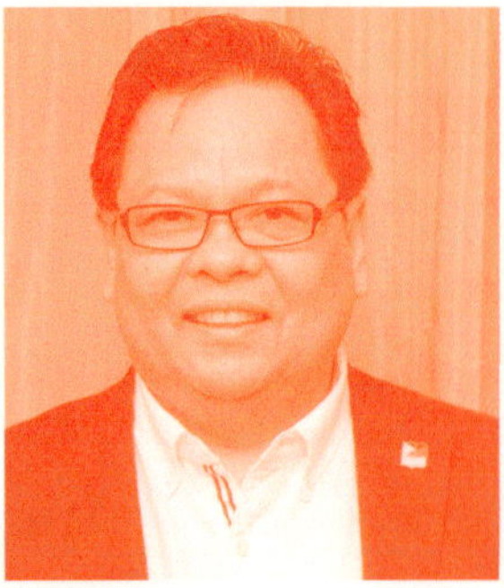
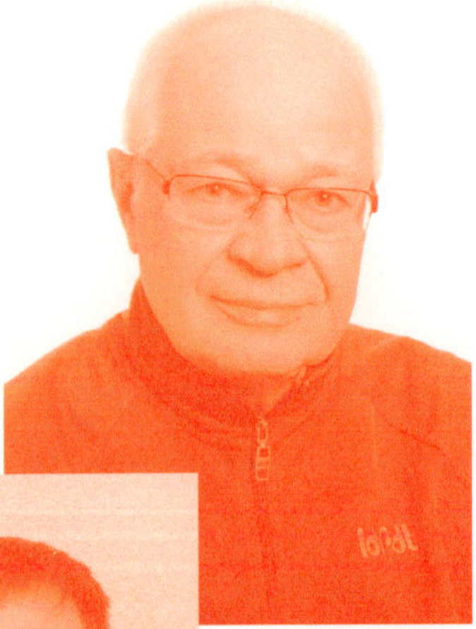
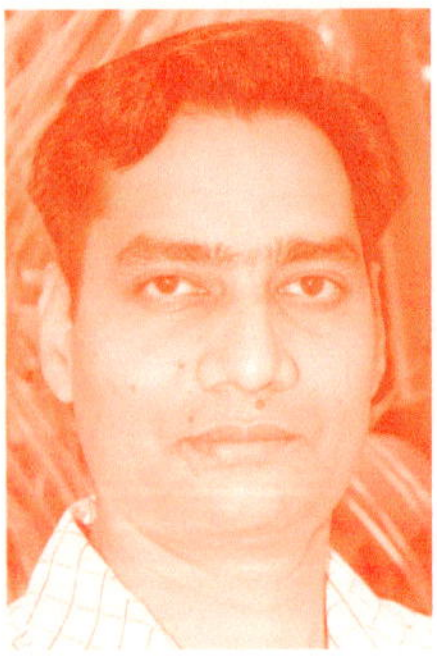
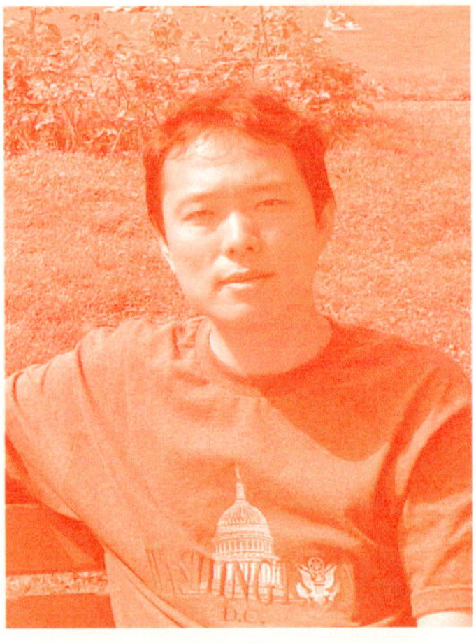
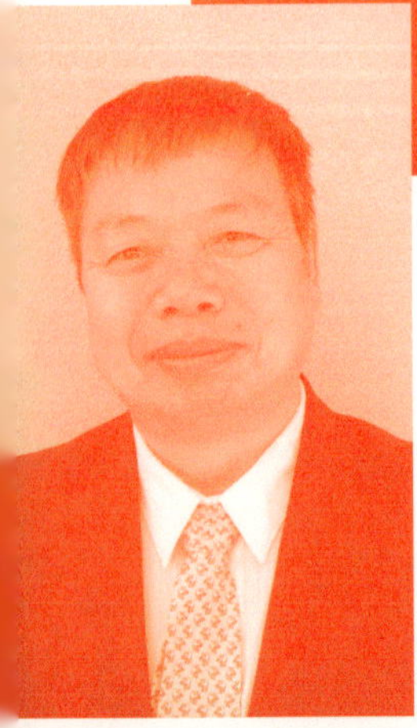
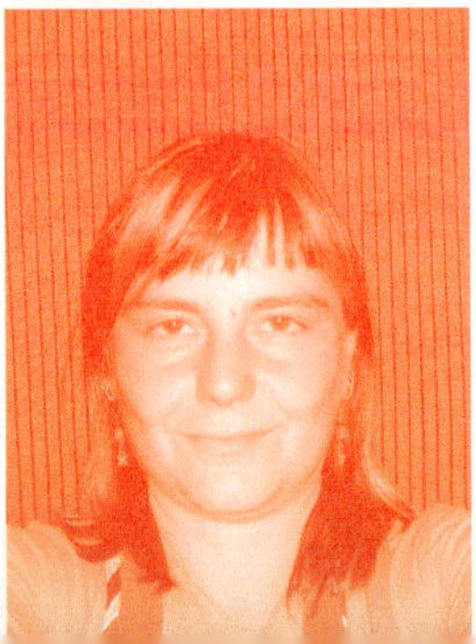

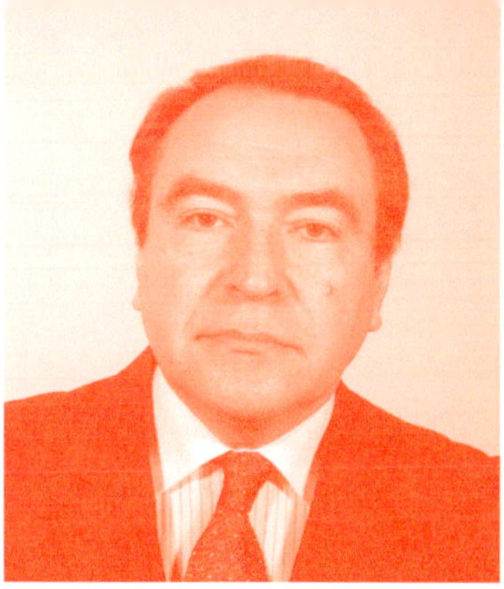

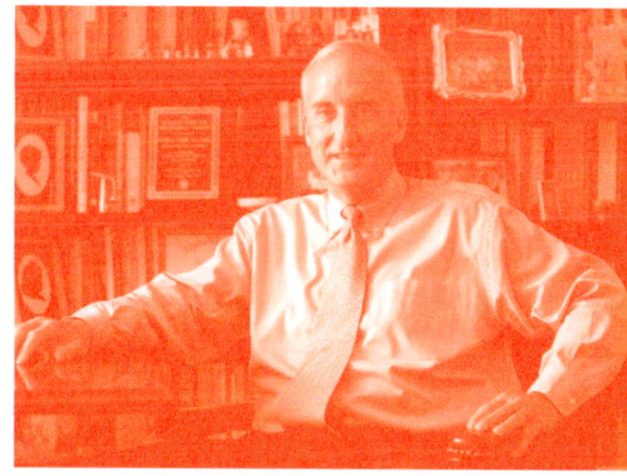

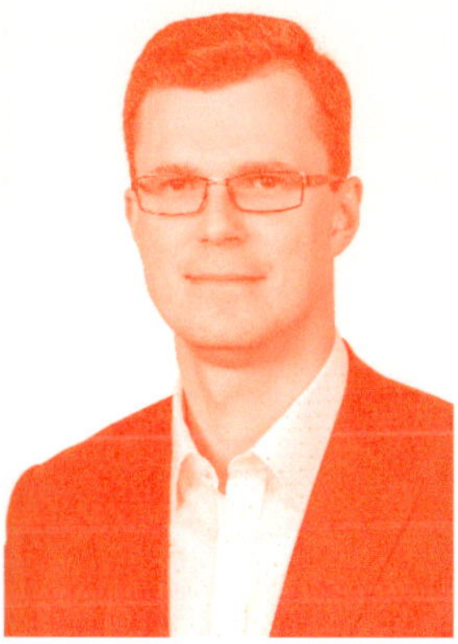

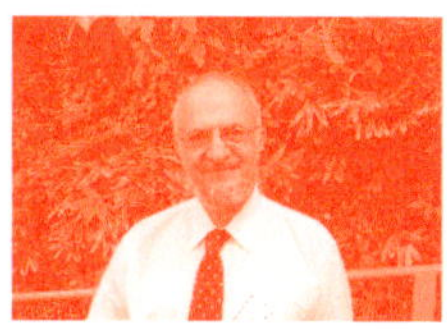

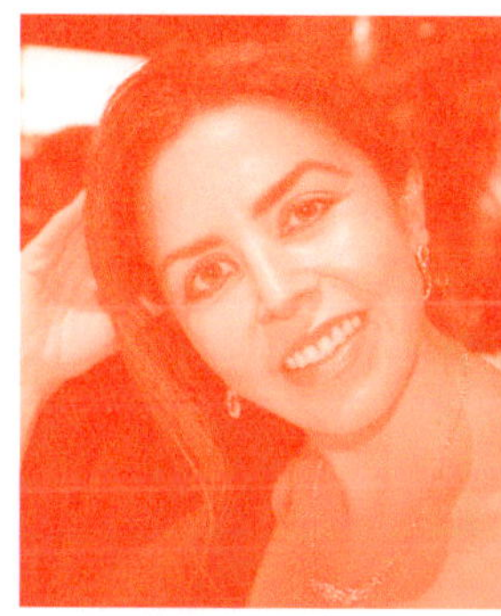

Supporting open minds since 2005

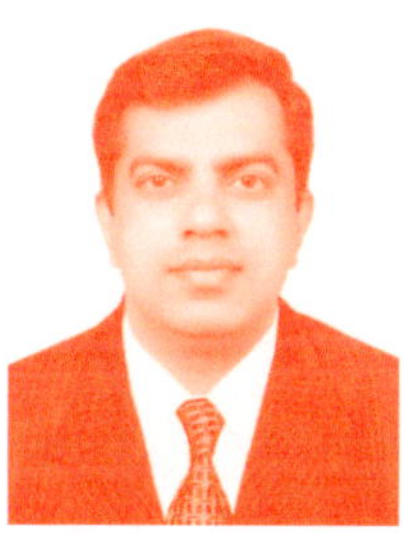

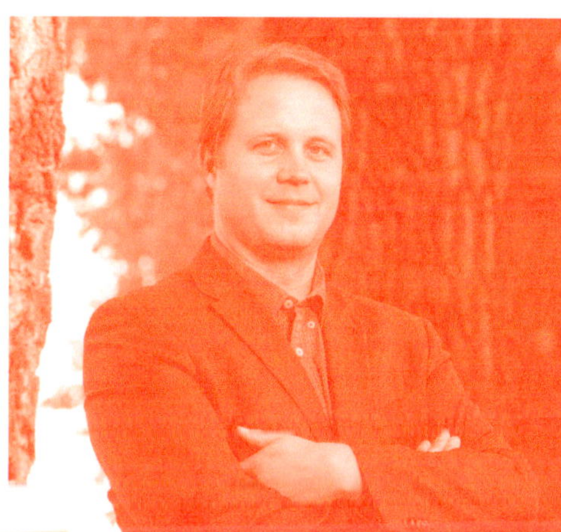

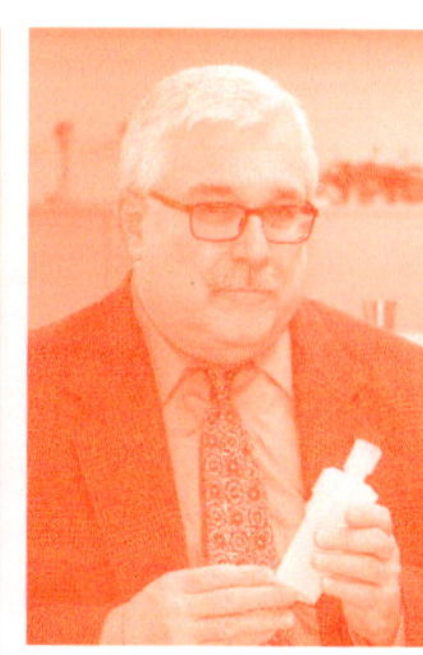

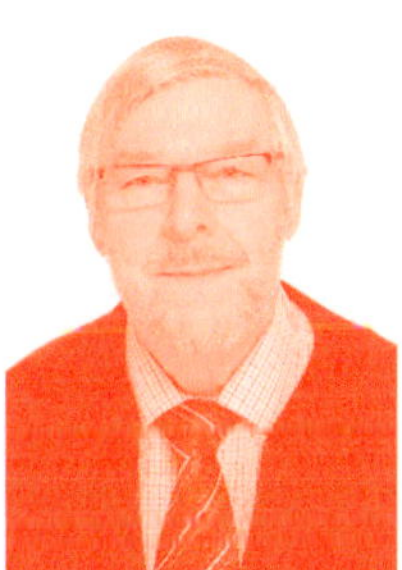

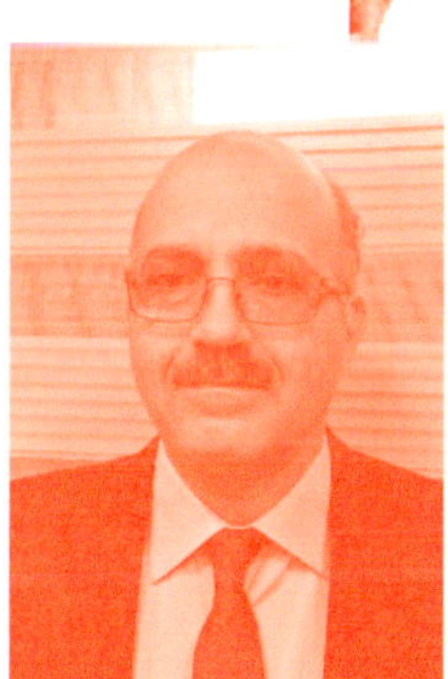

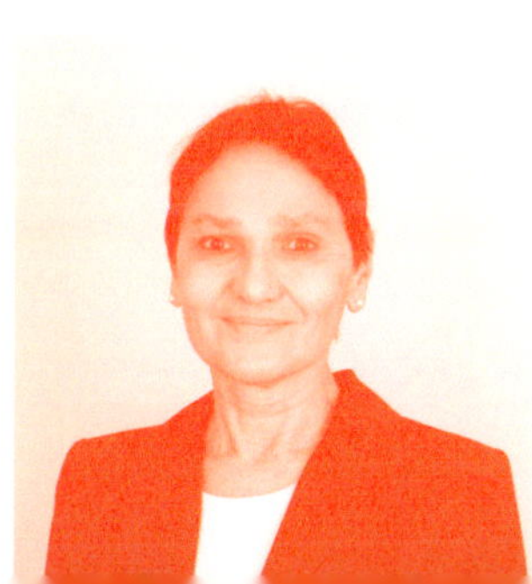

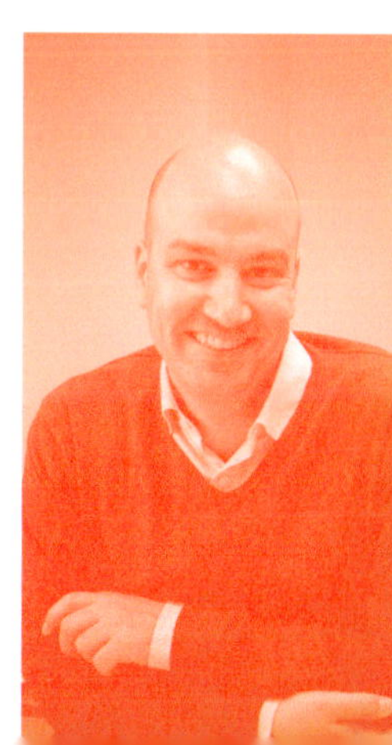

Current Cancer Treatment
http://dx.doi.org/10.5772/intechopen.83168
Edited by Mirjana Rajer and Eva Segelov

Contributors
Sumaira Kousar, Ayesha Siddiqua, Nusrat Shafiq, Amer Jamil, Sophia Frentzas, Ting-Yu Chen, Caroline Lum, Estelle M. Peyroux, Sharon T. Pattison, Silke Neumann, Matt J. Woodall, Sarah L. Young, Nick J. Shields, Deepti Sharma, Neha Sharma, Ee Shan Pang, Christophe Macri, Meredith O'Keeffe, Timothy Patton, Mariam Bafit, Begoña Díaz De La Noval, Fan Xu, Jie Chen, Liqiong Yang, Yuxi Duan, Tingting Pu, Sha Zheng, Fangfang Liu, Kun Huang, Greg Mirt, Riaz Tabassum, Tariq Mehmood

© The Editor(s) and the Author(s) 2020
The rights of the editor(s) and the author(s) have been asserted in accordance with the Copyright, Designs and Patents Act 1988. All rights to the book as a whole are reserved by INTECHOPEN LIMITED. The book as a whole (compilation) cannot be reproduced, distributed or used for commercial or non-commercial purposes without INTECHOPEN LIMITED's written permission. Enquiries concerning the use of the book should be directed to INTECHOPEN LIMITED rights and permissions department (permissions@intechopen.com).
Violations are liable to prosecution under the governing Copyright Law.

CC BY

Individual chapters of this publication are distributed under the terms of the Creative Commons Attribution 3.0 Unported License which permits commercial use, distribution and reproduction of the individual chapters, provided the original author(s) and source publication are appropriately acknowledged. If so indicated, certain images may not be included under the Creative Commons license. In such cases users will need to obtain permission from the license holder to reproduce the material. More details and guidelines concerning content reuse and adaptation can be found at http://www.intechopen.com/copyright-policy.html.

Notice
Statements and opinions expressed in the chapters are these of the individual contributors and not necessarily those of the editors or publisher. No responsibility is accepted for the accuracy of information contained in the published chapters. The publisher assumes no responsibility for any damage or injury to persons or property arising out of the use of any materials, instructions, methods or ideas contained in the book.

First published in London, United Kingdom, 2020 by IntechOpen
IntechOpen is the global imprint of INTECHOPEN LIMITED, registered in England and Wales, registration number: 11086078, 7th floor, 10 Lower Thames Street, London, EC3R 6AF, United Kingdom
Printed in Croatia

British Library Cataloguing-in-Publication Data
A catalogue record for this book is available from the British Library

Additional hard and PDF copies can be obtained from orders@intechopen.com

Current Cancer Treatment
Edited by Mirjana Rajer and Eva Segelov
p. cm.
Print ISBN 978-1-78985-967-6
Online ISBN 978-1-78985-968-3
eBook (PDF) ISBN 978-1-83880-998-0

For EU product safety concerns:
IN TECH d.o.o., Prolaz Marije Krucifikse Kozulić 3, 51000 Rijeka, Croatia, info@intechopen.com or visit our website at intechopen.com.

We are IntechOpen, the world's leading publisher of Open Access books

Built by scientists, for scientists

4,900+
Open access books available

123,000+
International authors and editors

140M+
Downloads

151
Countries delivered to

Our authors are among the
Top 1%
most cited scientists

12.2%
Contributors from top 500 universities

BOOK CITATION INDEX
CLARIVATE ANALYTICS
INDEXED

WEB OF SCIENCE™

Selection of our books indexed in the Book Citation Index
in Web of Science™ Core Collection (BKCI)

Interested in publishing with us?
Contact book.department@intechopen.com

Numbers displayed above are based on latest data collected.
For more information visit www.intechopen.com

Meet the editors

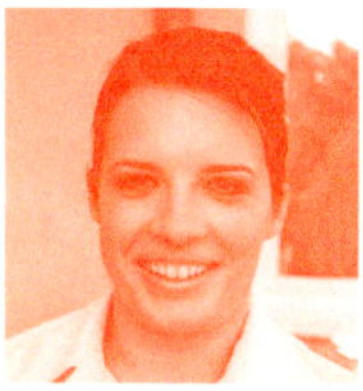

Assistant Professor Mirjana Rajer, MD, PhD, graduated from the Faculty of Medicine at the University of Ljubljana in 2001. For two years, she worked at the University Clinic Golnik, Slovenia. Currently, she works at the Institute of Oncology Ljubljana. Her main clinical work consists of treatment of lung cancer and mesothelioma patients. She is also involved as principal and co-investigator in several clinical trials of lung cancer, palliative care, and communication with cancer patients. She serves as an editor for national and international journals and is author of numerous published papers, book chapters, and books. Being a student mentor, Dr. Rajer is actively involved in education. She is an active member of the European Organisation for Research and Treatment of Cancer (EORTC), European Society for Medical Oncology (ESMO), *International Association for the Study of Lung Cancer* (IASLC), and the Central European Initiative against Lung Cancer.

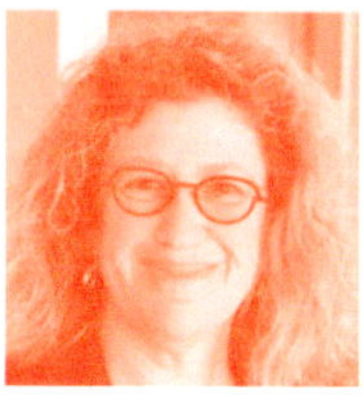

Eva Segelov, MBBS, PhD, FRACP, is Professor of Medicine at Monash University and Director of Oncology at Monash Health, Melbourne, Australia. She is a practicing medical oncologist with more than 20 years' experience, specializing in gastrointestinal cancer and neuroendocrine tumors, with an international reputation in clinical trials and translational research. Professor Segelov is a board member of the Australasian Gastrointestinal Trials Group; Gastrointestinal Chair of the Clinical Oncology Society of Australia; European Society of Medical Oncology faculty member for the CUP, Endocrine Tumours, and Others group; co-founder of the Commonwealth Neuroendocrine Tumour Society (CommNETS); Associate Editor of *Journal of Global Oncology* and a cancer editor for the *Journal of Visualized Experiments*. She heads a translational research laboratory specializing in interrogating clinical trial biospecimens. Professor Segelov has published more than 150 articles, expert reviews and book chapters and is a frequent invited speaker at national and international conferences. She is a member of the Australasian L'Oréal-UNESCO for Women in Science jury.

Contents

Preface

Cancer is the leading cause of death worldwide, and as such, research in this field remains one of the most important healthcare priorities. This book elucidates some of the new concepts in cancer research, including basic science and open questions in cancer treatment. Chapters cover a broad spectrum of currently very relevant topics, from biomarkers and immunotherapy to some unanswered questions in everyday clinical practice. Biomarkers are extremely important tools for early detection and prediction of cancer prognosis and response to therapeutic interventions. Authors comment on the value of miRNA as a biomarker, which seems to be a new and very promising one. In addition to biomarkers, two other hot topics are covered: angiogenesis and immunotherapy. There are many open questions regarding treatment with these two modalities. Angiogenesis has been a target for quite a few years, but there are still issues to address such as non-optimal therapeutic scenarios, lack of biomarkers and poor understanding of mechanisms of resistance. In recent years, immunotherapy has become one of the cornerstones of cancer treatment. Chapters describe both angiogenesis and immunotherapy as well as examine the influence of gastrointestinal microenvironement and the role of dendritic cells. Regarding cancer treatment, the recent trend is to try to deescalate treatment intensity and to spare patients avoidable side effects, of course with the same oncological results. Sentinel node biopsy for uterine cancer, as described in this book, is an important step toward this goal. Finally, the book addresses pediatric central nervous system tumors, which are the second most common childhood tumors, and reviews current treatment options and efforts to reduce morbidity and mortality.

I would like to thank all the authors and my co-editor, Prof. Eva Sgelov. They accomplished an excellent task. It was a privilege collaborating with them. I sincerely hope that this book will help readers, leading them to new horizons of cancer care and enlightening them to generate new research ideas.

Mirjana Rajer, MD, PhD
Assistant Professor,
Institute of Oncology Ljubljana,
Ljubljana, Slovenia

Eva Segelov
Professor,
MBBS (Hons 1) PhD FRACP,
Professor/Director of Oncology,
Monash Health and Monash University,
Australia
Board Member, Australasian Gastrointestinal Trials Group (AGITG)
Co-Founder, Commonwealth Neuroendocrine Tumour Collaboration
(CommNETS)

Section 1

Basic Science

Chapter 1

MicroRNA: A Signature for Cancer Diagnostics

Ayesha Siddiqua, Sumaira Kousar, Amer Jamil, Riaz Tabassum, Tariq Mehmood and Nusrat Shafiq

Abstract

Various tools and techniques are being used for the diagnosis of cancer, but not a sole technique provides powerful result at the very early stages of cancer. This provides the need for type of tools which could detect cancer at early stages so that survival rate could be augmented. There are various diagnostic ways to identify cancer, but in each case, there are always circumstances to compromise on the sensitivity. In this framework, a new and more advanced approach of diagnosis for cancer is microRNA (miRNA). miRNAs are conserved regions among humans and animals, and their synthesis takes place in the nucleus and cytoplasm. There are several types of microRNAs that could be upregulated and downregulated in various cancers. A cancer cell could be identified by measurement of the expression pattern of miRNA. By examining the expression level for different types of cancers, miRNA can be used as biomarker for early detection of cancer in human beings.

Keywords: microRNA, cancer biomarker, diagnostic, colorectal, upregulation, downregulation, breast cancer, cervical, liver, prostate

1. Introduction

MicroRNAs (miRNAs) are a small, non-coding, single-stranded RNA consisting of around 22 nucleotides [1]. More than 3% of the human genome (gene portion) encodes for microRNA, and their number is around 1000 [2–4]. This small RNA can regulate gene expression posttranscriptionally [5–7]. This small RNA can regulate gene expression posttranscriptionally by binding to its cognate RNA target at the 3^0 untranslated region (UTR) [8–11]. A small microRNA was discovered for the first time in *C. elegans* and is encoded by the Lin-4 gene [12] providing evidence for its evolutionary conservation. This conserved microRNA was found to be involved in many important biological processes including cell proliferation, growth, apoptosis, etc. [13, 14], and many cell-based factors have been known to regulate its expression [15]. The genes transcribing the miRNA are considered to belong to the set of tumor suppressor genes, and the serum level of miRNA can be detected [16, 17]. There are certain miRNAs that can behave as either oncomiRs (whose expression can cause the cancer) or tumor suppressor depending on the context "Several miRNAs cannot be clearly and unequivocally categorized as tumor suppressors or oncomiRs because data in our hands are quite intricate and conflicting since they could act as tumor suppressors in one scenario or as oncomiRs in the other" [18].

IntechOpen

2. Synthesis/biogenesis of miRNA

Synthesis of miRNA takes place in the nucleus as well as in the cytoplasm. Genes encoding miRNAs are present in the form of a cluster and contain introns (**Figure 1**). These genes are transcribed by polymerase II with the generation of the primary precursor pri-miRNA. This precursor miRNA consists of a 3′ poly-A tail and a 5′ end cap [19, 20] with a stem-loop structure. RNase 3 Drosha cleaves this structure with the help of its Pasha cofactor DGCR8. This resultant cleaved, precursor structure is known as pre-miRNA and consists of ~70–90 nucleotides [21]. This ~70 nt precursor is exported to the cytoplasm by Exportin-5.

In the cytoplasm, the whole pri-miRNA is recruited by a RNA-induced silencing complex (RISC) and is converted into mature miRNA. These are mediated by an RISC leaching complex (RLS), which is basically a multiprotein complex and consists of a double-stranded RNA domain protein (DICER), tar RNA-binding protein (TARB), and the Ago 2 protein. The RNAse 3 DICER along with its cofactor yields duplex miRNA (19–25 nucleotide duplex miRNA with 2 nucleotide overhangs at each 3′end). During the process of cleavage, two strands are formed, namely, a functional and a passenger strand. The functional strand along with the Ago protein (RISC) is involved in gene silencing function, while the passenger strand is degraded due to its instability. This miRISC incorporates one strand of miRNA (functional strand and guide strand) so that it takes the guidance from this complex to target mRNA (complementary) for its degradation or inhibition at the translational level [22]. miRNA is processed in the cytosol and transported to the blood. It is resistant to degradation because it is carried by complexes of lipoprotein inclusions [23] or in the form of exosomes [24, 25].

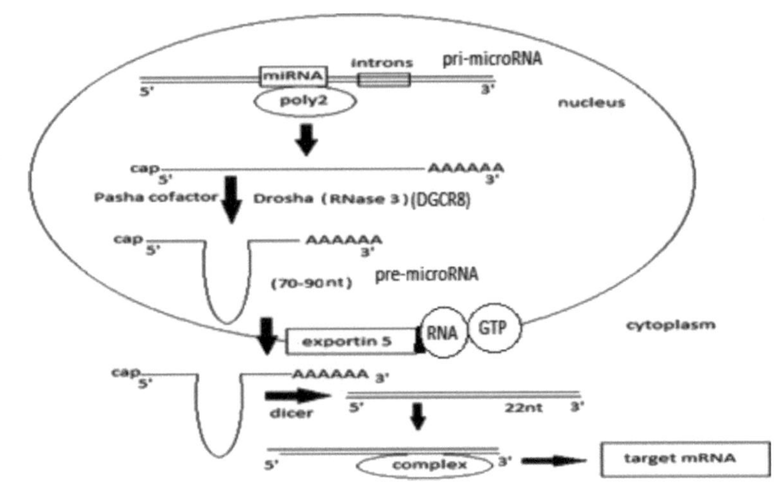

Figure 1.
Biogenesis of microRNA.

3. Mechanism of action

The mechanism of action of microRNA is such that it binds to its partial complementary sequence in the target mRNA (that codes for protein). Hence, the expression is repressed (**Figure 2**) and no product is synthesized [7].

In another scenario, the microRNA may bind to the complementary sequence of target mRNA that codes for protein and initiates RNA-mediated gene silencing, with the resultant cleavage of the target RNA (**Figure 3**) [26].

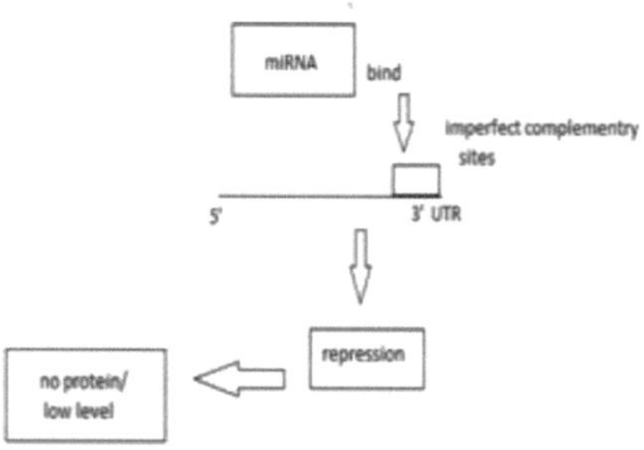

Figure 2.
Mechanism of action of miRNA.

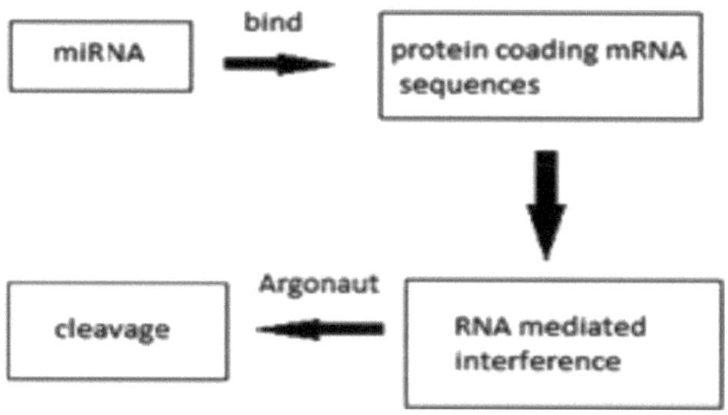

Figure 3.
Mechanism of miRNA.

4. Diagnosis of cancer

There are reported differences in the expression pattern of miRNA in normal and cancer cells [27]. Some miRNAs are overexpressed, while the others are downregulated in different kinds of cancers [28]. Due to its small size and resistance to RNase-mediated degradation, they have the potential as powerful biomarkers for cancer diagnosis [29]. miRNA expression is involved with the rearrangement of chromosomes, methylation of the promoter region, and transcriptional regulation. miRNA-mediated aberrations in one or more of these processes can culminate in alterations in protein and mRNA expression [30].

5. Types of miRNA and cancer according to organs

Different miRNAs are involved in different types of cancers:

5.1 Breast cancer

Breast cancer is the most prevalent form of cancer in women. Among 12.7 million cancer cases globally, breast cancer is most frequently diagnosed, that is, 23 and 14% deaths due to breast cancer have been reported [1, 31]. The alarmingly increasing mortality data coupled with increases in relapses warrants an improved molecular understanding of the etiology and mechanistic details that contribute to the chemoresistance. There are four subtypes (intrinsic) of breast cancer. These are $ErbB2^+$ (epidermal growth factor receptor 2-positive (also called HER2)), luminal A (hormone receptor positive for estrogen and progesterone, HER2), luminal B (hormone receptor positive for estrogen and progesterone and positive or negative for HER2), and basal like (hormone receptors negative for estrogen, progesterone, and HER2) showing its heterogeneity. Many of the microRNAs play a role in the inhibition of breast cancer. The upregulation of miR-21 (**Table 1**) results in the increased expression of BCL-2 protein and chemoresistance in breast cancer [38]. MiR-125b shows the resistance to chemotherapeutic agents 5-fluorouracil, and it has higher expression in the patients that are nonresponsive to this agent (**Table 2**). Many promote the prognosis of breast cancer by targeting the tumor suppressor at the gene level and activating the transcriptional factors that are oncogenic in nature [32, 38].

The Rab protein is a member of the Ras superfamily (**Figure 4**). This protein is a G-protein-coupled receptor and is involved in many cellular processes including fusion, budding, synthesis of vesicles, and motility [55]. A member of the Rab class is Rab11a, and this protein has many functions including cellular migration and phagocytosis [56]. In breast cancer there is overexpression of Rab11a protein [57] and is regulated by miRNA 320a. This miRNA can downregulate Rab11a protein, thereby mediating the inhibition of breast cancer progression.

MiR-320a has an important role in tumor suppression [58] and can be a biomarker for breast cancer. This miR-320a results in a 15% increase of cells in G0/G1,

Sr. no.	MicroRNAs	Potential targets	Function	Ref.
1	miR-10b	Homeobox D10	Promotes cellular invasion, migration, and metastasis by targeting the RhoC	[32]
2	miR-21	Programmed cell death protein 4, hypoxia-inducible factor-1α	Promotes cellular invasion, metastasis, epithelial-to-mesenchymal transition and migration	
		Phosphatase and tensin homolog, programmed cell death protein 4, tropomyosin 1	Promotes cellular invasion	[33]
		Metalloproteinase inhibitor 3	Promotes cellular invasion	[34]
3	miR-155 (chemosensitive determinant by targeting the FOXO3)	Suppressor of cytokine signaling 1	Promotes cell proliferation and growth	[35]
		Tumor protein p53 inducible nuclear protein	Promotes cell proliferation	[36]
		Forkhead box protein O3	Promotes cell proliferation and cell survival	[37, 38]
4	miR-373	CD44 (inversely correlated)	Promotes cellular invasion and migration	[39]
			Promotes cellular invasion and metastasis	[40]
5	miR-520c		Promotes cellular migration, invasion, and metastasis	[39]

Meta-analysis or Cochrane reviews documenting the involvement of a specific miRNA or a battery of miRNAs contributing to relapse or recurrence can be displayed as a separate table for each of the cancers.

Table 1.
MicroRNAs upregulating the breast cancer.

Sr. no.	MicroRNAs	Potential targets	Function	Ref.
1	miR-125b	Erythropoietin, erythropoietin receptors (positive correlation with ERBB2/HER2 expression)	Inhibition of cellular differentiation and proliferation	[41]
		Glutamyl aminopeptidase or aminopeptidase A, casein kinase 2-alpha, cyclin J, multiple EGF-like domains 9	Inhibition of cellular proliferation	[42]
		Receptor tyrosine-protein kinase erbB-2 (human epidermal growth factor receptor 2) (induction of miR cause the downregulation of ERBB2/ ERBB3)	Inhibition of invasion and migration	[43, 44]
2	miR-205	High-mobility group box 3 gene	Suppression of invasion and proliferation	[45, 46]
3	miR-17-92	Mitogen-activated protein kinase kinase kinase 2	Promotes the antitumoral activity of natural killer cells and reduction in metastasis	[47]
4	miR-206	Cyclin D2, connexin 43	Reduction in invasion, migration, and metastasis	[48]
5	miR-200	Zinc finger E-box binding homeobox 1/2, snail family zinc finger ½	Reduction in tumor growth, EMT through E-cadherin, and metastasis	[49]
6	miR-146b	Nuclear factor kappa B, signal transducer, and activator of transcription 3	Reduction in survival and metastasis via interleukin 6	[50]
7	miR-126	Insulin-like growth factor-binding protein 2, c-Mer tyrosine kinase, phosphatidylinositol transfer protein, cytoplasmic 1	Reduction in angiogenesis and metastasis	[51]
8	miR-335	SRY-related HMG-box 4, tenascin C	Suppression in migration and metastasis	[52]
9	miR-31	Ras homolog gene family	Targets various steps of metastasis and invasion for inhibition	[38]
		WAS protein family, member 3, Ras homolog gene family	Reduction in the metastasis and progression of cancer	[53]
		WAS protein family, member 3	Reduction in the metastasis and progression of cancer	[54]

Table 2.
MicroRNAs downregulating the breast cancer.

and the population of cells in the S phase is decreased. Apart from the G0/G1 cell cycle arrest, miR-320a also increases the activity of caspase resulting in the induction of apoptosis [59]. The potential target of miR-20 is Rab11a; it has two binding sites at the 3′UTR region for miR-320a and can mediate its posttranscriptional repression. This protein is also necessary for the activation of Akt via phosphatidylinositol-4-kinase (PI4K3) in breast cancer—a pro-survival signal [60]. Further, overexpression of Rab11a protein results in the reversal of cell cycle arrest and apoptosis mediated by miR-320a by targeting the MTDH at 3′UTR [61]. The gene coding for the Rab coupling protein (RCP) (a Rab11-FIP1C (Rab coupling protein))

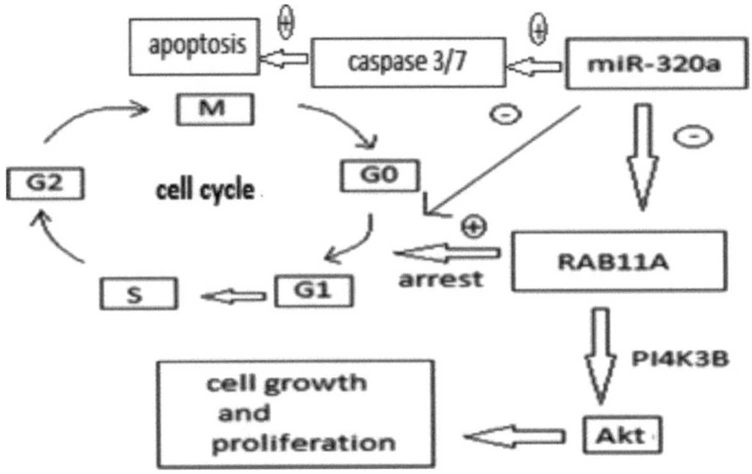

Figure 4.
MicroRNA and breast cancer.

is amplified in breast cancer and aids in the sorting of epidermal growth factor receptor (EGFR) [62, 63]. For the metastasis or migration of cancer, the cell critical factor is RCP which mediates this effect via cell surface integrin alpha-5-beta-1 demonstrating that Rab11a is a protein that is involved in the metastatic or invasive phenotype of breast cancer [64, 65].

5.2 Colorectal cancer

Colorectal cancer is the third most common cancer around the world. The incidence rate is increased up to 6% [66]. Survival rate can increase to 90%, if it is diagnosed at an early stage. Survival rate is inversely proportional to the stage of cancer [67].

In a study, the cluster of miR-17/miR-92 (chromosomal region 13q31.1 with miR-20a as one of its members). The region encompassing this cluster is under the regulation of the oncogenic Myc transcriptional factor and TGF-β [68, 69]. Overexpression converts a benign tumor to colorectal cancer [70].

Mir-20 acts as a potential colorectal cancer cell biomarker [71]. Induction of miR-20-mediated EMT is a critical factor contributing to the increases in tumor cell migration, metastasis, E-cadherin downregulation, and upregulation of matrix metalloproteinases (**Figure 5**) [72, 73]. This microRNA can cause a delay in TGF-β-mediated G1/S transition. However, cell cycle progression occurs due to an inactivating mutation in this pathway [74]. Normal TGF-β-mediated signaling can be a cytostatic response and inhibit tumorigenicity in colorectal cancer cells [75].

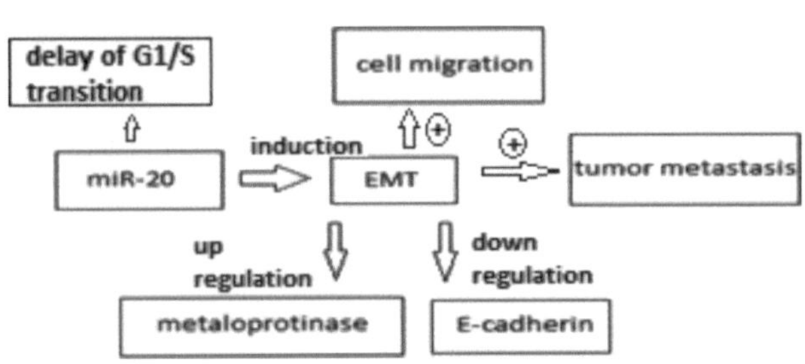

Figure 5.
MicroRNA and colorectal cancer.

miR-20 may be degraded by a bacterial strain that is dominant in the lumen of the bowel of colorectal patients. Hence, expression of miR-20a is reduced in patients having colorectal adenoma [76–78].

In another study, miR-34a modulates EMT and MET processes. There is methylation in CpG islands (cancer specific), and these are repressed by *IL-6/STAT3* pathway which is mediated by *interleukin-6 receptors (IL6R)* and *inactivation of TP53*. This results in downregulation of miR-34a [79]. miR-34a inhibits SIRT and activates *TP53*. A positive feedback loop has been suggested between miR-34a (**Table 3**) and TP53 [81]. In many cancers, TP53-inducible microRNA is miR-34a [82].

In another study, miR-200 is downregulated in primary colorectal cancer (invasive stage) correlatable with the disruption of the basement membrane [83]. The miR-200 family consists of five members and is encoded in two clusters. One cluster is present on chromosome 1 and encodes for miR-200a, miR-200b, miR-200c, and miR-141. The other cluster is present on chromosome 12 and encodes for miR-141. The potential target of miR-200 family is ZEB1/ZEB2 which is a repressor of CDH1 (**Table 4**). Expression of all members of this family can be repressed following methylation of CpG islands in the regulatory region of their genes [84, 85]. Strong expression of miR-200 results in metastatic colorectal cancer [83]. Another study shows that miR-155 and miR-21 are overexpressed in colorectal cancer [86]. In another study involving colorectal cancer patients, the expression of miR-195 and miR-497 is reduced [87].

5.3 Cervical cancer

Cervical cancer is the most common cause of death among women in the developing countries [88, 89]. Cervical cancer can cause the death of 270,000 women per year [90]. Human papillomavirus (HPV) is the causative agent, with the E6 and E7 proteins targeting p53 and pRb, respectively [91].

Sr. no.	MicroRNAs	Potential target	Function
1	miR-185	Ras homolog gene family, member A, and cell division control protein 42 homolog	Reduction in the proliferation, induction of cell cycle arrest at the G1 stage, and promotion of apoptosis
2	miR-192	cyclin-dependent kinase inhibitor 1	Regulating the p53
3	miR-215		
4	miR-34a	Tumor suppressor p53	Modulate the EMT transition

Table 3.
MicroRNAs suppressing the colorectal cancer [80].

Sr. no.	MicroRNAs	Potential target	Function
1	miR-130a	Mothers against decapentaplegic homolog 4 (SMAD4)	Enhances the cell proliferation and migration
2	miR-301a		
3	miR-454		
4	miR-200	Zinc finger E-box-binding homeobox ½	Promotes metastasis

Table 4.
MicroRNAs promoting the colorectal cancer [80].

Type of miRNA	Function	Ref.
miR-491-5p	Downregulated; suppress cervical cancer by telomerase reverse transcriptase and regulate the PI3K/AKT pathway	[92]
miR-142-3p	Inhibit the proliferation of cell Frizzled_7 receptor (FZD7)	[93]
miR-142-3p	Inhibit the growth of cell via downregulation of its FOXM1 target	[94]

Table 5.
AmiRNA involved in cervical cancer.

Several miRNAs are upregulated and downregulated during cervical cancer (**Table 5**). miR-135b is a biomarker for cervical cancer. Suppression of this biomarker results in the inhibition of cell growth.

Downregulation of miR-135b results in the percentage of G1 cells with a concomitant decrease in those in the S phase. The expression of cyclin-dependent kinases (p27 and p21) is increased and that of cyclin D1 is decreased. Cyclin D1 (nuclear protein) is responsible for the regulation of cells (proliferating) that are at the G1 phase of the cell cycle [72, 73].

There seems to be an inverse relationship between miR-135b and FOXO1 protein. When FOXO1 protein is downregulated, cervical cancer is promoted. When FOXO1 protein is expressed, then there is an increase in the p27 and p21 expression with a decrease in cyclin D1 level and cell cycle is arrested [95, 96]. So, when miR-135 is downregulated, FOXO1 is upregulated with the resultant inhibition of cell growth (**Figure 6**).

In cervical cancer, miR-196a is upregulated and its targets are $p27^{Kip}$ and FOXO1. It promotes the transition of cells from G1 phase to S phase, enhances the cellular proliferation by involving the PI3K/Akt pathway, and is involved in tumorigenesis [97].

In one study, miR-10a is overexpressed in cervical cancer (Long et al., 2012; [28]). The target of miR-10a is transmembrane protein type 1 close homolog of L1 (CHL1) that is downregulated. A decrease in CHL1 protein dysregulates PAK and MAPK pathways resulting in increases in cell growth followed by migration and invasion [98].

In another study, miR-21 is upregulated in cervical cancer, and it is located at the 17q23.21 locus (**Table 6**). The pri-miR-21 is transcribed by the intronic region of TMEM49 (protein-coding gene). This miRNA targets the p53 and Cdc25 (regulators of the expression of genes), TPM1 and RECK (suppressing the metastasis), and PTEN and PDCD4 (inducing the apoptosis of metastasized cell). Hence, decreases in this miRNA can result in the PDCD4 gene providing signals for the activation of the RAS pathway. This activation, in turn, activates the transcription factor AP-

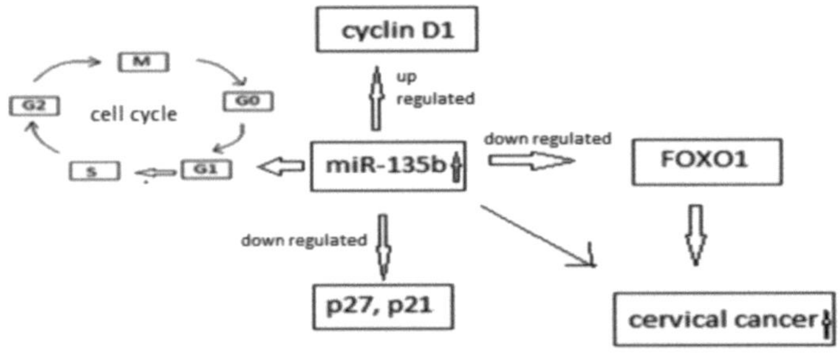

Figure 6.
MicroRNA and cervical cancer.

Sr. no.	MicroRNAs	Potential targets	Function	Ref.
1	miR-196a	Binds to the 3′UTR of $p27^{Kip}$ and FOXO1 and inhibits their translation	Increases in cell proliferation and tumorigenesis	[97]
2	miR-10a	Has an inverse relation with the expression of close homolog of L1 (CHL1) transmembrane protein type 1—a cell-adhesion protein	Cell growth followed by migration and invasion	[91]
3	miR-21	Negatively regulates p53 and Cdc25, TPM1 and RECK, and PTEN and PDCD4	Enhances the expression of genes associated with cell proliferation, metastasis, as well as those involved in the antiapoptosis effect	[91]
4	miR-886-5p	Negatively regulates the Bax gene	Dysregulation of the gene involved in apoptosis (miR-10a, miR-106b, miR-21, miR-135b, miR-141, miR146, miR-148a, miR-214, and miR-886-5p)	[91]
5	miR-20a	TNKS2 oncogene is upregulated (by binding at 3′UTR of mRNA of TNKS2 results in enhanced translation)	Migration, colony formation, and invasion	[91]

Table 6.
MicroRNAs activating the cervical cancer.

1gene. This AP-1 binds to a specific site on the promoter of miR-21 and as a result miR-21 gene is transcribed [99], thereby providing a plausible mechanism for a positive feedback loop.

It was reported that miR-886-5p targets and negatively regulates Bax gene expression via inhibition of translation, and hence, this form of control may be significant for the development of cervical cancer. When there is a death signal, the proapoptotic protein coded by Bax gene is inserted into the outer membrane of mitochondria. As a result, cytochrome C is released, and the initiator caspase-9 is subsequently activated with the initiation of apoptosis (**Table 7**) [91].

5.4 Liver cancer

Liver cancer is rising very rapidly globally with aflatoxins also contributing to its etiology. Specific miRNA may be expressed in the case of liver cancer. One of the

Sr. no.	MicroRNAs	Potential target	Function
1	miR-143	Target k-Ras, Bcl-2 and Macc1, specifically downregulation of Bcl-2	Inhibition of apoptosis and uncontrolled cell proliferation
2	miR-129-5p	Downregulates HPV18 E5 and E7 expression as well as inhibits the translation of SP-1 transcriptional factor	Suppressing the progression of cervical cancer
3	miR-34a	Cyclin E2 and D1, CDK6, E2F3, CDK4, E2F1, E2F5, P18, Bcl-2, and SIRT1	Aberrations in cell proliferation and differentiation—cell transformation

Table 7.
MicroRNAs suppressing cervical cancer [91].

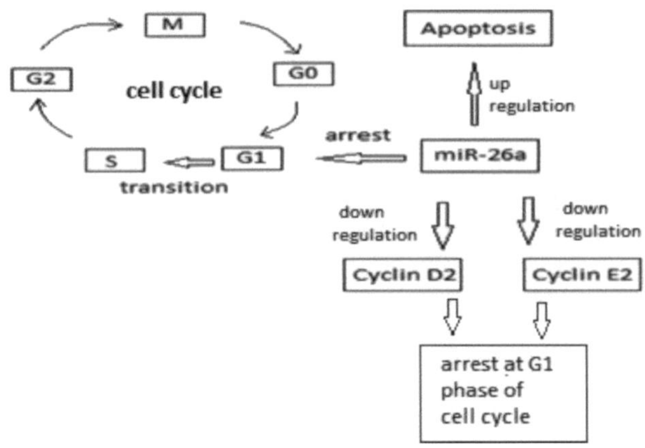

Figure 7.
MicroRNA and liver cancer.

miRNA biomarkers in liver cancer is miR-26a. Its expression is reduced in liver cancer unlike normal hepatic cells, where its expression level is increased [100].

miR-26a and miR-34a cause an increased number of cells in the G1 phase of the cell cycle, while there is a decrease in the cells in the S phase of the cell cycle. miR-26 causes cell cycle arrest at the G1 phase [84]. In the 3′UTR region of cyclins E2 and D2, there is a conserved binding site for miR-26a. miR-26a binds to these binding sites and represses the expression of both cyclins (**Figure 7**). miR-26 causes the induction of apoptosis in the tumor cells and suppresses hepatic cancer [101].

Kim et al. studied the expression of miR-31 in liver cancer (**Table 8**). The main target of miR-31 is CDK2 protein and HDAC2, with these proteins suppressed in the livers of normal individuals. There is an enhanced expression of CDK2 protein and HDAC2 in liver cancer. When HDAC2 is suppressed, $p21^{WAF1/Cip1}$ and $p16^{INK4A}$ are activated, and positive regulators of the cell cycle (cyclin D1, CDK2, and CDK4) are suppressed simultaneously [102].

In another study, the expression of miR-9 enhances the formation of tumor spheres in the liver. The direct target of the miR-9 is PPARA and CDH1 genes and regulates them via binding to the 3′UTR region of these genes. Upregulation of miR-9 enhances the level of vimentin (mesenchymal marker) and deregulates the CDH1 (**Table 9**). The transcriptional factor PPARA has been implicated in the metabolic homeostasis of the liver by regulating the nuclear factor-4 alpha (hepatocyte HNF4A) gene, which is a tumor suppressor. In liver cancer, miR-9 suppresses the CDH1 and also suppresses the PPARA at their mRNA level by binding to the 3′UTR of these genes [103].

In one study, there is overexpression of miR-525-3p in liver cancer, and its potential target is a zinc finger protein (Krüppel C2H2 type family) ZNF395. This

Sr. no.	MicroRNAs	Potential targets	Function	Ref.
1	miR-26a	Cyclin E2 and D2	The arrest of the cell cycle at G1 phase	[84]
2	miR-31	CDK2 protein and HDAC2	Suppress the positive regulators of cell cycle and promote those proteins involved in EMT-related processes	[102]

Table 8.
MicroRNAs suppressing the liver cancer.

Sr. no.	MicroRNAs	Potential targets	Function	Ref.
1	miR-9	Influences the PPARA/CDH1pathway	Suppress the tumor suppressor	[103]
2	miR-525-3p	Downregulates ZNF395	Enhances cell growth and prevent apoptosis	[104]

Table 9.
MicroRNAs activating the liver cancer.

zinc finger protein was originally a transcriptional factor and binds to the promoter region of the human papillomavirus (HPV). This protein mediates the regulation of PI3K/Akt pathway and causes the inhibition of cell growth via the induction of caspase-3 and the promotion of apoptosis. The expression of miR-525-3p enhances cell growth and prevention of apoptosis [104].

5.5 Prostate cancer

In countries in the West, prostate cancer is a more prevalent form of cancer among males with an increasing incidence rate [105]. Prostate cancer is the result of undesirable genomic alteration [106, 107]. CD9 is inactivated during prostate cancer and may cause its progression [108].

In the prostate cancer, serum level of miR-141 is elevated [109]. So it acts as the biomarker of prostate cancer. In the progression or repression of prostate cancer, miR-141 function is understood poorly [110]. One other study is done by Waltering et al. in which miR-141 is castrated and results in upregulation and activation (**Figure 8**). This causes the LNCaP cell growth to increase. This miRNA is also involved in the regulation of signaling of the androgen. This androgen has a crucial role in the growth of prostate cancer (castration-resistant and androgen-dependent). So it may be involved in the progression of prostate cancer [111, 112].

In a study involving prostate cancer, miR-888 was found to be upregulated. Its target is the tumor suppressors SMAD4 and RBL1. Binding of this miRNA to the 3′UTR causes their downregulation. RBL1 is the member of the RB (retinoblastoma) family and blocks the progression of cells at the G1-S phase following its binding and inhibition of the transcription factor E2F. SMAD4 protein binds to SMAD receptors and transduces the signal initiated by TGF-β/BMP ligands in order to regulate differentiation and cell growth [113].

In another study, there is the downregulation of miR-23a, b (**Table 10**). There is upregulation of the-Myc gene which causes the repression of these miRNAs at the transcriptional level. Mitochondrial glutaminase protein is expressed in the prostate

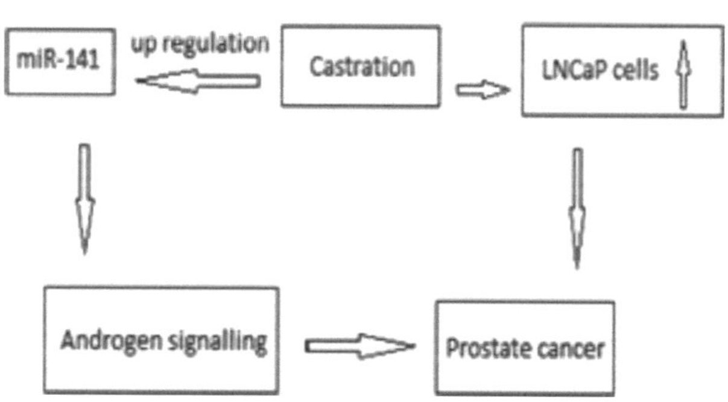

Figure 8.
miRNA and prostate cancer.

Sr. no.	MicroRNAs	Potential targets	Function	Ref.
1	miR-141	LNCaP cells	Promote cell growth Decreased growth in response to anti-miR-141 treatment	[112]
2	miR-888	Downregulates SMAD4 and RBL1	G1-S phase transition	[113]

Table 10.
MicroRNAs activating the prostate cancer.

cancer cells. Consequently, glutamine catabolism is increased, providing a growth advantage to the cancer cells [114].

In another study, miR-34a is suppressed in prostate cancer. The target of miR-34a is deacetylase sirtuin (SIRT1) and cyclin-dependent kinase 6 (CDK6). CDK6 regulates cyclin D, which, in turn, regulates cell cycle progression and G1-S phase transition, while p53 protein-dependent apoptosis is regulated by SIRT1 via deacetylation and stabilization of p53. The target of the p53 gene is miR-34a. It is suggested that there is a positive feedback loop in which SIRT1 mediates the activation of miR-34a via stabilization of p53 and induces the apoptosis and blocks the cell cycle transition. This activation of p53 causes the upregulation of miR-34a which in turn suppresses the SIRT1 (**Table 11**) [114].

5.6 Lung cancer

The leading cause of death around the world is lung cancer by tobacco smoke. This environmental lifestyle-related factor may cause undesirable epigenetic and genetic modifications [115]. The key role in lung cancer is the alteration and mutation in tumor suppressor genes (p53 and *RB/p16pathway)* and less frequent is the genetic alteration of *FHIT*, *K-ras*, *MYO18B*, and *PTEN* [116].

Five miRNAs were differentially expressed in lung cancer tissues, and these include miR-21, miR-155, miR-145, miR-17-3p, and hsa-let-7a-2. Specifically, hsa-miR-155 levels were increased, while that of hsa-let-7a-2 was downregulated [117].

There is a functional interaction of let-7 with the Ras as a target gene is overexpressed associated with protein kinase and resulting intracellular pathway of signaling [118]. The molecular mechanism is unclear involving miRNA in lung cancer. Alteration in the somatic genes resulted in the defective miRNA expression in lung cancer. This reduced expression of miRNA (has-let-7a-2) in the lung cancer is due to epigenetic modification and results in the silencing of tumor suppressor gene and many others (**Figure 9**) [119, 120]. The expression of hsa-miR-21 is upregulated in cancer cell and causes the inhibition of product of gene which initiates apoptosis and causes lung cancer [121]. In a report miR-17~92 cluster is overexpressed in the lung cancer. This cluster consists of six miRNAs.

Sr. no.	MicroRNAs	Potential targets	Function
1	miR-23a,b	Glutaminase protein (indirect)	Glutamine catabolism
2	miR-34a	SIRT1 and CDK6	Progression of cell cycle, G1-S phase transition, and antiapoptosis

Table 11.
MicroRNAs suppressing the prostate cancer [114].

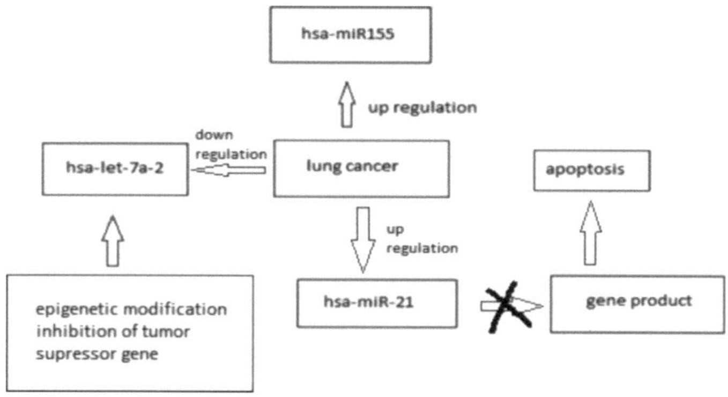

Figure 9.
miRNA and lung cancer.

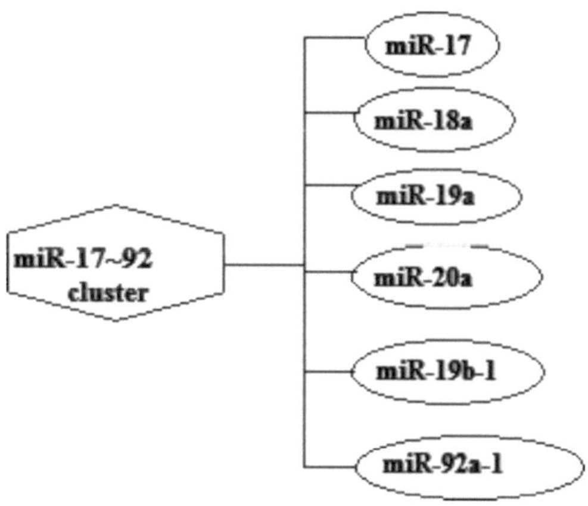

This cluster in lung cancer is transactivated via MYC and members of the E2F family. The direct target of this cluster is HIF-1α. Upregulation of MYC causes the downregulation of HIF-1α and affects proliferation of cell in normoxia without affecting the hypoxic condition. Overexpression of this cluster causes knockdown of retinoblastoma gene and results in the formation of reactive oxygen species. Another direct target of this cluster is RAS-related protein 14 (RAB-14), and it is downregulated by this cluster and results in the initiation and development of cancer [122].

In another study, miR-21 is upregulated in the lung cancer. Its direct target is tumor suppressor gene PTEN that is repressed by overexpression of miR-21 (**Table 12**), which results in cell growth enhancement and non-small cell lung carcinoma invasion [123]. miR-21 is upregulated by RAS via PI3K and RAF/MAPK pathways [122].

In another study, miR-34 is downregulated in the lung cancer. This miRNA is directly regulated by p53 and regulates the apoptosis and arrest of the cell cycle in cancer [81].

The miR-34/miR-499 is downregulated in lung cancer and its direct target is E2F and p53 (**Table 13**). Both miRNAs suppress the E2F and upregulate the p53 via SIRT1 so cell growth is increased [124].

The miR-15/miR-16 is downregulated in lung cancer. There is upregulation of cyclin D1 with the downregulation of miR-15/miR-16. The overexpression of miR-15/miR-16 causes the arrest of the cell cycle at G1 phase [122]

Sr. no.	MicroRNAs	Potential targets	Function	Ref.
1	let-7	Ras	Protein kinase-associated signaling pathway	[118]
2	miR-17~92	HIF-1α and RAB14	ROS and initiation and development of cancer	[122]
3	miR-21	PTEN	Cell growth enhancement and invasion	[122]

Table 12.
MicroRNAs activating the lung cancer.

Sr. no.	MicroRNAs	Potential targets	Function	Ref.
1	miR-34	p53	Regulate the apoptosis and arrest of cell cycle	[81]
2	miR-34/miR-499	E2F and p53	Cell growth and proliferation	[124]
3	miR-15/miR-16	Cyclin D1	The arrest of the cell cycle at the G1 phase	[122]

Table 13.
MicroRNAs suppressing the lung cancer.

5.7 Gastric cancer

The second malignancy that is widely prevailed is the gastric cancer which results in 12% deaths around the world [125]. Gastric cancer is the result of a series of steps. When transforming growth factor (TGF-beta) resistance is developed and E2F1 is upregulated, then gastric cancer is developed [126, 127].

In gastric cancer, there is upregulation of cluster of miR-106b-25 present on Mcm gene [128]. The transition of the G1/S phase of the cell cycle is targeted by Mcm gene. It ensures that DNA is replicated only one time when replication fork is assembled on the DNA during each cycle [129]. When cells exit from the mitosis, then expression of cluster of miR-106b-25 is activated by E_2F1 (**Figure 10**) and gains the reentry in the G1 phase of the cell cycle. The cell cycle inhibitor is p21 [130].

The cytokine TGF-beta causes the cell cycle arrests by activating p21 and causes the apoptosis [131]. As this cytokine is activated it causes the downregulation of miR-106b-25 cluster, reduces the expression of E2F1, causes the cell cycle arrest at G1/S phase of cell cycle, and causes the induction of apoptosis. The key target of miR-93 and miR-106b is E2F1 [132]. The key target of miR-25, the biomarker of gastric cancer, is TGF-beta cytokine [133]. The target of cytokine in mediating the apoptosis is Bim protein that in turn causes the activation of proapoptotic Bax and Bad molecules acting as an antagonist of Bcl2 and BclXL antiapoptotic factors (**Figure 11**) [134].

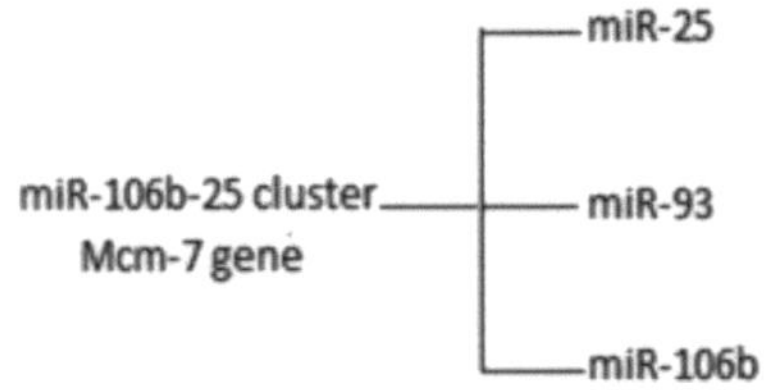

Figure 10.
miR-106b-25 cluster.

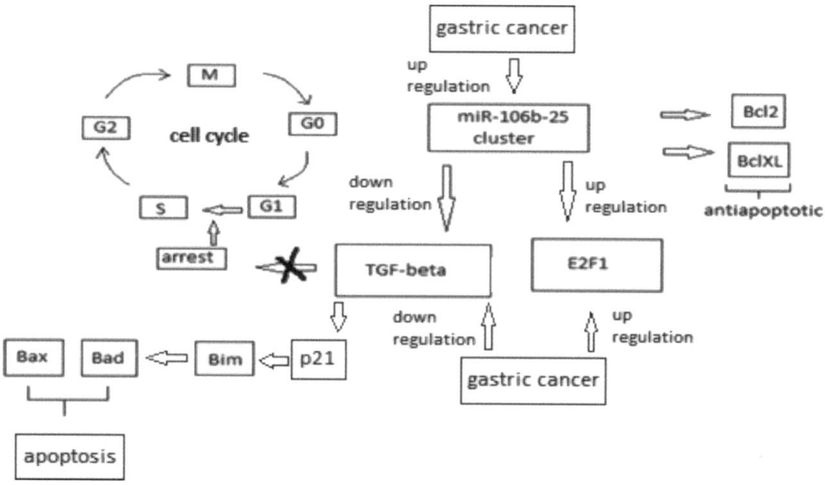

Figure 11.
miRNA and gastric cancer.

Lim found that miR-196b is upregulated in the gastric cancer (**Table 14**). This miRNA is present in chromosome 9 at HOXA cluster. There is a positive association of expression of miR-196b with the expression of HOXA10. Unmethylation of CpG islands results in the expression of miR-196b. The HOXA10 expression results in hematopoietic stem cell proliferation and progenitor cell proliferation leading to the development of cancer via expression of genes that codes for integrin-β3, TGFβ2, and dual-specificity protein phosphatase 4 [135].

We studied miR-375 is downregulated in gastric cancer (**Table 15**). Its expression in cancer cell causes the decrease in cell viability by downregulation of PDK1 and JAK2 revealing that miR-375 is a tumor suppressor in gastric cancer [136, 137].

In another study, miR-135a is a tumor suppressor in gastric cancer. Upregulation of miR-135a causes the suppression of gastric cancer via suppression of proliferation of cell via E2F, metastasis, and EMT. In gastric cancer, lymph node metastasis is associated with proliferation, metastasis, and EMT which is suppressed by overexpression of miR135a [138].

Sr. no.	MicroRNAs	Potential targets	Function	Ref.
1	miR-106b-25	E2F1	Antiapoptosis and cell proliferation	[132]
2	miR-196b	HOXA10	Progenitor and hematopoietic stem cell proliferation	[135]

Table 14.
MicroRNAs activating the gastric cancer.

Sr. no.	MicroRNAs	Potential targets	Function	Ref.
1	miR-375	PDK1 and JAK2	Decrease the cell viability	[136, 137]
2	miR-135a	E2F	Suppress cell proliferation, metastasis, and EMT	[138]

Table 15.
MicroRNAs suppressing the gastric cancer.

5.8 Bladder cancer

In males, bladder cancer is an important malignancy present in two forms that are muscle invasive and non-muscle invasive (benign) [139]. There are two microRNAs associated with bladder cancer. They are miR-21 and miR-129 [140].

In the bladder cancer, miR-129 and miR-21 both are upregulated. The direct target of miR-21 is the tumor suppressor genes that are TPM1 and PTEN (**Figure 12**) [141, 142]. The known targets of miR-129 are the genes involved in the regulation of transcription and processing of miRNA that are TAMTA1 and EIF2CA [143]. The mir-129's pathway of death effectors leads to the tumor as its target is also SOX4 [144].

According to one study, miR-19a is frequently upregulated in the bladder cancer. The expression of miR-19a is related to PTEN expression (**Table 16**). PTEN is a tumor suppressor gene. When miR-19a is overexpressed, it causes the downregulation of PTEN and increases the cell level of phosphatidylinositol-3,4,5-trisphosphate in AKT/PKB pathway. When growth factors are released, then the AKT pathway is initiated and cell growth is increased [145].

Zhang studied that miR-125b is downregulated in bladder cancer. The expression of miR-135b causes the inhibition of formation of colony and development of cancer via suppression of E2F3 which is overexpressed in bladder cancer [74].

In another study angiogenesis in the bladder cancer is suppressed by miR-34a (**Table 17**). The target of miR-34a is CD44 and causes the suppression of CD44 when upregulated which results in the regulation of transcription of the various

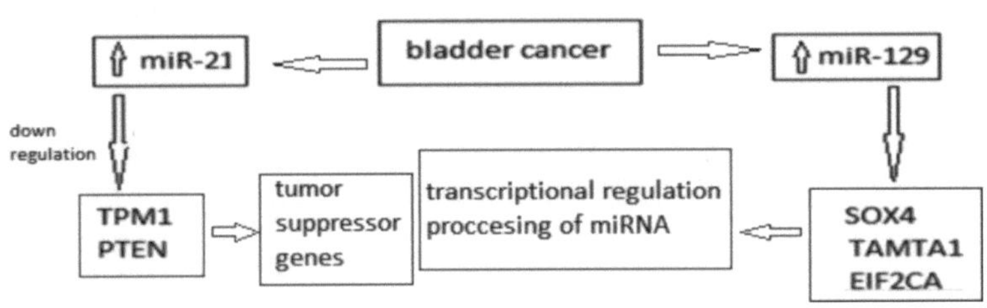

Figure 12.
miRNA and bladder cancer.

Sr. no.	MicroRNAs	Potential targets	Function	Ref.
1	miR-129	TAMTA1 and EIF2CA	Regulation of transcription	[143]
2	miR-21	TPM1 and PTEN	Growth of tumor cell	[141]
3	miR-19a	PTEN	Increase in the cell growth	[145]

Table 16.
MicroRNAs activating the bladder cancer.

Sr. no.	MicroRNAs	Potential targets	Function	Ref.
1	miR-125b	E2F3	Inhibition of formation of colony and development of cancer	[74]
2	miR-34a	CD44	Inhibition of invasion, metastasis, migration, tube formation, and angiogenesis	[146]

Table 17.
MicroRNAs suppressing the bladder cancer.

genes in bladder cancer. Over expression of miR-34a causes the inhibition of invasion, metastasis, migration, tube formation, and angiogenesis by targeting the CD44 [146].

5.9 Glioblastoma

Glioblastoma is the tumor of astrocytes, star-shaped cells that form the supportive tissues (glue-like) of the brain. This is readily metastasizing tumor because it is surrounded by large blood vessels. Glioblastoma is a complex and heterogeneous tumor that comprises on neoplastic cells, endothelial cells, stemlike cells, neural precursor cells, microglia, reactive extracellular components, and peripheral immune cells [147].

The biomarker in glioblastoma is miR-21 that is upregulated in this cancer (**Figure 13**). It mediates its effect in two ways: acting at the translational level and acting at the transcription level. It binds the 3′UTR region of the target gene (for apoptosis) [148] and causes the inhibition of transcription of apoptotic genes by decreasing the stability. It also resists the caspases 3 and 7 that are important apoptotic agents so apoptosis does not occur [149].

Upregulation of miR-221 and miR-222 was in glioma cells. These two miRNAs present as a cluster on Xp11.3 and have the same target. Functional studies revealed that there is an association of these two miRNAs with the progression of the cell cycle. Their direct target is cyclin-dependent kinase 1B/p27. The overexpression of these miRNAs cause the activation of quiescent glioblastoma cells and the progression of these cells from G1 phase to S phase of the cell cycle. miR-221/miR-222 also targets the p57 and p27 (inhibitors of cell-dependent kinase) to prevent the quiescence at G1 phase and cause their entry to S phase of the cell cycle. The miR-221/miR-222 also targets the PUMA, a proapoptotic protein, to prevent the apoptosis (**Table 18**) [150].

Another biomarker miR-128 is found to be downregulated in glioblastoma. The expression of miR-128 causes the regulation of proliferation of glioblastoma multiform (GBM) cells via targeting the PDGFR-α and EGFR, the oncogenic kinases

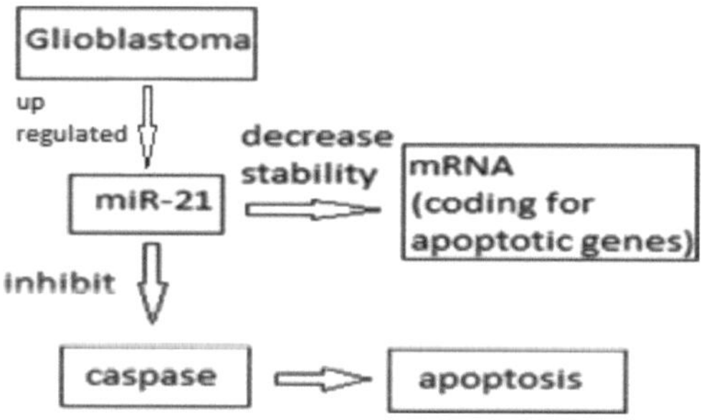

Figure 13.
miRNA and glioblastoma.

Sr. no.	MicroRNAs	Potential targets	Function	Ref.
1	miR-21	Caspases 3 and 7	Antiapoptotic	[149]
2	miR-221/miR-222	Cyclin-dependent kinase 1B/p27	Prevent the apoptosis	[150]

Table 18.
MicroRNAs activating the glioblastoma.

(receptor tyrosine kinases) (**Table 19**). It suppresses the GBM by enhancing the differentiation of neuronal cells. It also targets the signaling molecules in the PI3-kinase/AKT pathway which causes the tumor cell proliferation [147].

In other study miR-7 is downregulated in glioblastoma. Its target is EGFR and causes the inhibition of AKT pathways and EGFR and results in the reduction of cell viability of GBM via direct binding to mRNA of EGFR or via targeting to IRS1 and IRS2 (insulin receptor substrate). The major regulators EGFR and IRS are at upstream site of AKT pathway [151].

5.10 B cell chronic lymphocytic leukemia

This is the cancer of B lymphocytes (antibodies), and it is a prevalent form of leukemia in the adult around western countries [152].

In B cell leukemia, the expression of three microRNAs is seen as cancer biomarker. These are miR-15a, miR-16-1, and miR-19a (**Figure 14**). Two microRNAs are present at 13q14.3 chromosomal location; these are miR-15a and 16-1 [153]. The expression of these two is decreased in this leukemia, whereas the expression of miR-19a is increased [152]. The region encoding for miR-15a and miR-16-1 was deleted. This leads to the presence of the genes of IgV_H that were mutated [154]. The potent target of miR-19a is PTEN, and there is down-expression of this PTEN gene; hence its protein is not properly synthesized because the promoter of the gene is hypermethylated [155].

The miR-16-1 and miR-15a (located on chromosome 13) are downregulated in B cell lymphocytic leukemia (**Table 20**). These miroRNAs target the p53 gene which

Sr. no.	MicroRNAs	Potential targets	Function	Ref.
1	miR-128	PDGFR-α and EGFR	Enhancing the differentiation of neuronal cells	[147]
2	miR-7	EGFR	Reduction of cell viability	[151]

Table 19.
MicroRNAs suppressing the glioblastoma.

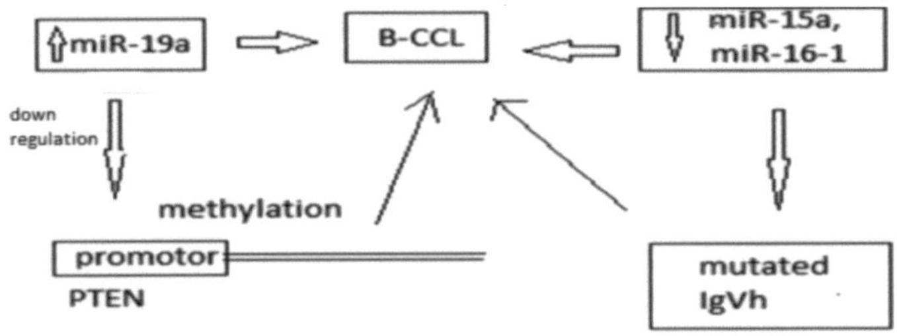

Figure 14.
miRNA and B cell lymphocytic leukemia.

Sr. no.	MicroRNAs	Potential targets	Function	Ref.
1	miR-15a	p53	Prevent the apoptosis and cell survival is increased	[153]
2	miR-16-1	p53	Prevent the apoptosis and cell survival is increased	[156]

Table 20.
MicroRNAs suppressing the B cell lymphocytic leukemia.

is a tumor suppressor gene. When these miRNAs are downregulated, then the expression of p53 is reduced or inhibited, and expression of BCL-2 is increased which prevent the apoptosis and cell survival is increased [156].

In one study, miR-17/miR-92 cluster is overexpressed in the B cell lymphocytic leukemia (**Table 21**). The direct target of this cluster is PTEN and Bim. The PTEN is a tumor suppressor gene, and Bim is proapoptotic protein. Overexpression of this cluster causes prevention of apoptosis and progression of tumor [157].

In other study, miR-155 is overexpressed in the B cell lymphocytic leukemia [159]. The potential target for miR-155 is SHIP1. Expression of miR-155 causes the alteration of BCR response in signaling pathway via the modulation of SHIP1 expression in chronic lymphocytic leukemia. Scr homology-2 domain comprising the inositol 5-phosphatase is encoded by SHIP1. This phosphatase causes the inhibition of BCR signaling and surface immunoglobulin [158].

5.11 Pancreatic cancer

Pancreatic tumor is most of the time identified at the last stages when therapy does not save life. Li et al. characterize the pancreatic cancer stem cells (PCSCs) for the very first time [160].

In one study, there is overexpression of miR-1290 in pancreatic cancer. The direct target of miR-1290 is FoxA1 which has an effect on the transition of epithelial mesenchyma. The overexpression of miR-1290 results in the growth of cell and invasion [94].

In another study there is overexpression of miR-194 in pancreatic cancer. The target of miR-194 is DACH1 and results in the formation of the colony, the proliferation of cell, and migration (**Table 22**), so miR-194 causes the progression of the tumor [161].

The growth and differentiation of the cell are regulated by LIN28, a protein that binds to the RNA [162]. The protein that is encoded by LIN28 is 25 kDa and has two binding sites for RNA: cold shock domain (CSD) and a pair of zinc fingers. In pancreatic cancer, the expression of LIN28 is increased which in turn suppresses the biosynthesis of family let-7 of microRNA (**Figure 15**). This family targets the genes involved in the growth and differentiation regulation [163]. This LIN28 causes the inhibition by binging to the loop present at the terminal region of let-7 family, so

Sr. no.	MicroRNAs	Potential targets	Function	Ref.
1	miR-19a	PTEN	Cause the tumor	[155]
2	miR-17/miR-92	PTEN and Bim	Prevention of apoptosis and progression of tumor	[157]
3	miR-155	SHIP1	Inhibition of BCR signaling and surface immunoglobulin	[158]

Table 21.
MicroRNAs activating the B cell lymphocytic leukemia.

Sr. no.	MicroRNAs	Potential targets	Function	Ref.
1	miR-1290	FoxA1	Cell growth and invasion	[94]
2	miR-194	DACH1	Progression of tumor	[161]

Table 22.
MicroRNAs activating the pancreatic cancer.

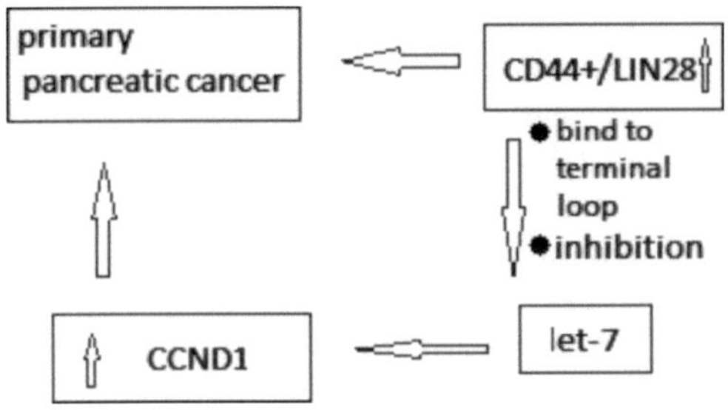

Figure 15.
miRNA and pancreatic cancer.

their processing is blocked [45, 46, 164]. This family is involved in the regulation of tumor by cyclin D1 (CCND1) inhibition [165, 166].

In one study there is downregulation of miR-145 in pancreatic cancer. The decreased expression of miR-145 is due to activation of the K-ras gene. Expression of miR-145 causes the inhibition of expression of insulin growth factor-1 receptors (**Table 23**). Its expression causes the downregulation of genes related to cancer (SET, MCM2, SPTBN1). These genes cause growth and carcinogenesis of pancreatic cancer [161].

5.12 Acute myeloid leukemia

In the myeloid leukemia, malignant blast cells are synthesized in comparison to mononuclear cells of healthy bone marrow [167]. In myeloid leukemia the hypermethylation of the DNA is involved in tumor suppression [168]. In one study, there is overexpression of miR-204 in acute myeloid leukemia. The target of miR-204 is MEIS1 and HOXA 10 genes which disturbs the differentiation of myeloid cells. Its overexpression causes tumorigenesis [169].

In another study, miR-125b (located on chromosome 1) is overexpressed in acute myeloid leukemia. The target of miR-125b is BCL2-antagonist/killer 1 (Bak1) which enhance the proliferation of AML cell and prevent the apoptosis [169].

In another study, miR-155 (located on chromosome 21) is overexpressed in the acute myeloid leukemia. This miR-155 is located in B cell integration cluster (BIC) gene. This BIC correlated to MYC to initiate lymphomas. Overexpression of miR-155 causes the inhibition of WEE1, a regulator of the cell cycle, and hMLH1, hMLH6, and hMLH4, the genes for mismatch repair (**Table 24**). The result of this inhibition is increased in mutation rate in progenitor and hematopoietic stem cells [169].

The known biomarker for the acute myeloid leukemia is miR-29b [167]. miR-29b causes the hypomethylation of the DNA. Sp1 transcriptional factor has the binding site for both miR-29b and DNMT1. In DNMT, it binds to its promoter and 3′UTR for miR-29b of Sp1 (specificity protein 1). Binding to the 3′UTR causes the reduced expression of Sp1, so DNMT (DNA methyltransferase) expression is also

Sr. no.	MicroRNAs	Potential targets	Function	Ref.
1	let-7 family	cyclin D1 (CCND1)	Regulation of tumor	[166]
2	miR-145	K-ras	Growth and carcinogenesis	[161]

Table 23.
MicroRNAs suppressing the pancreatic cancer.

Sr. no.	MicroRNAs	Potential targets	Function
1	miR-204	MEIS1 and HOXA	Tumorigenesis
2	miR-125b	Bak1	Enhance proliferation and prevent apoptosis
3	miR-155	WEE1, hMLH1, hMLH6, and hMLH4	Increase mutation rate in progenitor and hematopoietic stem cells

Table 24.
MicroRNAs activating the acute myeloid leukemia [169].

reduced (**Figure 16**). In acute myeloid leukemia, miR-29b results in the apoptosis when it directly targets the MCL (induced myeloid leukemia cell differentiation protein) [170]. So the expression of miR-29b is reduced in acute myeloid leukemia which leads to cancer progression as apoptosis has been decreased with reduced expression of miR-29b (**Table 25**).

5.13 Ovarian cancer

In ovarian cancer, the biomarker that is used is miR-214 and it is upregulated in cancer. It binds to the 3′UTR region of phosphatase and tensin analog (PTEN) gene and causes its hypermethylation. So this is inactivated. The direct target of PTEN is Akt protein kinase B and mediates its activation by the help of PI4K3B [171]. Akt causes the downstream effects such as activation of glycogen synthase. So when PTEN is inhibited, it activates the expression of Akt. This miR-214 resists the cisplatin-mediated cell death, so it is antiapoptotic in nature (**Figure 17**). Cisplatin is an important factor in mediating cell death [172].

In a study, there is overexpression of Hsa-miR-182 in ovarian cancer. The potential target of Hsa-miR-182 is forkhead box 3 (FOXO3) and forkhead box 1 (FOXO1) which promote the differentiation and inhibition of growth (acting as a tumor suppressor). These tumor suppressor genes are suppressed, and growth and proliferation of ovarian cell are increased (**Table 26**) [173].

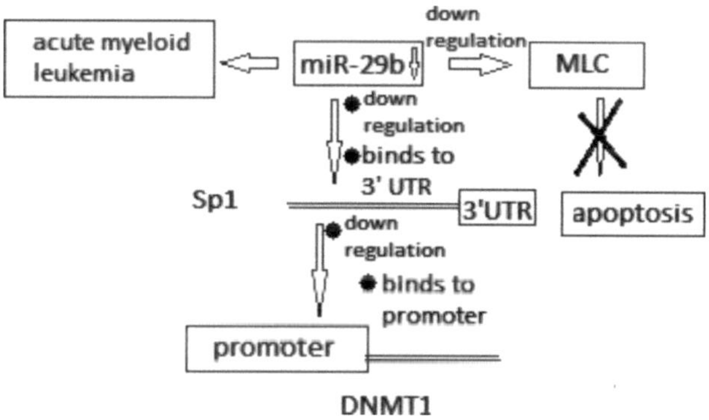

Figure 16.
miRNA and acute myeloid leukemia.

Sr. no.	MicroRNAs	Potential targets	Function
1	miR-29b	DNMT	Apoptosis
2	miR-29b	MCL protein	Apoptosis

Table 25.
MicroRNAs suppressing the acute myeloid leukemia [170].

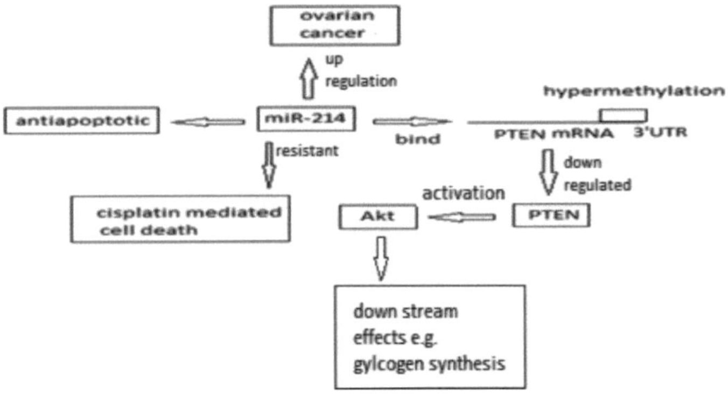

Figure 17.
miRNA and ovarian cancer.

Sr. no.	MicroRNAs	Potential targets	Function	Ref.
1	miR-214	PTEN	Antiapoptosis	[172]
2	Hsa-miR-182	FOXO3 and FOXO1	Increased proliferation and growth	[173]

Table 26.
MicroRNAs activating the ovarian cancer.

Sr. no.	MicroRNAs	Potential targets	Function	Ref.
1	miR-200	ZEB1 and ZEB2	Prevent the EMT, metastasis, invasion, and migration	[174]
2	miR-506	SNAI2, CDK4/ CDK6-FOXM1 axis	Inhibition of cell invasion and migration and proliferation; initiates the senescence	[175]

Table 27.
MicroRNAs suppressing the ovarian cancer.

In another study, there is downregulation of miR-200 family in ovarian cancer. The direct target of miR-200 is zinc finger E-box-binding homeobox 1 and 2 (ZEB1 and ZEB2). It prevents the EMT, metastasis, invasion, and migration of tumor cell. Interleukin-8 and CXCL1 (released from tumor epithelial cells) are also the target of miR-200 and prevent the angiogenesis of tumor cell [174].

In another study there is downregulation of miR-506 in ovarian cancer, so there is cell migration invasion of the cancer cell. When this miRNA is overexpressed, it causes the expression of E-cadherin and results in inhibition of cell invasion and migration and proliferation of ovarian cancer and, via targeting SNAI2 (E-cadherin transcriptional factor), prevents the EMT induction by *TGF-β* (**Table 27**). The miR-506 directly targets the CDK4/CDK6-FOXM1 axis and initiates the senescence [175].

6. Conclusion

MicroRNAs (miRNAs) could be used as potential tool for early detection of cancer. It may upregulate or downregulate multiple targets through various mechanisms. It is upregulated as an oncogene (miRNA) and downregulated as a tumor suppressor. microRNA targets the PTEN, interferon (tumor suppressor genes), and also to the cell cycle along with the regulation of these genes [172]. MicroRNA is of vital importance because of its resistance to degradation and could be a potential candidate for clinical applications. However, its expression level can be screened in the serum/plasma (blood) by high-throughput sequencing technology. Further research for identification of novel microRNA will warrant the development of microRNA-related cancer prognosis [176–180].

Abbreviations

miRISC	microRNA-associated RNA-induced silencing complex
DGCR8	DiGeorge syndrome chromosomal [or critical] region 8
EGFR	epidermal growth factor receptor
FOXO1	forkhead box protein O1
PTEN	phosphatase and tensin homolog
TPM1	tropomyosin alpha-1 chain
SOX4	SRY-related HMG-box
CCND1	cyclin-D1
DNMT	DNA methyltransferase
MCL	induced myeloid leukemia cell differentiation protein Mcl-1
PKB	Akt (protein kinase B)

Author details

Ayesha Siddiqua[1], Sumaira Kousar[1,2]*, Amer Jamil[1], Riaz Tabassum[1], Tariq Mehmood[1] and Nusrat Shafiq[2]

1 Department of Biochemistry, University of Agriculture, Faisalabad, Pakistan

2 Department of Biochemistry, Government College Women University, Faisalabad, Pakistan

*Address all correspondence to: sumairakausar@gcwuf.edu.pk

IntechOpen

© 2020 The Author(s). Licensee IntechOpen. This chapter is distributed under the terms of the Creative Commons Attribution License (http://creativecommons.org/licenses/by/3.0), which permits unrestricted use, distribution, and reproduction in any medium, provided the original work is properly cited. CC BY

References

[1] Hong L, Pan F, Jiang H, Zhang L, Liu Y, Cai C, et al. miR-125b inhibited epithelial-mesenchymal transition of triple-negative breast cancer by targeting MAP2K7. OncoTargets and Therapy. 2016;**9**:2639-2648

[2] Mirnezami AH, Pickard K, Zhang L, Primrose JN, Packham G. MicroRNAs: Key players in carcinogenesis and novel therapeutic targets. European Journal of Surgical Oncology. 2009;**35**:339-347

[3] Berezikov E, Guryev V, van de Belt J, Wienholds E, Plasterk RH, Cuppen E. Phylogenetic shadowing and computational identification of human microRNA genes. Cell. 2005;**120**:21-24

[4] Bentwich I, Avniel A, Karov Y, Aharonov R, Gilad S, Barad O, et al. Identification of hundreds of conserved and nonconserved human microRNAs. Nature Genetics. 2005;**37**:766-770

[5] Qu J, Li M, Zhong W, Hu C. Prognostic role of microRNA-25 in cancers: Evidence from a meta-analysis. International Journal of Clinical and Experimental Medicine. 2015;**8**: 12921-12927

[6] Kosaka N, Lguchi H, Ochiya T. Circulating microRNA in body fluid: A new potential biomarker for cancer diagnosis and prognosis. Cancer Science. 2010;**101**:2087-2092

[7] Paranjape T, Slack FJ, Weidhaas JB. MicroRNAs: Tools for cancer diagnostics. Gut. 2009;**58**:1546-1554

[8] Ghosh A, Ghosh A, Datta S, Dasgupta D, Das S, Ray S, et al. Hepatic miR-126 is a potential plasma biomarker for detection of hepatitis B virus infected hepatocellular carcinoma. International Journal of Cancer. 2016;**138**:2732-2744

[9] Li C, Liu Z, Yang K, Chen X, Zeng Y, Liu J, et al. miR-133b inhibits glioma cell proliferation and invasion by targeting Sirt1. Oncotarget. 2016;7:36247-36254

[10] Shah JS, Soon PS, Marsh DJ. Comparison of methodologies to detect low levels of Hemolysis in serum for accurate assessment of serum microRNAs. PLoS One. 2016;**11**:0153200

[11] Pillai RS. MicroRNA function: Multiple mechanisms for tiny RNA. RNA. 2005;**11**(2):1753-1761

[12] Lee RC, Feinbaum RL, Ambros V. The *C. elegans* heterochronic gene lin-4 encodes small RNAs with antisense complementarity to lin-14. Cell. 1993;**75**: 843-854

[13] Bartel DP. MicroRNAs: Genomics, biogenesis, mechanism and function. Cell. 2004;**116**:281-297

[14] Kim VN, Han J, Siomi MC. Biogenesis of small RNAs in animals. Nature Reviews Molecular Cell Biology. 2009;**10**:126-139

[15] Lee YS, Dutta A. MicroRNAs in cancer. Annual Review of Pathology. 2009;**4**:199-227

[16] Nishida-Aoki N, Ochiya T. Interactions between cancer cells and normal cells via miRNAs in extracellular vesicles. Cellular and Molecular Life Sciences. 2015;**72**:1849-1861

[17] Zhou X, Ji G, Chen H, Jin W, Yin C, Zhang G. Clinical role of circulating miR-223 as a novel biomarker in early diagnosis of cancer patients. International Journal of Clinical and Experimental Medicine. 2015;**9**: 16890-16898

[18] Oliveto S et al. Role of microRNAs in translation regulation and cancer. World Journal of Biological Chemistry. 2017;**8**(1):45-56

[19] Lee Y, Jeon K, Lee JT, Kim S, Kim VN. MicroRNA maturation: Stepwise processing and subcellular localization. EMBO Journal. 2002;**21**:4663-4670

[20] Lee Y, Kim M, Han J, Yeom KH, Lee S, Baek SH, et al. MicroRNA genes are transcribed by RNA polymerase II. EMBO Journal. 2004;**23**:4051-4060

[21] Lee Y, Ahn C, Han J, Choi H, Kim J, Yim J, et al. The nuclear RNase III Drosha initiates microRNA processing. Nature. 2003;**425**:415-419

[22] Hammond SM, Bernstein E, Beach D, Hannon GJ. An RNA-directed nuclease mediates post-transcriptional gene silencing in drosophila cells. Nature. 2000;**404**:293-296

[23] El-Hefnawy T, Raja S, Kelly L, Bigbe WL, Kirkwood JM, Luketich JD, et al. Characterization of amplifiable, circulating RNA in plasma and its potential as a tool for cancer diagnostics. Clinical Chemistry. 2004;**50**:564-573

[24] Valadi H, Ekstrom K, Bossios A, Sjostrand M, Lee JJ, Lotvall JO. Exosome mediated transfer of mRNAs and microRNAs is a novel mechanism of genetic exchange between cells. Nature Cell Biology. 2007;**9**:654-659

[25] Hayes N, Chayama K. MicroRNAs as biomarkers for liver disease and hepatocellular carcinoma. International Journal of Molecular Sciences. 2016;**17**: 1-17

[26] Yekta K, Shih IH, Bartel DP. MicroRNA-directed cleavage of HOXB8 mRNA. Science. 2004;**304**:594-596

[27] Lu J, Getz G, Miska EA, Alvarez-Saavedra E, Lamb J, Peck D, et al. MicroRNA expression profiles classify human cancers. Nature. 2005;**435**: 834-838

[28] Volinia S, Calin GA, Liu CG, Ambs S, Cimmino A, Petrocca F, et al. A microRNA expression signature of human solid tumors defines cancer gene targets. Proceedings of the National Academy of Sciences. 2006;**103**: 2257-2261

[29] Waldman SA, Terzic A. Translating MicroRNA discovery into clinical biomarkers in cancer. Journal of the American Medical Association. 2007; **297**:1923-1925

[30] Chen CZ. MicroRNAs as oncogenes and tumor suppressors. The New England Journal of Medicine. 2005;**353**: 1768-1771

[31] Jemal A, Bray F, Center MM, Ferlay J, Ward E, Forman D. Global cancer statistics. A Cancer Journal for Clinicians. 2011;**61**:69-90

[32] Tang J, Ahmad A, Sarkar FH. The role of microRNAs in breast cancer migration, invasion and metastasis. International Journal of Molecular Sciences. 2012;**13**:13414-13437

[33] Qi L, Bart J, Tan LP, Platteel I, Sluis T, Huitema S, et al. Expression of miR-21 and its targets (PTEN, PDCD4, TM1) in flat epithelial atypia of the breast in relation to ductal carcinoma in situ and invasive carcinoma. BMC Cancer. 2009; **9**:163

[34] Song B, Wang C, Liu J, Wang X, Lv L, Wei L, et al. MicroRNA-21 regulates breast cancer invasion partly by targeting tissue inhibitor of metalloproteinase 3 expression. Journal Experimental Clinical Cancer Reseaech. 2010;**29**(1):29

[35] Jiang S, Zhang HW, Lu MH, He XH, Li Y, Gu H, et al. MicroRNA-155 functions as an OncomiR in breast cancer by targeting the suppressor of cytokine signaling 1 gene. Cancer Research. 2010;**20**(8):3119-3127

[36] Zhang CM, Zhao J, Deng HY. MiR-155 promotes proliferation of

human breast cancer MCF-7 cells through targeting tumor protein 53-induced nuclear protein 1. Journal of Biomedical Sciences. 2013;**20**:79

[37] Kong W, He L, Coppola M, Guo J, Esposito NN, Coppola D, et al. MicroRNA-155 regulates cell survival, growth, and chemosensitivity by targeting FOXO3a in breast cancer. Journal of Biological Chemistry. 2010; **285**:17869-17879

[38] Schooneveld EV, Wildiers H, Vergote I, Vermeulen PB, Dirix LY, Laere SJV. Dysregulation of microRNAs in breast cancer and their potential role as prognostic and predictive biomarkers in patient management. Breast Cancer Research. 2015;**17**:21

[39] Huang GQ, Gumireddy K, Schrier M, le Sage C, Nagel R, Coukos G, et al. The microRNAs miR-373 and miR-520c promote tumour invasion and metastasis. Nature Cell Biology. 2008; **10**:202-210

[40] Yan GR, Xu SH, Tan ZL, Liu L, He QY. Global identification of miR-373-regulated genes in breast cancer by quantitative proteomics. Proteomics. 2011;**11**:912-920

[41] Ferracin M, Bassi C, Pedriali M, Pagotto S, D'Abundo L, Zagatti B, et al. miR-125b targets erythropoietin and its receptor and their expression correlates with metastatic potential and ERBB2/HER2 expression. Molecular Cancer. 2013;**12**:130

[42] Feliciano A, Castellvi J, ArteroCastro A, Leal JA, Romagosa C, HernandezLosa J, et al. miR-125b acts as a tumor suppressor in breast tumorigenesis via its novel direct targets ENPEP, CK2-α, CCNJ, and MEGF9. PLoS One. 2013;**8**:e76247

[43] Scott GK, Goga A, Bhaumik D, Berger CE, Sullivan CS, Benz CC. Coordinate suppression of ERBB2 and ERBB3 by enforced expression of micro-RNA miR-125a or miR-125b. Journal of Biological Chemistry. 2007;**282**: 1479-1486

[44] Wang S, Huang J, Lyu H, Lee CK, Tan J, Wang J, et al. Functional cooperation of miR-125a, miR-125b, and miR-205 in entinostat-induced downregulation of erbB2/erbB3 and apoptosis in breast cancer cells. Cell Death & Disease. 2013;**21**(4):e556

[45] Liu J, Mao Q, Liu Y, Hao X, Zhang S, Zhang J. Analysis of miR-205 and miR-155 expression in the blood of breast cancer patients. Chinese Journal of Cancer Research. 2013a;**25**:46-54

[46] Liu T, Huang Y, Liu J, Zhao Y, Jiang L, Huang Q, et al. MicroRNA-122 influences the development of sperm abnormalities from human induced pluripotent stem cells by regulating TNP2 expression. Stem Cells and Development. 2013b;**22**:1839-1850

[47] Jiang H, Wang P, Li X, Wang Q, Deng Z-B, Zhuang X, et al. Restoration of MiR-17/20a in Solid Tumor Cells Enhances the Natural Killer Cell Antitumor Activity by Targeting Mekk2. Cancer Immunology Research. 2014;**2**(8):789-799

[48] Li Y, Hong F, Yu Z. Decreased expression of microRNA-206 in breast cancer and its association with disease characteristics and patient survival. The Journal of International Medical Research. 2013;**41**:596-602

[49] Roy SS, Gonugunta VK, Bandyopadhyay A, Rao MK, Goodall GJ, Sun LZ, et al. Significance of PELP1/HDAC2/miR-200 regulatory network in EMT and metastasis of breast cancer. Oncogene. 2014;**33**:3707-3716

[50] Xiang M, Birkbak NJ, Vafaizadeh V, Walker SR, Yeh JE, Liu S, Kroll Y, Boldin M, Taganov K, Groner B, Richardson AL, and Frank DA. STAT3

Induction of MiR-146b Forms a Feedback Loop to Inhibit the NF-κB to IL-6 Signaling Axis and STAT3-Driven Cancer Phenotypes. Science Signal. 2014;**7**(310):ra11

[51] Png KJ, Halberg N, Yoshida M, Tavazoie SF. A microRNA regulon that mediates endothelial recruitment and metastasis by cancer cells. Nature. 2012; **481**:190-194

[52] Zhang S, Kim K, Jin UH, Pfent C, Cao H, Amendt B, et al. Aryl hydrocarbon receptor agonists induce microRNA-335 expression and inhibit lung metastasis of estrogen receptor negative breast cancer cells. Molecular Cancer Therapeutics. 2012;**11**:108-118

[53] Augoff K, McCue B, Plow EF, Sossey-Alaoui K. miR-31 and its host gene lncRNA LOC554202 are regulated by promoter hypermethylation in triple-negative breast cancer. Molecular Cancer. 2012;**11**:5

[54] Sossey-Alaoui K, Downs-Kelly E, Das M, Izem L, Tubbs R, Plow EF. WAVE3, an actin remodeling protein, is regulated by the metastasis suppressor microRNA, miR-31, during the invasion-metastasis cascade. International Journal of Cancer. 2011; **129**:1331-1343

[55] Stenmark H. Rab GTPases as coordinators of vesicle traffic. Nature Reviews Molecular Cell Biology. 2009; **10**:513-525

[56] Kelly EE, Horgan CP, McCaffrey MW. Rab11 proteins in health and disease. Biochemical Society Transactions. 2012;**40**:1360-1367

[57] Palmieri D, Bouadis A, Ronchetti R, Merino MJ, Steeg PS. Rab11a differentially modulates epidermal growth factor-induced proliferation and motility in immortal breast cells. Breast Cancer Research and Treatment. 2006; **100**:127-137

[58] Yang H, Yu J, Wang L, Ding D, Zhang L, Chu C, et al. miR-320a is an independent prognostic biomarker for invasive breast cancer. Oncology Letters. 2014;**8**:1043-1050

[59] Schneider JG, Alosi JA, McDonald DE, McFadden DW. Pterostilbene inhibits lungs cancer through induction of apoptosis. Journal of Surgical Research. 2010;**161**:18-22

[60] Morrow AA, Alipour MA, Bridges D, Yao Z, Saltiel AR, Lee JM. The lipid kinase PI4KIII beta is highly expressed in breast tumors and activates Akt in cooperation with Rab11a. Molecular Cancer Research. 2014;**12**: 1492-1508

[61] Yu J, Wang J, Zhang L, Yang H, Wang L, Ding D, et al. MicroRNA-320a inhibits breast cancer metastasis by targeting metadherin. Oncotarget. 2016; **7**(25):38612-38625

[62] Peden AA, Schonteich E, Chun J, Junutula JR, Scheller RH, Prekeris R. The RCP-Rab11 complex regulates endocytic protein sorting. Molecular Biology of the Cell. 2004;**15**:3530-3541

[63] Gelsi-Boyer V, Orsetti B, Cervera N, Finetti P, Sircoulomb F, Rouge C, et al. Comprehensive profiling of 8p11-12 amplification in breast cancer. Molecular Cancer Research. 2005;**3**: 655-667

[64] Zhang J, Liu X, Datta A, Govindarajan K, Tam WL, Han J, et al. RCP is a human breast cancer-promoting gene with Ras-activating function. The Journal of Clinical Investigation. 2009;**119**:2171-2183

[65] Caswell PT, Chan M, Lindsay AJ, McCaffrey MW, Boettiger D, Norman JC. Rab-coupling protein coordinates recycling of alpha5beta1 integrin and EGFR1 to promote cell migration in 3D microenvironments. Journal of Cell Biology. 2008;**183**:143-155

[66] Siegel R, Desantis C, Jemal A. Colorectal cancer statistics. A Cancer Journal for Clinicians. 2014;**64**:104-117

[67] Smith RA, Eschenbach ACV, Wender R, Levin B, Byers T, Rothenberger D, et al. American Cancer Society guidelines for the early detection of cancer: Update of early detection guidelines for prostate, colorectal, and endometrial cancers. Also: Update 2001—Testing for early lung cancer detection. A Cancer Journal for Clinicians. 2001;**51**:38-75

[68] O'Donnell KA, Wentzel EA, Zeller KI, Dang CV, Mendell JT. c-Myc-regulated microRNAs modulate E2F1 expression. Nature. 2005;**435**:839-843

[69] Sokolova V, Fiorino A, Zoni E, Crippa E, Reid JF, Gariboldi M, et al. The effects of miR-20a on p21: Two mechanisms blocking growth arrest in TGF-β-responsive colon carcinoma. Journal of Cellular Physiology. 2015;**230**: 3105-3114

[70] Diosdado B, van de Wiel MA, Terhaar Sive Droste JS, Mongera S, Postma C, Meijerink WJHJ, et al. MiR-17-92 cluster is associated with 13q gain and c-myc expression during colorectal adenoma to adenocarcinoma progression. British Journal of Cancer. 2009;**101**:707-114

[71] Luo X, Burwinkel B, Tao S, Brenner H. MicroRNA signatures: Novel biomarker for colorectal cancer. American Association for Cancer Research. 2011;**20**:1272-1286

[72] Xu T, Jing C, Shi Y, Miao R, Peng L, Kong S, et al. MicroRNA-20a enhances the epithelial-to-mesenchymal transition of colorectal cancer cells by modulating matrix metalloproteinases. Experimental and Therapeutic Medicine. 2015a;**10**(10):683-10688

[73] Xu Y, Zhao S, Cui M, Wang Q. Down-regulation of microRNA-135b inhibited growth of cervical cancer cells by targeting FOXO1. International Journal of Clinical and Experimental Pathology. 2015b;**8**:10294-10304

[74] Zhang GJ, Li Y, Zhou H, Xiao HX, Zhou T. miR-20a is an independent prognostic factor in colorectal cancer and is involved in cell metastasis. Molecular Medicine Reports. 2014;**10**: 283-291

[75] Wang J, Sun L, Myeroff L, Wang X, Gentry LE, Yang J, et al. Demonstration that mutation of the type II transforming growth factor beta receptor inactivates its tumor suppressor activity in replication error-positive colon carcinoma cells. The Journal of Biological Chemistry. 1995; **270**:22044-22049

[76] Zhong CY, Sun WW, Ma Y, Zhu H, Yang P, Wei H, et al. Microbiota prevents cholesterol loss from the body by regulating host gene expression in mice. Scientific Reports. 2015;**5**:10512

[77] Schaubeck M, Clavel T, Calasan J, Lagkouvardos I, Haange SB, Jehmlich N, et al. Dysbiotic gut microbiota causes transmissible Crohn's disease-like ileitis independent of failure in antimicrobial defence. Gut. 2015;**65**:225-237

[78] Yau TO, Wu CW, Tang C, Chen Y, Fang J, Dong Y, et al. microRNA-20a in human faeces as a non-invasive biomarker for colorectal cancer. Oncotarget. 2016;**7**:1559-1568

[79] Siemens H, Jackstadt R, Hunten S, Kaller M, Menssen A, Gotz U, et al. miR-34 and SNAIL form a double-negative feedback loop to regulate epithelial-mesenchymal transitions. Cell Cycle. 2011;**10**(24):4256-4271

[80] Cekaite L, Eide PW, Lind GE, Skotheim RI, Lothe RA. MicroRNAs as growth regulators, their function and biomarker status in colorectal cancer. Oncotarget. 2016;**7**(6):6476-6505

[81] He L, He X, Lim LP, De Stanchina E, Xuan Z, Liang Y, et al. A microRNA component of the p53 tumour suppressor network. Nature. 2007; **447**(7148):1130-1134

[82] Bieging KT, Mello SS, Attardi LD. Unravelling mechanisms of p53-mediated tumour suppression. Nature Review Cancer. 2014;**14**(5):359-370

[83] Davalos V, Moutinho C, Villanueva A, Boque R, Silva P, Carneiro F, et al. Dynamic epigenetic regulation of the microRNA-200 family mediates epithelial and mesenchymal transitions in human tumorigenesis. Oncogene. 2012;**31**(16):2062-2074

[84] Chen L, Zheng J, Zhang Y, Yang L, Wang J, Ni J, et al. Tumor-specific expression of microRNA-26a suppresses human hepatocellular carcinoma growth via cyclin-dependent and -independent pathways. Molecular Therapy. 2011; **19**(8):1521-1528

[85] Paterson EL, Kazenwadel J, Bert AG, Khew- Goodall Y, Ruszkiewicz A, Goodall GJ. Down- regulation of the miRNA-200 family at the invasive front of colorectal cancers with degraded basement membrane indicates EMT is involved in cancer progression. Neoplasia. 2013;**15**(2):180-191

[86] Oster B, Linnet L, Christensen LL, Thorsen K, Ongen H, Dermitzakis ET, et al. Group Colofol Steering. Laurberg S et al. Non-CpG island promoter hypomethylation and miR-149 regulate the expression of SRPX2 in colorectal cancer. International Journal of Cancer. 2013;**132**(10):2303-2315

[87] El-Murr N, Abidi Z, Wanherdrick K, Svrcek M, Gaub MP, Flejou JF, et al. MiRNA genes constitute new targets for microsatellite instability in colorectal cancer. PLoS One. 2012;7(2):e31862

[88] Nandakumar A, Ramnath T, Chaturvedi M. The magnitude of cancer cervix in India. Indian Journal of Medical Research. 2009;**130**:219-221

[89] Denny L. Cervical cancer: Prevention and treatment. Discovery Medicine. 2012;**14**:125-131

[90] Cuzick J, Arbyn M, Sankaranarayanan R, Tsu V, Ronco G, Mayrand MH, et al. Overview of human papillomavirus-based and other novel options for cervical cancer screening in developed and developing countries. Vaccine. 2008;**26**(supplement 10):K29-K41

[91] Díaz-González SM, Deas J, Benítez-Boijseauneau O, Gómez-Cerón C, Bermúdez-Morales VH, Rodríguez-Dorantes M, et al. Utility of microRNAs and siRNAs in cervical carcinogenesis. BioMed Research International. 2015; **2015**:374924

[92] Zhao Q, Zhai XY, Liu HQ, Shi YA, Li XB. MicroRNA-491-5p suppresses cervical cancer cell growth by targeting Htert. Oncology Reports. 2015;**34**: 979-986

[93] Deng B, Zhang Y, Zhang S, Wen F, Miao Y, Guo K. MicroRNA-142-3p inhibits cell proliferation and invasion of cervical cancer cells by targeting FZD7. Tumour Biology. 2015;**36**: 8065-8073

[94] Li XR, Chu HJ, Lv T, Wang L, Kong SF, Dai SZ. miR-342-3p suppresses proliferation, migration and invasion by targeting FOXM1 in human cervical cancer. FEBS Letters. 2014;**588**: 3298-3307

[95] Greer EL, Brunet A. FOXO transcription factors at the interface between longevity and tumor suppression. Oncogene. 2005;**24**: 7410-7425

[96] Huang H, Regan KM, Lou Z, Chen J, Tindall DJ. CDK2-dependent phosphorylation of FOXO1 as an

apoptotic response to DNA damage. Science. 2006;**314**:294-297

[97] Hou T, Ou J, Zhao X, Huang X, Huang Y, Zhang Y. MicroRNA-196a promotes cervical cancer proliferation through the regulation of FOXO1 and p27Kip1. British Journal of Cancer. 2014;**110**:1260-1268

[98] Long MJ, Wu FX, Li P, Liu M, Li X, Tang H. MicroRNA-10a targets CHL1 and promotes cell growth, migration and invasion in human cervical cancer cells. Cancer Letters. 2012;**324**(2): 186-196

[99] Sekuklu SD, Donoghue MTA, Spillane C. miR-21 as a key regulator of oncogenic processes. Biochemical Society Transactions. 2009;**37**(4): 918-925

[100] Kota J, Chivukula RR, Donnell KA, Wentzel EA, Montgomery LC, Hwang HW, et al. Therapeutic microRNA delivery suppresses tumorigenesis in a murine liver cancer model. Cell. 2009; **137**:1005-1017

[101] Gaur A, Jewell DA, Liang Y, Ridzon D, Moore JH, Chen C, et al. Characterization of microRNA expression levels and their biological correlates in human cancer cell lines. Cancer Research. 2007;**67**:2456-2468

[102] Kim HS, Lee KS, Bae HJ, Eun JW, Shen Q, Park SJ, et al. MicroRNA-31 functions as a tumor suppressor by regulating cell cycle and epithelial-mesenchymal transition regulatory proteins in liver cancer. Oncotarget. 2015;**6**(10):8089-8102

[103] Drakaki A, Hatziapostolou M, Polytarchou C, Vorvis C, Poultsides GA, Souglakos J, et al. Functional microRNA high throughput screening reveals miR-9 as a central regulator of liver oncogenesis by affecting the PPARA-CDH1 pathway. BMC Cancer. 2015;**15**: 542

[104] Pang F, Zha R, Zhao Y, Wang Q, Chen D, Zhang Z, et al. MiR-525-3p enhances the migration and invasion of liver cancer cells by downregulating ZNF395. PLoS One. 2014;**9**(3):e90867

[105] Gronberg H. Prostate cancer epidemiology. Lancet. 2003;**361**:859-864

[106] Meeker AK, Hicks JL, Platz EA, March GE, Bennett CJ, Delannoy MJ. Telomere shortening is an early somatic DNA alteration in human prostate tumorigenesis. Cancer Research. 2002; **62**:6405-6409

[107] Dong JT, Isaacs WB, Isaacs JT. Molecular advances in prostate cancer. Current Opinion in Oncology. 1997;**9**: 101-107

[108] Wang JC, Begin LR, Berube NG, Chevalier S, Aprikian AG, Gourdeau H, et al. Down-regulation of CD9 expression during prostate carcinoma progression is associated with CD9 mRNA modification. Clinical Cancer Research. 2007;**13**:2354-2361

[109] Yaman AF, Kovancilar M, Dizdar Y, Darendeliler E, Holdenrieder S, Dalay N. Investigation of miR-21, miR-141, and miR-221 in blood circulation of patients with prostate cancer. Tumor Biology. 2011;**32**:583-588

[110] Kim WT, Kim WJ. MicroRNAs in prostate cancer. Prostate International. 2013;**1**:3-9

[111] Massard C, Fizazi K. Targeting continued androgen receptor signaling in prostate cancer. Clinical Cancer Research. 2011;**17**:3876-3883

[112] Waltering KK, Porkka KP, Jalava SE, Urbanucci A, Kohonen PJ, Latonen LM. Androgen regulation of micro-RNAs in prostate cancer. Prostate. 2011; **71**:604-614

[113] Lewis H, Lance R, Troyer D, Beydoun H, Hadley M, Orians J, et al.

miR-888 is an expressed prostatic secretions-derived microRNA that promotes prostate cell growth and migration. Cell Cycle. 2014;**13**(2): 227-239

[114] Saini S, Majid S, Dahiya R. Diet, MicroRNAs and Prostate Cancer. Pharmaceutical Research. 2010;**27**(6): 1014-1026

[115] Travis WD, Brambilla E, Harris CC, Muller-Hermelink HK, editors. World Health Organization Classification of Tumours, Pathology and Genetics: Tumours of the Lung, Pleura, Thymus and Heart. Lyon: IARC Press; 2004. pp. 12-15

[116] Minna JD, Roth JA, Gazdar AF. Focus on lung cancer. Cancer Cell. 2002; **1**:49-52

[117] Yanaihara N, Caplen E, Bowman E, Seike M, Kumamoto K, Yi M, et al. Unique microRNA molecular profiles in lung cancer diagnosis and prognosis. Cancer Cell. 2006;**9**:189-198

[118] Johnson SM, Grosshans H, Shingara J, Byrom M, Jarvis R, Cheng A, et al. RAS is regulated by the let-7 microRNA family. Cell. 2005;**120**: 635-647

[119] Eberharter A, Becker PB. Histone acetylation: A switch between repressive and permissive chromatin. Second in review series on chromatin dynamics. EMBO Reports. 2002;**3**:224-229

[120] Jones PA, Baylin SB. The fundamental role of epigenetic events in cancer. Nature Reviews Genetics. 2002; **3**:415-428

[121] Calin GA, Ferracin M, Cimmino A, Di Leva G, Shimizu M, Wojcik SE, et al. A microRNA signature associated with prognosis and progression in chronic lymphocytic leukemia. The New England Journal of Medicine. 2005;**353**: 1793-1801

[122] Qi J, Mu D. MicroRNAs and lung cancers: from pathogenesis to clinical implications. Front Medicine. 2012;**6**(2): 134-155

[123] Zhang JG, Wang JJ, Zhao F, Liu Q, Jiang K, Yang GH. MicroRNA-21 (miR-21) represses tumor suppressor PTEN and promotes growth and invasion in non-small cell lung cancer (NSCLC). Clinica Chimica Acta. 2010;**411**(11-12): 846-852

[124] Lize M, Klimke A, Dobbelstein M. MicroRNA-449 in cell fate determination. Cell Cycle. 2011;**10**(17):2874-2882

[125] Uemura N, Okamoto S, Yamamoto S, Matsumura N, Yamaguchi S, Yamakido M, et al. Helicobacter pylori infection and the development of gastric cancer. Helicobacter pylori infection and the development of gastric cancer. The New England Journal of Medicine. 2001;**345**:784-789

[126] Ju HR, Jung U, Sonn CH, Yoon SR, Jeon JH, Yang Y, Lee KN, Choi I. Aberrant signaling of TGF-beta1 by the mutant Smad4 in gastric cancer cells. Cancer Letters 2003;**196**:197-206

[127] Park K, Kim SJ, Bang YJ, Park JG, Kim NK, Roberts AB, et al. Genetic changes in the transforming growth factor beta (TGFbeta) type II receptor gene in human gastric cancer cells: Correlation with sensitivity to growth inhibition by TGF-beta. Proceedings of the National Academy of Sciences. 1994; **91**:8772-8776

[128] Kim YK, Kim VK. Processing of intronic microRNAs. EMBO Journal. 2007;**26**:775-783

[129] Blow JJ, Hodgson B. Replication licensing—Defining the proliferative state. Trends in Cell Biology. 2002;**12**: 72-78

[130] Mattioli E, Vogiatzi P, Sun A, Abbadessa G, Angeloni G, D'Ugo D,

et al. Immunohistochemical analysis of pRb2/p130, VEGF, EZH2, p53, p16 (INK4A), p27(KIP1), p21(WAF1), Ki-67 expression patterns in gastric cancer. Journal of Cellular Physiology. 2007;**210**:183-191

[131] Brink VD, Offerhaus GJ. The morphogenetic code and colon cancer development. Cancer Cell. 2007;**11**: 109-117

[132] Petrocca F, Visone R, Onelli MR, Shah MH, Nicoloso MS, Martino ID, et al. E2F1-regulated microRNAs impair TGFbeta-dependent cell-cycle arrest and apoptosis in gastric cancer. Cancer Cell. 2008;**13**:272-286

[133] Ohgushi M, Kuroki S, Fukamachi H, O'Reilly LA, Kuida K, Strasser A, et al. Transforming growth factor beta-dependent sequential activation of Smad, Bim, and caspase-9 mediates physiological apoptosis in gastric epithelial cells. Molecular and Cell Biology. 2005;**25**:10017-10028

[134] Gross A, McDonnell JM, Korsmeyer SJ. BCL-2 family members and the mitochondria in apoptosis. Genes & Development. 1999;**13**: 1899-1911

[135] Lim JY, Yoon SO, Seol S-Y, Hong SW, Kim JW, Choi SH, et al. Overexpression of miR- 196b and HOXA10 characterize a poor-prognosis gastric cancer subtype. World Journal of Gastroenterology. 2013;**19**(41): 7078-7088

[136] Wu C, Li M, Hu C, Duan H. Clinical significance of serum miR-223, miR-25 and miR-375 in patients with esophageal squamous cell carcinoma. Molecular Biology Reports. 2014a;**41**(3):1257-1266

[137] Wu H-H, Lin W-C, Tsai KW. Advances in molecular biomarkers for gastric cancer: miRNAs as emerging novel cancer markers. Expert Reviews in Molecular Medicine. 2014b;**16**:e1

[138] Shin JY, Kim YI, Cho SJ, Lee MK, Kook MC, Lee JH, et al. MicroRNA 135a suppresses lymph node metastasis through down-regulation of ROCK1 in early gastric cancer. PLoS One. 2014;**9**: e85205

[139] Cookson MS, Herr HW, Zhang ZF, Soloway S, Sogani PC, Fair WR. The treated natural history of high risk superficial bladder cancer: 15-year outcome. Journal of Urology. 1997;**158**: 62-67

[140] Dyrskjot L, Ostenfeld MS, Bramsen JB, Silahtaroglu AN, Lamy P, Ramanathan R, et al. Genomic profiling of microRNAs in bladder cancer: miR-129 is associated with poor outcome and promotes cell death in vitro. Cancer Research. 2009;**69**:4851-4860

[141] Meng F, Henson R, Wehbe-Janek H, Ghoshal K, Jacob ST, Patel T. MicroRNA-21 regulates expression of the PTEN tumor suppressor gene in human hepatocellular cancer. Gastroenterology. 2007;**133**:647-658

[142] Zhu S, Si ML, Wu H, Mo YY. MicroRNA-21 targets the tumor suppressor gene tropomyosin 1 (TPM1). Journal of Biological Chemistry. 2007; **282**:14328-14336

[143] Liao R, Sun J, Zhang L. MicroRNAs play a role in the development of human hematopoietic stem cells. Journal of Cellular Biochemistry. 2008;**104**: 805-817

[144] Aaboe M, Birkenkamp-Demtroder K, Wiuf C. SOX4 expression in bladder carcinoma: Clinical aspects and in vitro functional characterization. Cancer Research 2006;**66**:343-442.

[145] Feng Y, Liu J, Kang Y, He Y, Liang B, Yang P, et al. miR-19a acts as an oncogenic microRNA and is up-regulated in bladder cancer. Journal of Experimental Clinical Cancer Research. 2014;**33**(1):67

[146] Yu G, Yao W, Xiao W, Li H, Xu H, Lang B. MicroRNA-34a functions as an anti-metastatic microRNA and suppresses angiogenesis in bladder cancer by directly targeting CD44. Journal of Experimental Clinical Cancer Research. 2014;**33**(1):779

[147] Rooj AK, Mineo M, Godlewski J. MicroRNA and extracellular vesicles in glioblastoma: Small but powerful. Brain Tumor Pathology. 2016;**33**:77-88

[148] Cheng AM, Byrom MW, Shelton J, Ford LP. Antisense inhibition of human miRNAs and indications for an involvement of miRNA in cell growth and apoptosis. Nucleic Acids Research. 2005;**33**:1290-1297

[149] Chan JA, Krichevsky AM, Kosik K. Glioblastoma cells MicroRNA-21 is an antiapoptotic factor in human. Cancer Research. 2005;**65**:6029-6033

[150] Brower JV, Clark PA, Lyon W, Kuo JS. MicroRNAs in cancer: glioblastoma and glioblastoma cancer stem cells. Neurochemistry International. 2014;**77**: 68-77

[151] Kefas B, Godlewski J, Comeau L, Li Y, Abounader R, Hawkinson M, et al. microRNA-7 Inhibits the Epidermal Growth Factor Receptor and the Akt Pathway and Is Down-regulated in Glioblastoma. Cancer Research. 2008; **68**:10

[152] Calin GA, Liu CG, Sevignani C, Ferracin M, Felli N, Dumitru CD, et al. MicroRNA profiling reveals distinct signatures in B cell chronic lymphocytic leukemias. Proceedings of the National Academy of Sciences of the United States of America. 2004;**101**:11755-11760

[153] Calin GA, Dumitru CD, Shimizu M, Bichi R, Zupo S, Noch E, et al. Frequent deletions and down-regulation of micro-RNA genes miR15 and miR16 at 13q14 in chronic lymphocytic leukemia. Proceedings of the National Academy of Sciences of the United States of America. 2002;**99**:15524-15529

[154] Oscier DG, Gardiner A, Mould SJ, Glide S, Davis ZA, Ibbotson RE, et al. Multivariate analysis of prognostic factors in CLL: Clinical stage, IGVH gene mutational status, and loss or mutation of the p53 gene are independent prognostic factors. Blood. 2002;**100**:1177-1184

[155] Soria JC, Lee HY, Lee JI, Wang L, Issa JP, Kemp BL, et al. Lack of PTEN expression in non-small cell lung cancer could be related to promoter methylation. Clinical Cancer Research. 2002;**8**:1178-1184

[156] Balatti V, Pekarky Y, Croce CM. Role of microRNA in chronic lymphocytic leukemia onset and progression. Journal of Hematology Oncology. 2015;**8**:12

[157] Xiao C, Srinivasan L, Calado DP, Patterson HC, Zhang B, Wang J, et al. Lymphoproliferative disease and autoimmunity in mice with increased miR-17-92 expression in lymphocytes. Nature Immunology. 2008;**9**:405-414

[158] Balatti V, Acunzo M, Pekarky Y, Croce CM. Novel mechanisms of regulation of miRNAs in CLL. Trends Cancer. 2016;**2**(3):134-143

[159] Fulci V, Chiaretti S, Goldoni M, Azzalin G, Carucci N, Tavolaro S. Quantitative technologies establish a novel microRNA profile of chronic lymphocytic leukemia. Blood. 2007; **109**(11):4944-4951

[160] Li C, Heidt DG, Dalerba P, Burant CF, Zhang L, Adsay V, et al. Identification of pancreatic cancer stem cells. Cancer Research. 2007;**67**:1030-1037

[161] Li Y, Sarkar FH. MicroRNA Targeted Therapeutic Approach for Pancreatic Cancer. International Journal of Biological Sciences. 2016;**12**(3): 326-337

[162] Lei XX, Xu J, Ma W, Qiao C, Newman MA, Hammond SM, et al. Determinants of mRNA recognition and translation regulation by Lin28. Nucleic Acids Research. 2012;**40**:3574-3584

[163] Peng S, Chen LL, Lei XX, Yang L, Lin H, Carmichael GG, Huang Y. Genome-wide studies reveal that Lin28 enhances the translation of genes important for growth and survival of human embryonic stem cells. Stem Cells. 2011;**29**:496-504

[164] Qin W, Ren Q, Liu T, Huang Y, Wang J. MicroRNA-155 is a novel suppressor of ovarian cancer-initiating cells that targets CLDN1. FEBS Letters. 2013;**587**:1434-1439

[165] Qiu C, Ma Y, Wang J, Peng S, Huang Y. Lin28-mediated post-transcriptional regulation of Oct4 expression in human embryonic stem cells. Nucleic Acids Research. 2010;**38**: 1240-1248

[166] Shao Y, Zhang L, Cui L, Lou W, Wang D, Lu W, et al. LIN28B suppresses microRNA let-7b expression to promote CD44+/LIN28B+ human pancreatic cancer stem cell proliferation and invasion. American Journal of Cancer Research. 2015;**5**:2643-2659

[167] Garzon R, Liu S, Fabbri M, Liu Z, Heaphy CEA, Callegari E, et al. MicroRNA-29b induces global DNA hypomethylation and tumor suppressor gene reexpression in acute myeloid leukemia by targeting directly DNMT3A and 3B and indirectly DNMT1. Blood. 2009;**113**:6411-6418

[168] Toyota M, Kopecky KJ, Toyota MO, Jair KW, Willman CL, Issa JP. Methylation profiling in acute myeloid leukemia. Blood. 2001;**97**:2823-2829

[169] Yeh CH, Moles R, Nicot C. Clinical significance of microRNAs in chronic and acute human leukemia. Molecular Cancer. 2016;**15**(1):37

[170] Garzon R, Pichiorri F, Marcucci G, Kornblau S, Andreeff M, Croce C. MicroRNA-29b targets MCL-1 and is down-regulated in chemotherapy-resistant acute myeloid leukemia (AML). Blood. 2007;**110**:717

[171] Testa JR, Bellacosa A. AKT play a central role in tumorigenesis. Proceedings of the National Academy of Sciences of the United States of America. 2001;**98**:10983-10985

[172] Yang H, Kong W, He L, Zhao JJ, O'Donnell JD, Wang J, et al. MicroRNA expression profiling in human ovarian cancer: miR-214 induces cell survival and cisplatin resistance by targeting PTEN. Cancer Research. 2008;**68**: 425-433

[173] Delfino KR, Rodriguez-Zas SL. Transcription Factor-MicroRNA-Target Gene Networks Associated with Ovarian Cancer Survival and Recurrence. PLoS One. 2013;**8**(3):e58608

[174] Kinose Y, Sawada K, Nakamura K, Kimura T. The Role of MicroRNAs in Ovarian Cancer. Biomed Research International. 2014;**2014**:249393

[175] Liu G, Sun Y, Ji P, Li X, Cogdell D, Yang D, et al. MiR-506 suppresses proliferation and induces senescence by directly targeting the CDK4/6-FOXM1 axis in ovarian cancer. The Journal of Pathology. 2014;**233**(3):308-318

[176] Baek D, Villen J, Shin C, Camargo FD, Gygi SP, Bartel DP. The impact of microRNAs on protein output. Nature. 2008;**455**:64-71

[177] Chen L, Bourguignon LY. Hyaluronan-CD44 interaction promotes c-Jun signaling and miRNA21 expression leading to Bcl-2 expression and chemoresistance in breast cancer cells. Molecular Cancer. 2014;**13**:52

[178] Mei M, Ren Y, Zhou X, Yuan XB, Han L, Wang GX, et al. Downregulation

of miR-21 enhances chemotherapeutic effect of taxol in breast carcinoma cells. Technology in Cancer Research & Treatment. 2010;**9**:77-86

[179] Zhou M, Liu Z, Zhao Y, Ding Y, Liu H, Xi Y, et al. MicroRNA-125b confers the resistance of breast cancer cells to paclitaxel through suppression of pro-apoptotic Bcl-2 antagonist killer 1 (Bak1) expression. The Journal of Biological Chemistry. 2010;**285**: 21496-21507

[180] Hayashita Y, Osada H, Tatematsu Y, Yamada H, Yanagisawa K, Tomida S, et al. A polycistronic microRNA cluster, miR-17-92, is overexpressed in human lung cancers and enhances cell proliferation. Cancer Research;**65**: 9628-9632

Chapter 2

Angiogenesis and Its Role in the Tumour Microenvironment: A Target for Cancer Therapy

Sophia Frentzas, Caroline Lum and Ting-Yu Chen

Abstract

The process of angiogenesis refers to the growth of new blood vessels from existing ones. Tumours can produce factors in the micro-environment which act on blood vessels to promote angiogenesis. It is therefore considered to be fundamental in tumour progression and metastatic dissemination. This neovascularization can be regulated by numerous endogenous factors in the tumour micro-environment. As a result, anti-angiogenic therapies have been developed in the hope of targeting this process to reduce tumour growth and progression. However, only a proportion of patients respond to therapy, indicating the presence of treatment resistance in some. In this chapter, we aim to highlight the process of angiogenesis and to review pivotal evidence for the use of anti-angiogenic therapies thus far (alone and in combination with other agents). Finally, we will illustrate recent evidence for the discovery of biomarkers for anti-angiogenic therapies and potential mechanisms of resistance to such agents.

Keywords: angiogenesis, tumour microenvironment, blood vessels, growth factor, stroma, anticancer therapies, biomarkers, resistance mechanisms

1. Introduction

Angiogenesis is a process that is important to the growth of cancers. It refers to when new blood vessels sprout from existing ones. This multi-step process is imperative to the physiological maintenance of the body such as tissue repair [1]. It is also thought to be a critical process that tumours depend on for the delivery of oxygen and nutrients, in order to facilitate growth and progression [2]. Both pro-angiogenic factors and anti-angiogenic factors play a role in modulating tumour neovascularisation. Notably, vascular endothelial growth factors (VEGF) and catecholaminergic signalling pathways have been shown to be key factors in angiogenesis, invasion and metastases [3]. Investigations into catecholaminergic signalling from the sympathetic nervous system have shown to increase VEGF and matrix metalloprotease (MMP) levels, promoting tumour growth, invasion and metastasis [4]. Since tumour angiogenesis requires the up-regulation of these factors, anti-angiogenic agents have now been developed. A multitude of trials have investigated the effect of anti-angiogenic agents on the progression of cancer as well as combination therapies to improve the current standard of care. However, not all patients respond to these, leading to studies that aim at elucidating the mechanisms of resistance.

IntechOpen

2. The role of VEGF in tumour angiogenesis

Angiogenesis is considered to be a fundamental event in tumour progression and metastatic dissemination and is [2] regulated by numerous endogenous factors that stimulate or inhibit neovascularisation [3]. One of the most studied pathways is the vascular endothelial growth factor (VEGF) family of ligands and their receptors [5]. In humans and mice, the VEGF family consists of 5 members: VEGF-A, -B, -C, -D and placental growth factor (PIGF). These ligands demonstrate variable specificity for the three VEGF receptors (VEGFR1, VEGFR2, VEGFR3) [3, 5]. The predominant member of the VEGF family involved in tumourigenesis is VEGF-A and will be referred to as simply 'VEGF' from herein.

One of the most important stimuli for tumour angiogenesis is hypoxia, which can occur when a rapidly growing tumour exceeds the ability of the local vasculature to supply its needs. Hypoxia-inducible factor 1 (HIF-1) is a heterodimeric transcription factor, made up of two DNA binding proteins (HIF-1α and HIF-1β), which induces the transcription of many genes, including VEGF [6]. In the presence of adequate oxygen concentrations, HIF-1α is ubiquitinated and subsequently degraded by the proteasome. However, under hypoxic conditions, HIF-1α is stabilised and persistently dimerises with the other subunit, HIF-1β, to form the HIF-1 heterodimer. The stabilised HIF-1 is then able to bind the VEGF promoter, leading to persistent transcription of the VEGF gene [7]. The expression of VEGF is also stimulated by oncogenes, including Ras, c-Src, Bcr-Abl and p53 [8]. A multitude of studies have shown that VEGF is overexpressed in the majority of solid tumours and that it is a key driver of sprouting angiogenesis [9]. Furthermore, it has been demonstrated in multiple xenograft models that VEGF inhibition supresses tumour growth [10].

3. Signalling in the VEGF pathway

Binding of VEGF to the extracellular domain of VEGFR2 causes receptor dimerisation and phosphorylation of the receptor on tyrosine residues within the

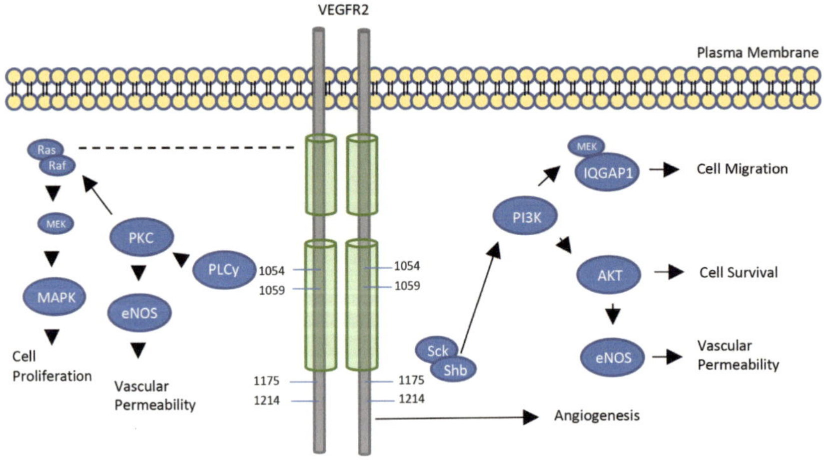

Figure 1.
Signalling from VEGFR2. The signalling cascades downstream of VEGFR2 have been the best studied and are illustrated here. VEGF binding to VEGFR2 induces dimerisation of VEGFR2 and phosphorylation of tyrosine residues (indicated by the four-digit numbers in the illustration). Pathways activated include the Ras-Raf-MEK-ERK pathway, PLCγ/PKC pathway and the PI3K/Akt pathway. Activation of downstream signalling from VEGF receptors exerts control over multiple processes required for angiogenesis including endothelial cell proliferation, migration, tube formation and vascular permeability.

intracellular domain (**Figure 1**) [11]. The Y1054 and Y1059 residues, which lie within the kinase domain, become phosphorylated in response to VEGF stimulation. These positively regulate the intrinsic kinase activity of the intracellular domain and signal to phospholipase-Cγ (PLCγ), which in turn leads to VEGFR2 internalisation [12]. The Y1175 and Y1214 residues lie in the carboxyl terminal tail. These residues become highly phosphorylated in response to VEGF. Y1214 signalling leads to endothelial cell migration and Y1175 signalling leads to PLCγ and extracellular related kinase 1/2 (ERK1/2) activation that is required for DNA synthesis and cell proliferation [13]. Activation of ERK1/2 requires the Ras-Raf-MEK-ERK1/2 signalling cascade but may also require the PLCγ/PKC/PKD pathway [14]. The roles of Y951 and Y996 residues, which lie in the kinase insert region, have not been definitively determined, but Y951 phosphorylation has been shown to increase endothelial cell migration and proliferation via both the PLC-γ and PI3K pathways [15].

4. Sprouting angiogenesis

According to the established dogma, VEGF released by tumours stimulates the growth of new vessels in the following way. The VEGF diffuses through the tissue and activates endothelial cells located in local blood vessels. Firstly, VEGF receptor activation induces the selection of sprouting endothelial cells. Proteinases such as urokinase-type plasminogen activator, uPA, and members of the matrix metalloproteinase (MMP) family mediates the dissolution of the vascular basement membrane and extracellular matrix to facilitate the infiltration of sprouting endothelial cells into the surrounding tissue [16]. Next, endothelial proliferation, migration and branching allows for the formation of new vessels. This is followed by sprout fusion and lumen formation where vessels fuse together to form a network. Finally, there is perfusion and maturation. This is where the stabilisation of new blood vessels forms a functionally perfused system, which is mediated by the recruitment of pericytes to surround the newly formed endothelial tubes; recruitment of pericytes prevents further endothelial cell proliferation and migration and also suppresses vessel leakage [17].

5. VEGF immunomodulation

Multiple possible mechanisms exist regarding immunosuppressive effects of VEGF on the tumour microenvironment. Firstly, due to the effect of VEGF on tumour vasculature, T cell migration from lymph nodes to the microenvironment may be impaired. Furthermore, the ability of T cells to migrate through vessels is negatively affected by VEGF through the down regulation of vascular endothelial selectins, adhesion molecules and promotion of Fas ligand expression. Secondly, VEGF binding to its receptor on myeloid derived suppressor cells within the tumour microenvironment results in STAT 3 signalling, with subsequent promotion of Treg cells and the down regulation of tumour specific T cells [18]. Additionally, the binding of VEGF to VEGFR2 has effects including reduced activation of cytotoxic CD8+ and CD4+ T cells, as well as the upregulation of inhibitory receptors including PD1 and CTLA4 [19]. The interaction of VEGF with VEGFR may also upregulate the programmed death ligand 1 (PDL1) on dendritic cells (DCs) [20]. Furthermore, the binding of VEGF to VEGFR1 on dendritic cells has the effect of inhibiting dendritic cell maturation [20].

6. The development of anti-angiogenic therapies

Given the key role VEGF is proposed to play in tumour angiogenesis, it is unsurprising that it has become a major drug target. Various drugs designed to inhibit VEGF signalling have been developed, including VEGF neutralising antibodies (e.g. bevacizumab), novel fusion proteins which bind pro-angiogenic growth factors (e.g. aflibercept) and VEGF receptor tyrosine kinase inhibitors (e.g. sunitinib) [5, 21]. Such agents have shown promise in the treatment of several malignancies, including mCRC, metastatic renal cell carcinoma (mRCC), metastatic lung cancer, hepatocellular carcinoma (HCC) and pancreatic neuroendocrine tumours (PNET) [22].

6.1 Bevacizumab

Bevacizumab (Avastin®) is a recombinant humanised monoclonal antibody that binds to the VEGF-A isoform of human VEGF specifically and prevents the VEGF from activating the VEGF receptor [23].

6.1.1 Bevacizumab in metastatic CRC

Trials with bevacizumab as a single agent in metastatic colorectal cancer (mCRC) failed to demonstrate activity, but early Phase I trials demonstrated that it has the potential to be combined with many chemotherapy agents [24]. In the advanced setting, several randomised Phase II and III clinical trials clearly demonstrated that bevacizumab improves response rates (ORR), progression free survival (PFS) and overall survival (OS) in mCRC, when added to standard chemotherapy in the first line setting [25, 26], and the second line setting [27] (**Table 1**). In February 2004, the US Food and Drug Administration (FDA) approved bevacizumab for the treatment of mCRC in combination with 5-fluorouracil-based chemotherapy regimens based on a pivotal Phase III study which demonstrated significant PFS and OS survival benefit [25]. Of clinical importance, bevacizumab in combination with a fluoropyrimidine has also demonstrated efficacy in elderly patients with mCRC [26].

Despite these data, only a small proportion of patients benefit from the addition of bevacizumab, and furthermore, some studies have demonstrated only an increase in PFS, with no increase in ORR or OS (**Table 1**) [28]. Additionally, even those who respond initially to bevacizumab combined with chemotherapy will inevitably develop resistance and relapse [29].

In the setting of colorectal liver-only metastasis (CRLM), it has been well demonstrated that preoperative chemotherapy improves outcome and metastatectomy rates [30]. With this in mind, and on the basis that bevacizumab can improve ORR, several groups set out to evaluate its role in the preoperative CRLM setting. Findings from a small non-randomised controlled trial of neoadjuvant conventional chemotherapy with bevacizumab in high-risk CRLM patients alluded to an improvement of CRC liver metastasis rate to 40% [31]. Data from retrospective, inter-trial studies have also suggested that the addition of bevacizumab to chemotherapy significantly improves pathological response in CRLM compared to when chemotherapy is administered alone [32]. Subgroup post hoc analyses extracted from large randomised controlled trials of unselected patients have failed to show significant improvements in resection rates with the addition of bevacizumab [33]. Without prospective randomised trials however, it is difficult to make conclusions regarding the efficacy of chemotherapy versus chemotherapy combined with bevacizumab in the CRLM setting.

The role of continuing bevacizumab beyond first progression in advanced colorectal cancer has also been examined. The results of two non-randomised

Study	Tumour	Treatment groups	ORR (%)	mPFS (months)	HR and significance for PFS	mOS (months)	HR and significance for survival
Hurwitz et al., 2004[1] Phase 3 N=813	mCRC	Irino + bolus 5FU + LV + Bev	44.8	10.6	0.54 P<0.001	20.3	0.66 P<0.001
		Irino + bolus 5FU + LV + placebo	34.8	6.2		15.6	
Kabbinavar et al., 2005[2] Phase 2 N=209	mCRC	Bolus 5FU + LV + Bev	26	9.2	0.5 P=0.0002	16.6	0.79 P=0.16
		Bolus 5FU + LV	15.2	5.5		12.9	
Saltz et al., 2008[3] Phase 3 N= 1401	mCRC	XELOX + Bev Or FOLFOX + Bev	49	9.4	0.83 P=0.0023	21.3	0.89 P=0.077
		XELOX Or FOLFOX	47	8		19.9	
Cunningham et al., 2013[4] Phase 3 N=280	mCRC	Cape + Bev	19	9.1	0.53 P<0.0001	20.7	0.79 P=0.18
		Cape	10	5.1		16.8	

Bev: bevacizumab; Cape: capecitabine; FOLFOX: Bolus 5-fluorouracil plus infusional 5-fluorouracil plus LV plus oxaliplatin; FU: fluorouracil; HR: hazard ratio; Irino: irinotecan; LV: leucovorin; mCRC: metastatic colorectal cancer; met: metastatic; mOS: medial overall survival; mPFS: median progression free survival; N: number of participants; ORR: objective response rate; PFS: progression free survival; XELOX: Capecitabine plus oxaliplatin; 5FU: 5-fluorouracil.

Table 1.
Studies investigating bevacizumab in metastatic colorectal cancer in the first line.

observational cohort studies (BRiTE and ARIES) demonstrated a significant correlation between the use of bevacizumab beyond progression and substantial improvement in OS [34, 35]. Benefit of treatment beyond progression following first line treatment was later confirmed in a prospective randomised trial [36].

The efficacy of bevacizumab has also been evaluated in the adjuvant setting in CRC patients. Two large randomised studies compared survival between the following arms: adjuvant chemotherapy alone for 6 months versus adjuvant chemotherapy in combination with bevacizumab for 6 months (followed by bevacizumab alone for 6 months). Both studies demonstrated that at 1 year there was an improvement in PFS in the bevacizumab arm. However, no significant difference in OS was observed between treatment arms when assessed at 3 or 5 years [37, 38]. In fact, an analysis at 5 years in the AVANT study demonstrated a possible detrimental effect on survival with the addition of bevacizumab, documenting a higher number of relapses and deaths due to disease progression [37].

6.1.2 Bevacizumab in other tumour types

Bevacizumab in combination with cytotoxic chemotherapy has also shown significant clinical efficacy in other tumour types.

In advanced non-squamous non-small cell lung cancer (NSCLC), two randomised controlled phase III trials demonstrated significant benefit in PFS when bevacizumab was added to platinum-based doublet chemotherapy [39, 40], but only one study reported an increase in OS [40]. To further understand this discrepancy, a recent meta-analysis pooling data from several studies including the aforementioned two, deduced a modest but significant improvement in OS [41]. More recently in metastatic non-squamous NSCLC, the Impower150 phase 3 clinical trial investigated treatment with bevacizumab plus platinum doublet chemotherapy with or without the PDL1 inhibitor atezolizumab. Treatment with atezolizumab, bevacizumab and chemotherapy compared with bevacizumab and chemotherapy resulted in a significant improvement in PFS at 6 months (66.9% vs. 36.5%) and at 12 months (56.1% vs. 18%) [42]. In an interim analysis of OS, an improvement was again seen (**Table 2**) [42].

In advanced ovarian cancer, in the first- and second-line settings, the efficacy of bevacizumab has been assessed when added to platinum-based chemotherapy doublets. Two pivotal first line phase III studies utilising the same chemotherapy doublet (ICON7/AGO-OVAR and GOG-0218 trials) demonstrated a significant improvement in PFS [43]. An updated survival analysis failed to show a significant survival benefit [43].

Bevacizumab has been investigated in glioblastoma multiforme (GBM), in the recurrent setting following first line treatment with temozolamide and radiation therapy. In this setting bevacizumab monotherapy is ineffective, however in combination with lomustine it has resulted in improvement in PFS but not OS [44]. Bevacizumab has also been investigated in the first line setting with chemoradiation in a large randomised placebo controlled trial, but failed to improve outcomes [45].

Earlier phase III trials in RCC have demonstrated efficacy of bevacizumab in combination with sorafenib, sunitinib and interferon alpha (**Table 2**). More recently, bevacizumab has been combined with atezolizumab in metastatic RCC. A phase III randomised trial confirmed significant improvement in PFS for bevacizumab combined with atezolizumab compared with sunitinib monotherapy but mature OS data are still awaited [46].

Despite such encouraging results, bevacizumab has thus far failed to make a significant impact in several other indications, including metastatic breast cancer (mBC), melanoma, pancreatic cancer and prostate cancer. Interestingly, in breast cancer, pooled data from four large clinical trials demonstrated that it neither prolonged OS, nor delayed disease progression significantly, leading the FDA to revoke its initial approval of bevacizumab for mBC [47]. The variation in impact that bevacizumab has, not only across tumour types, but also within a single tumour type, is curious and needs to be better understood.

6.2 Ramucirumab

Ramucirumab is a fully human IgG1 monoclonal antibody that binds to the extracellular domain of VEGFR-2, blocking VEGF from activating the receptor [48]. Clinical efficacy and tolerability have been demonstrated in a number of preclinical studies and more recently in phase III trials. In the refractory metastatic gastric and gastro-oesophageal junction (GOJ) adenocarcinoma setting, ramucirumab significantly improved median OS compared with placebo but this only represented an absolute improvement of 1.4 months [49]. In the second line setting of advanced gastric and GOJ adenocarcinoma, the combination of ramucirumab and paclitaxel has become standard treatment based on the results of the pivotal RAINBOW trial showing significant improvement in OS compared with paclitaxel and placebo [50]. Ramucirumab has not shown benefit in the first line setting including combination with chemotherapy [51].

Ramucirumab has also been investigated in metastatic NSCLC but does not yet have an established role for this indication. After progression on first line platinum based chemotherapy, there was a small but statistically significant benefit in median OS of ramucirumab added to docetaxel [52]. Early results of the RELAY phase 3 clinical trial investigating ramucirumab in combination with erlotinib in the first

Study	Tumour	Treatment groups	ORR (%)	mPFS (months)	HR and significance for PFS	mOS (months)	HR and significance for survival
Sandler et al 2006[5] Phase N= 878	Recurrent/ advanced NSCLC 1L	Carbo + pacli + Bev	35	6.2	0.66 P<0.001	12.3	0.79 P=0.003
		Carbo + Bev	15	4.5		10.3	
Reck et al., 2009[6] Reck et al., 2010 [7](updated analysis) Phase 3 N= 1043	Advanced NSCLC 1L	Cisplatin + gem + Bev 7.5mg/kg	37.8	6.7	Bev 7.5mg/kg vs placebo 0.75 P=0.0003	13.6	Bev 7.5mg/kg vs placebo 0.93 P=0.42
		Cisplatin + gem + Bev 15mg/kg	34.6	6.5	Bev 15mg/kg vs placebo 0.85 P=0.0456	13.4	Bev 15mg/kg vs placebo 1.03 P=0.761
		Cisplatin + gem + placebo	21.6	6.1		13.1	
Socinski et al., 2018 Phase 3 N= 1202	Met NSCLC 1L	Atezolizumab + Carbo + pacli (ACP)	NA	NA	0.62* P<0.001 (ABCP vs BCP)	NA	ABCP vs BCP 0.78 P=0.02
		Carbo + pacli + bev (BCP)	48*	6.8* 6.8** 6.1***	0.51** P<0.001	14.7*	
		Atezo + Carbo + pacli + Bev (ABCP)	63.5*	8.3* 11.3** 9.7***	0.59***	19.2*	
Rini et al., 2008[8] Phase 3 N=732	mRCC 1L	Bev + IFN	25.5	8.5	0.71 P<0.0001	NA	NA
		IFN	13.1	5.2			
Escudier et al 2007[9] Phase 3 N=903	mRCC 2L	Sorafenib	57	5.5	0.44 P<0.001	19.3	0.77 P=0.02
		Placebo	34	2.8		15.9	
Motzer et al., 2009[10] (updated analysis) Phase 3 N=750	mRCC 1L	Sunitinib	47	11	0.42 P<0.001	26.4	0.821 P=0.051
		IFN-α	12	5		21.8	

Bev: bevacizumab; C: cycle; Carbo: carboplatin; chemo: chemotherapy; gem: gemcitabine; HR: hazard ratio; IFN: interferon; mOS: medial overall survival; mPFS: median progression free survival; mRCC: metastatic renal cell carcinoma; N: number of participants; NA: not available; NR: not reached; NSCLC: non-small cell lung cancer; ORR: objective response rate; pacli: paclitaxel; PFS: progression free survival; PD-L1: programmed deat- ligand 1.

* *Population with wild type (WT) genotype*

** *WT population with high expression of an effector T-cell*

*** *Patients with EGFR and ALK mutations*

Table 2.
Studies investigating anti-VEGF agents in NSCLC and RCC.

line setting of metastatic EGFR mutated NSCLC have indicated an improvement in PFS however formal publication of the study findings are awaited.

Ramucirumab has also been investigated in urothelial cancers. In a phase III trial of ramucirumab plus docetaxel compared with docetaxel plus placebo in patients with advanced urothelial carcinoma who had received platinum-based chemotherapy, there was a statistically significant improvement in median PFS (4.07 months vs. 2.76 months) [53].

6.3 Aflibercept

Aflibercept is a recombinant fusion protein that binds to VEGF-A, VEGF-B and placental growth factor (PLGF), all of which have been implicated in angiogenesis and/or the survival of newly formed blood vessels [54]. As it binds to additional pro-angiogenic targets (compared to bevacizumab which binds only VEGF-A), aflibercept may provide further anti-angiogenic effects compared to targeting VEGF-A alone. In preclinical studies, it demonstrated a broad range of anti-tumour and anti-angiogenic activity both alone and in combination with chemotherapy, which was also observed in phase I clinical trials [55]. Recently, a large randomised phase III clinical trial (VELOUR) in advanced CRC patients, receiving second line therapy, demonstrated that the addition of aflibercept to systemic chemotherapy significantly improved outcomes compared to chemotherapy alone [56]. Based on this data, aflibercept was recently approved for use in the second line setting in mCRC when given in combination with chemotherapy. Importantly, results from a subanalysis of VELOUR showed that there was no significant impact of prior exposure to bevacizumab, illustrating the benefit that it provides as a multiple angiogenic factor trap, in a setting where resistance to bevacizumab may have developed [57].

6.4 Receptor tyrosine kinase inhibitors (TKIs)

Several small molecule inhibitors of VEGF receptor tyrosine kinase activity now have an established role in the treatment of certain tumour types, including mRCC, HCC and advanced CRC. These small molecule inhibitors readily diffuse through the cell membrane to compete for ATP binding to the intracellular tyrosine kinase domain of VEGF receptor 2.

6.4.1 Sunitinib

Sunitinib is an orally active multi-kinase inhibitor, which targets VEGFR1–3, PDGFRα/β, c-Kit and FLT3 [58]. Xenograft models have clearly demonstrated that as well as inhibiting new blood vessel formation, sunitinib also induces regression of newly formed immature vessels and significantly stunts tumour growth [59]. Furthermore, immunohistochemical studies performed on human tissue derived from mRCC patients treated with sunitinib have demonstrated that this agent can induce a reduction in tumour vessel density [60].

In terms of outcome in the clinical setting, sunitinib initially showed efficacy, as a single agent, for second-line therapy in single-arm, Phase II studies in mRCC [61]. Patients treated with sunitinib showed promising outcomes in terms of ORR, response duration, PFS and OS. A pivotal Phase III study was subsequently conducted comparing sunitinib with interferon-α as a first-line treatment in mRCC, which demonstrated improved OS, PFS and ORR in the sunitinib arm [62]. Based on such data, sunitinib was approved by the FDA in 2006 for the first line treatment of mRCC. Other TKI's, with similar target specificity (sorafenib, pazopanib, cabozantinib and axitinib) also have activity in mRCC. Combination with immunotherapeutic agents has also shown promising results and we are seeing the treatment algorithm for mRCC change rapidly. In a recent landmark phase 3 trial of advanced RCC in the first line setting, axitinib was combined with the PD1 inihibitor pembrolizumab and compared with sunitinib monotherapy (KEYNOTE-426). The results are promising with a significant improvement in PFS and ORR with axitinib and pembrolizumab, however more mature OS data are awaited [63].

The role of such TKIs has also being evaluated in mCRC. The anti-tumour and anti-angiogenic effects of sunitinib have been well documented in a series of CRC xenograft tumour models [64]. In the clinical setting, however, sunitinib employed either as a single agent or with combination chemotherapy, has failed to demonstrate favourable outcome, both for ORR and PFS [65].

6.4.2 Regorafenib

Recently, another TKI called regorafenib has created a lot of interest in advanced CRC. This agent inhibits VEGFR1-3, PDGFRα/β, KIT, RET, FGFR1 and Tie2. It is also a potent inhibitor of Raf-1 and suppresses both wild-type and V599E mutant BRAF activity *in vitro* and in mouse models [66]. Significant anti-tumour and anti-angiogenic effects in CRC xenograft models, both as a single agent and in combination with irinotecan chemotherapy have been reported [67]. In the clinical setting, the Phase III CORRECT trial demonstrated significant benefit for OS and PFS in advanced CRC patients, when it was used as a single agent compared to best supportive care, in a population who had failed previous standard therapy [68]. Based on this data, regorafenib was approved by the FDA as a multikinase inhibitor for metastatic colorectal cancer in the third line setting in 2012.

Regorafenib also has clinical utility in gastrointestinal stromal tumours (GIST) where it is currently employed in the third line setting after imatinib and sunitinib. This indication followed from a phase 3 randomised trial, demonstrating significantly improved PFS for regorafenib compared with placebo (4.8 months vs. 0.9 months) [69]. There was no significant difference in OS, however this trial did allow for crossover which likely impacted on this finding [69].

Regorafenib has FDA approval for second line treatment of HCC following the positive results of the phase 3 RESORCE clinical trial. Compared with placebo, regorafenib demonstrated survival benefit [70].

7. Potential mechanisms of synergy between bevacizumab and chemotherapy

Early phase clinical trials have demonstrated that bevacizumab, in combination with systemic cytotoxic chemotherapy, can potentiate treatment efficacy when given concomitantly [71]. In fact, in most clinical settings, with the exception of ovarian cancer where bevacizumab has been observed to have single agent activity [72], bevacizumab has only shown significant activity when it is combined with cytotoxic chemotherapy and the same is true for aflibercept [21].

It has been well-established that the tumour vasculature is dysfunctional and leaky, resulting in enhanced interstitial fluid pressure and thus preventing effective delivery of chemotherapy [73]. Evidence from preclinical studies showed that bevacizumab can 'normalise' the chaotic tumour vasculature, achieving reduced vessel tortuosity, reduced leakiness and reduced interstitial fluid pressure. Based on these studies, it was proposed that bevacizumab works in combination with chemotherapy to improve chemotherapy delivery [71, 73], which is now a widely accepted notion amongst many clinicians.

However, this concept is also highly controversial, with some work even refuting the normalisation hypothesis. For example, one group demonstrated that bevacizumab persistently reduced both tumour perfusion and chemotherapy delivery when NSCLC patients were treated with bevacizumab-containing chemotherapy [74]. Therefore, other potential explanations for synergy between bevacizumab and chemotherapy must be considered. Current alternative theories based mostly on preclinical data include: (1) direct synergy between the anti-angiogenic effects of bevacizumab and potential anti-angiogenic effects of chemotherapy [75], (2) targeting of VEGF signalling directly in cancer cells by bevacizumab [21], (3) chemotherapy may inhibit resistance to bevacizumab, because chemotherapy suppresses the tumour recruitment of myeloid cells that have been implicated in resistance to bevacizumab [76], (4) bevacizumab may prevent tumour rebound that may occur during breaks in chemotherapy [76].

It should be noted that vessel normalisation facilitated by anti-angiogenic agents may provide therapeutic benefit through other mechanisms, which are independent of chemotherapy delivery. For example, in glioblastoma patients, vessel normalisation induced by single agent VEGF-targeted therapy may prolong survival due to other effects, such as oedema control or improved tumour oxygenation [77].

There are two other curious observations that have yet to be properly explained. Firstly, the synergistic effect of adding bevacizumab to chemotherapy does not occur in all tumour types. For example, the addition of bevacizumab does not lead to improvements in outcome in advanced breast cancer [78]. Secondly, VEGFR TKIs show single agent activity without the need for co-administration of chemotherapy [21].

Recent insight into these two curious observations has been reported. A study examining both clinical and mouse tumour tissue specimens demonstrated that tumour types utilising a vasculature surrounded by a well-developed stroma (e.g. mCRC, NSCLC) respond better to bevacizumab when it is added to chemotherapy as opposed to tumour types that utilise a vasculature without a well-developed intervening stromal component (e.g. mRCC, PNET) which respond better to VEGF TKIs alone [79]. This suggests that tumour cell interactions with different stromal components may influence response to different anti-angiogenic agents and how they synergise with concomitant drugs. However, there is still much work to be done in order to understand the mechanisms involved.

8. Synergy of anti-angiogenic agents with immunomodulatory therapy

A series of pre-clinical studies have shown that the use of anti-angiogenic agents along with immune checkpoint inhibitors (ICI) as a combination therapy has a synergistic and enhanced effect on the tumour when compared to either ICI therapy or anti-angiogenic therapy alone. Immunotherapy has emerged as a promising treatment option for many cancer types, offering hope for patients with the demonstration of improved outcomes including durable responses in some. Unfortunately, there are still many patients that either have short lived responses to such therapies or none at all. To overcome resistance mechanisms, combinations of immunotherapy with other treatments including VEGF inhibitors are being explored.

Since 2013, pre-clinical investigations in mice with various tumours have indicated that the combination of ICI and anti-angiogenic agents results in prolonged overall survival [80]. It has been observed that the VEGF can cause the upregulation of immune checkpoint molecules such as PD-1 and as a result, the use of anti-VEGF agents has been seen to reduce the expression of PD-1 on cytotoxic T lymphocytes [81]. Thus, the combination of using both anti-VEGF agents as well as anti-PD-1 agents could have a synergistic effect on inhibiting further tumour development [81]. Through the encouraging findings of pre-clinical investigations, many clinical studies have recently or are still in the process of investigating this.

There are a multitude of clinical studies supporting the role of bevacizumab in the positive immune modulation of the tumour microenvironment and its beneficial effects when combined with the immune checkpoint PD1/PDL1 and

CTLA4 inhibitors. In a study investigating melanoma patients treated with ipilimumab plus bevacizumab versus ipilimumab alone, the results showed that the combination therapy increased circulating CD4+ and CD8+ T cells compared with ipilimumab monotherapy [82]. The investigation showed that there was a greater median overall survival in patients undergoing combination therapy (25.1 months) compared to those who underwent the ipilimumab alone treatment (10.1 months) [82]. Furthermore, a separate study of patients with RCC investigating the effect that bevacizumab plus atezolizumab had versus bevacizumab alone found that the combination therapy demonstrated a reduction in neovasulature-related gene expression and decreased microvascular density. The treatment was also associated with an increased tumour infiltration of CD8+ T cells as demonstrated by immunohistochemical staining of cells [83]. This study also demonstrated that MHC Class I is upregulated as a result of the treatment and that both intratumoural CD8+ T cells and macrophages increased as well.

In a phase II study involving patients with RCC, as compared with sunitinib monotherapy, atezolizumab and bevacizumab demonstrated improvements in PFS in patients with an immunosuppressive tumour microenvironment [84]. Whilst it was also discovered that the use of atezolizumab failed to generate an anti-tumour immune response (possibly due to myeloid-induced immune suppression), the addition of bevacizumab to atezolizumab was found to be able to overcome this suppression [84].

Both pre-clinical and clinical studies have shown that anti-angiogenic agents and immunomodulatory therapies have a synergistic affect in reducing tumour growth and a multitude of clinical trials are currently investigating this synergy further. Thus, there is promise in the use of a combination therapy with anti-angiogenic agents and immunomodulatory agents to improve on patient prognosis.

9. Potential predictive biomarkers for anti-angiogenic agents

In view of the variable outcomes seen in the clinic, there is a need for the development of validated predictive biomarkers of response for anti-angiogenic therapy. In this way, patients who will derive benefit from such agents could be appropriately selected, whilst those that will not derive benefit (either at the outset or during therapy) could be selected for alternative, more effective therapy. Such a strategy would not only improve clinical outcomes but would also reduce the unnecessary burden of (a) toxicity to the patient, and (b) cost to the economy. Despite extensive international research in this field, there is currently no biomarker which predicts benefit or resistance to anti-angiogenic agents that is approved for routine clinical practice. The following are amongst several which have been investigated in the clinical setting.

9.1 Circulating biomarkers

Circulating biomarkers are an attractive tool for patients and clinicians as 'liquid biopsies' are relatively non-invasive and easy to perform, as compared with tissue biopsies of tumour with associated risks and potential technical difficulties depending on tumour site. VEGF levels have been studied as a potential biomarker with high levels associated with poorer outcomes [85]. Findings regarding its utility as a predictive biomarker have been more inconsistent [85]. An analysis of four randomised phase 3 trials investigated circulating VEGF level as a prognostic and predictive biomarker in mCRC, lung cancer and RCC which included bevacizumab in the treatment regimen. Tumour specimens were also tested for VEGF level. This found that higher baseline circulating VEGF levels were associated with poorer clinical outcomes but levels did not predict response to bevacizumab [86]. There is early evidence from small and exploratory studies to suggest soluble VEGFR-1, with higher levels being associated with poorer outcomes with anti-angiogenic treatments, however larger studies are required to confirm these findings [87].

Other potential circulating biomarkers have also been investigated. In mCRC, elevated IL-8 levels at baseline were associated with a shorter PFS in patients treated with chemotherapy (FOLFIRI) and bevacizumab [88]. Elevated LDH and neutrophil levels have been found to independently predict poorer survival in patients treated with chemotherapy plus bevacizumab [89]. A promising predictive biomarker for response to bevacizumab based therapy in CRC appears to be circulating endothelial cells, with studies showing that patients with lower circulating endothelial cells at baseline undergoing treatment with bevacizumab based therapy had improved PFS [90].

9.2 Levels of tumour VEGF isoforms

Levels of VEGF expression in a tumour could be a determinant of responsiveness to anti-VEGF therapy. Some small studies have demonstrated a relationship between baseline VEGF expression and response, however these findings have not been consistently replicated in large clinical trials and are often more informative as prognostic rather than predictive biomarkers [91]. Data from more recent prospective studies, however, have shown more consistency in the use of VEGF as a biomarker. A large randomised trial in patients with advanced breast cancer treated with bevacizumab demonstrated a significant association between high circulating levels of VEGF and survival benefit [78]. VEGF expression in tumours was investigated in the large phase III clinical trial of bevacizumab plus chemotherapy in mCRC, but this failed to predict outcomes [92].

There are multiple reasons why using VEGF expression as a biomarker could be problematic: (1) advanced tumours express numerous pro-angiogenic factors in addition to VEGF which could confer resistance to bevacizumab irrespective of the amount of VEGF produced [93], (2) differences in the intensity of VEGF expression might be too small to be clinically relevant, (3) hypoxia, which is promoted by anti-angiogenic therapy, is an important inducer of VEGF expression and might, therefore, lead to increased VEGF production in the presence of bevacizumab treatment; indeed, anti-angiogenic agents have been shown to induce expression of VEGF even in tumour naïve hosts [94], (4) variations in methodology across centres (including sample handling, the use of different scoring systems and non-validated antibodies) have a significant effect on biomarker trial results [95], (5) it is very challenging to standardise cut-offs for low and high VEGF levels, due to: (a) different methods used to measure VEGF at different centres and (b) differences in biology that occur between racial groups, tumour types and different stages of disease [95].

9.3 Levels of alternative pro-angiogenic growth factors

Studies which have investigated other single circulating factors (such as FGF2, and r soluble VEGFR2) have also yielded contradictory and unsatisfactory conclusions [96]. Interestingly, however, recent clinical work in mRCC patients treated with anti-angiogenic TKIs suggests that profiling multiple circulating factors in the blood could have a more powerful prognostic and predictive role than assessing levels of single factors alone [97]. In this study, when patients with mRCC were treated with the TKI pazopanib, a biomarker signature of six factors (HGF, interleukin 6 and interleukin 8, osteopontin, VEGF and TIMP1) was able to distinguish a sub-group of patients that derived a significantly greater overall survival benefit from this agent.

9.4 VEGF polymorphisms

Polymorphisms in VEGF or VEGF receptors have been proposed to predict outcome from anti-angiogenic therapy. As these are generally binary in nature, they are attractive biomarkers since they may be easier to measure and apply prospectively. In metastatic breast cancer, polymorphisms in VEGF and VEGFR2 were analysed in several retrospective subset analyses in patients treated with chemotherapy, with or without bevacizumab. Two polymorphisms within the VEGF promoter/5′ untranslated region, VEGF alleles −2578AA and −1154AA, were significantly associated with improved OS in the bevacizumab plus paclitaxel group when compared to the −2578CA/−2578CC and −1154GA/−1154GG alleles. In contrast, they did not have prognostic power for OS in the chemotherapy-only arm [98]. The predictive power of the −2578AA and −1154AA VEGF alleles was also reported in a retrospective subset analysis of patients with metastatic colorectal cancer that received either FOLFIRI (leucovorin, fluorouracil, and irinotecan) plus bevacizumab or XELIRI (capecitabine and irinotecan) plus bevacizumab [99].

More recently, the role of VEGFR1 polymorphisms was studied in a large meta-analysis pooling DNA data from two phase III trials in patients with advanced pancreatic cancer treated with bevacizumab. VEGFR1 −1213AC/−1213CC alleles were significantly associated with poor outcome in patients receiving bevacizumab when compared to VEGFR1 −1213AA alleles [100]. To understand how this VEGFR1 polymorphism functionally affects VEGFR1 expression and how it might explain its correlation with poor outcome in patients receiving bevacizumab, Lambrechts and colleagues performed an *in vitro* study where the mutant codon of Tyr1213 was transiently overexpressed in HEK293T cells. Lysates from these cells demonstrated a significant increase in expression and signalling of VEGFR1 compared to HEK293T cells harbouring the wild type codon, thus providing a biological rationale for the role of this polymorphism as a negative predictive marker of response [100]. A significant correlation of the VEGFR −1213 with poor outcome was also corroborated by a subsequent study in patients with mRCC treated with sunitinib [101].

9.5 Radiological parameters

Functional clinical imaging, taking into account tumour vasculature or metabolic activity by utilising CT, MRI or PET scanning, either prior to commencing treatment or following brief exposure of patients to therapy, may be a useful tool for predicting response or resistance to anti-angiogenic therapy [102]. For conventional cytotoxic chemotherapy, imaging has been employed to assess therapy response based on change in tumour size, as defined by RECIST (Response Evaluation Criteria In Solid Tumours). However, biological agents, such as bevacizumab and TKIs, may be cytostatic in terms of their mechanism of action, thus size may not be the only parameter that needs to be considered when assessing response and outcome. Examination of various parameters such as blood flow and tumour morphology may provide additional important predictive information.

9.5.1 Baseline vascular perfusion on imaging

Several studies have examined pre-treatment levels of tumour perfusion and whether they can predict outcome. For example, enhanced levels of vessel perfusion at baseline (measured by contrast-assisted tumour enhancement) in mRCC patients treated with VEGF TKIs has been shown to predict for response and survival [103].

9.5.2 Changes in vascular characteristics on imaging

Early alterations in features of the tumour vasculature on imaging after a short period of therapy have also been shown to be associated with response and outcome. For example, in studies of mRCC patients treated with anti-angiogenic TKIs, response criteria that measured both a significant reduction in tumour vascular perfusion and a significant reduction in tumour size were more predictive of outcome compared to change in lesion size alone [104].

Although the use of the above radiological criteria may seem promising as predictors of response and outcome, there are associated challenges that need to be considered before incorporating them into clinical practice. These include, (a) diversity in the methodologies used to assess potential surrogate radiological biomarkers of response between studies and across centres, and (b) insufficient comprehension of how certain radiological features correlate with the underlying tumour biology.

10. Measuring the clinical response to anti-angiogenic agents

Currently, the efficacy of any anti-neoplastic therapy is assessed by several outcome measures, which include (a) effective downsizing of tumours on clinical imaging (to facilitate curative surgery or consolidative radiotherapy for localised disease and to reduce the symptomatic burden of disease in the metastatic setting), (b) prolongation of the interval where a patient is either disease-free or progression-free, and (c) prolongation of survival.

Conventional assessment of residual tumour volume after cytotoxic chemotherapy has traditionally been performed with the use of size-based criteria (overall response rate, ORR, by RECIST). This was based on evidence that there is good correlation between radiological information and residual viable tumour (pathological response) and good correlation with progression-free (PFS) and overall survival (OS) in patients treated with cytotoxic chemotherapy [105]. However, with the advent of biological therapies, such as bevacizumab, the value of utilising RECIST on its own as a surrogate for outcome has been questioned and new imaging criteria have been proposed [102].

10.1 RECIST criteria

For anti-angiogenic therapy employed in advanced malignant disease, retrospective clinical meta-analyses have (a) highlighted the pitfalls and limitations of using RECIST alone in the assessment of response and progression, and (b) highlighted a disassociation of RECIST from time-related endpoints of PFS and OS [105].

This curiosity was provoked by several large randomised clinical trials investigating the effect of adding bevacizumab to conventional chemotherapy in different tumour types. These have consistently demonstrated that significant improvements in PFS and OS were incongruent with modest increases in ORRs [25, 28, 40]. In their CRC meta-analysis, Grothey and colleagues specifically examined the impact of tumour response to bevacizumab (ORR) on treatment benefit (PFS, OS) and concluded that patients who did not attain a positive response according to RECIST (i.e. stable disease) in fact showed significant benefit from bevacizumab, which was of the same magnitude as responding patients (i.e. complete or partial response) [105].

Moreover, similar concepts have consistently featured in several Phase I and II clinical trials employing antiangiogenic agents, and other molecular targeted therapies. These studies corroborate that there is little value in utilising ORR alone, particularly in predicting whether an agent will ultimately have truly meaningful effects on pathological response or in prolonging survival [106]. The underlying reason for these incongruent observations with bevacizumab and other molecular targeted therapies may be because such agents are cytostatic rather than cytotoxic [107].

10.2 Morphological response criteria

There has been growing interest in how the appearance of lesions on clinical imaging can be utilised to accurately assess the effect of bevacizumab on tumour volume and how this appearance may correlate with other clinical end-points. In a small retrospective colorectal liver only metastasis (CRLM) patient cohort treated with bevacizumab and chemotherapy, Chun and colleagues demonstrated that novel morphological response criteria predicted more accurately for OS and pathological response than RECIST (**Figure 2**) [108]. This was subsequently validated in a larger patient population which included patients who were treated with and without bevacizumab [109]. Not only were the morphological response criteria superior to RECIST in predicting major pathological response and OS, further analyses confirmed that the morphological response criteria did not correlate with responses measured according to RECIST. Moreover, there was a significantly higher incidence of optimal responses (measured by morphological response criteria) in the patient cohort receiving bevacizumab with chemotherapy compared to the chemotherapy alone cohort [109]. These data suggest that (a) morphological response criteria and RECIST measure different biological parameters, and (b) the use of morphological response criteria represents a more sensitive tool for measuring tumour response and time-related endpoints of survival for bevacizumab. Similar findings were reported in a retrospective study of non-small cell lung cancer patients treated with bevacizumab and concomitant chemotherapy [110].

10.3 Pathological response criteria

Radiological assessment alone may not accurately reflect response to therapy because simple, unidimensional imaging parameters may overestimate or underestimate downstaging of tumour burden [111]. Furthermore, in the case of adding anti-angiogenic therapy to chemotherapy, although it has been suggested that proposed morphological imaging characteristics can accurately predict tumour response and clinical outcome, such scoring methods have not yet been validated for conventional use in clinical practice and may also be too subjective. Scoring of pathological response may therefore be a better alternative or perhaps an adjunct in assessing residual viable tumour. Moreover, in the case of preoperative chemotherapy or radiotherapy in settings such as rectal cancer and oesophageal cancer, pathological response has also been shown to correlate significantly to disease-free survival (DFS) and OS [112].

Several methodologies incorporating various parameters for scoring pathological response in resected CRLMs, treated with and without bevacizumab, have been proposed. It is still not clear from the current literature which of these classification methods may be superior.

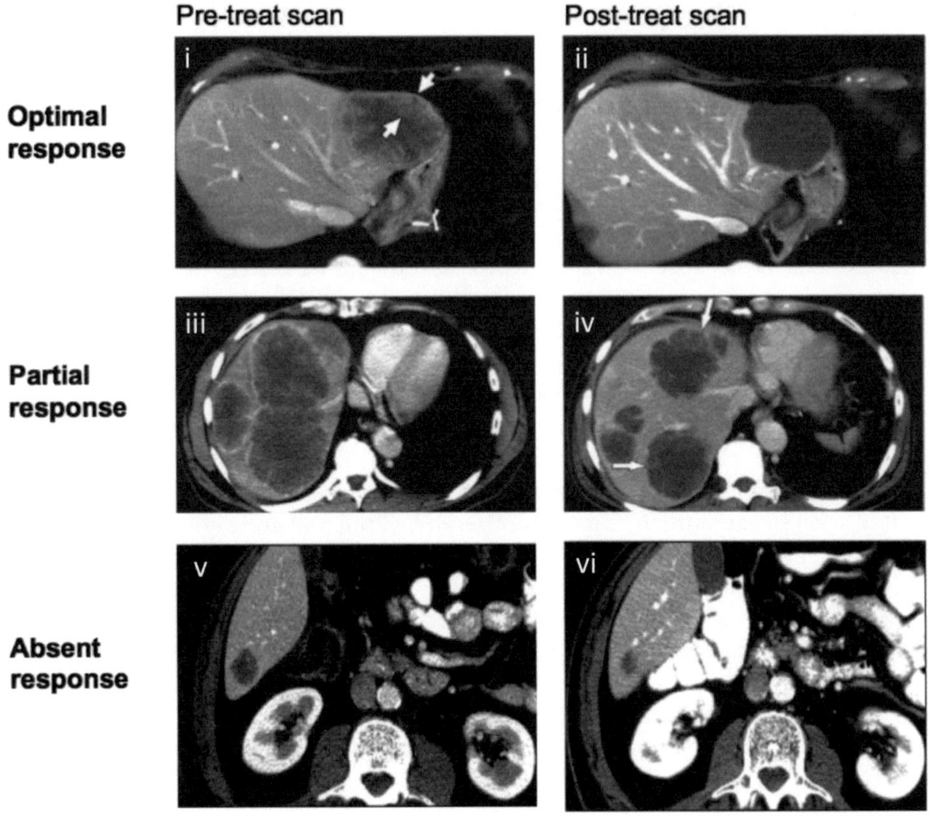

Figure 2.
Morphological response criteria on contrast-enhanced CT (CECT) scans as a predictor of outcome (i) and (ii) CECT performed in a 43-year old patient before and after 10 cycles of bevacizumab containing chemotherapy demonstrating an optimal response (OR). (i) Before therapy, the liver metastasis presented with profound heterogeneous attenuation, a hyperattenuated peripheral rim and a thick, poorly defined tumour-liver interface ('group 3' metastasis). (ii) After therapy, the same liver metastasis shows complete resolution of these features (i.e. it is homogeneous, of low attenuation, with a thin, sharply defined tumor-liver interface). Change in size of lesion is minimal. (iii) and (iv) CECT of the liver performed in a 67-year old patient before and after 2 cycles of bevacizumab-containing chemotherapy demonstrating a partial response (PR). (iii) Before therapy, the liver metastas is presented with features of a 'group 3' metastasis. (iv) After therapy, the same liver metastasis shows moderate resolution of these features (i.e. it has a moderate degree of heterogeneous attenuation, a moderately defined tumor-liver interface with a slight hyperattenuating peripheralrim ('group 2' metastasis)). (v) and (vi) CECT of the liver performed in a 56-year old patient before and after 2 cycles of bevacizumab-containing chemotherapy demonstrating an absent response (AR). (v) Before therapy, the liver metastasis presented with features of a 'group 3' metastasis. (vi) After therapy, the same liver metastas is shows a decrease in tumour size without change in attenuation or tumour-liver interface ('group 3' metastasis). Changes in tumour morphology on CECT have been shown to correlate more significantly with survival than the use of RECIST citeria in CRLM patients treated with bevacizumab-containing chemotherapy.

10.3.1 Percentage viable tumour

Microscopic assessment of the percentage residual viable tumour on haematoxylin & eosin-stained sections of resected tissue has been employed as a predominant parameter in assessing the efficacy of different pre-operative chemotherapy regimens in tumour types such as oesophageal, gastric and rectal adenocarcinomas [113]. Based on this methodology, Ribero and colleagues modified this scoring system for application in CRLMs treated preoperatively, with or without bevacizumab [114]. A semi-quantitative estimation of the percentage area of residual viable tumour cells relative to total tumour surface area within each CRLM metastasis was made with the analysis of four tumour cell viability subsets (<25%, 25–49%,

50–75%, >75%). This retrospective study confirmed that the addition of bevacizumab to chemotherapy yielded an incrementally greater decrease in residual viable cells within these CRLMs in comparison to those treated with chemotherapy alone but no correlation with imaging, or other clinical end-points, was made [114].

10.3.2 Tumour regression grade (TRG)

Mandard and colleagues were one of the first to establish a five-point histological scoring system for pathological response. This was based on cytological and stromal changes on haematoxylin & eosin-stained sections of primary oesophageal squamous cell carcinomas treated with chemoradiotherapy prior to resection [115].

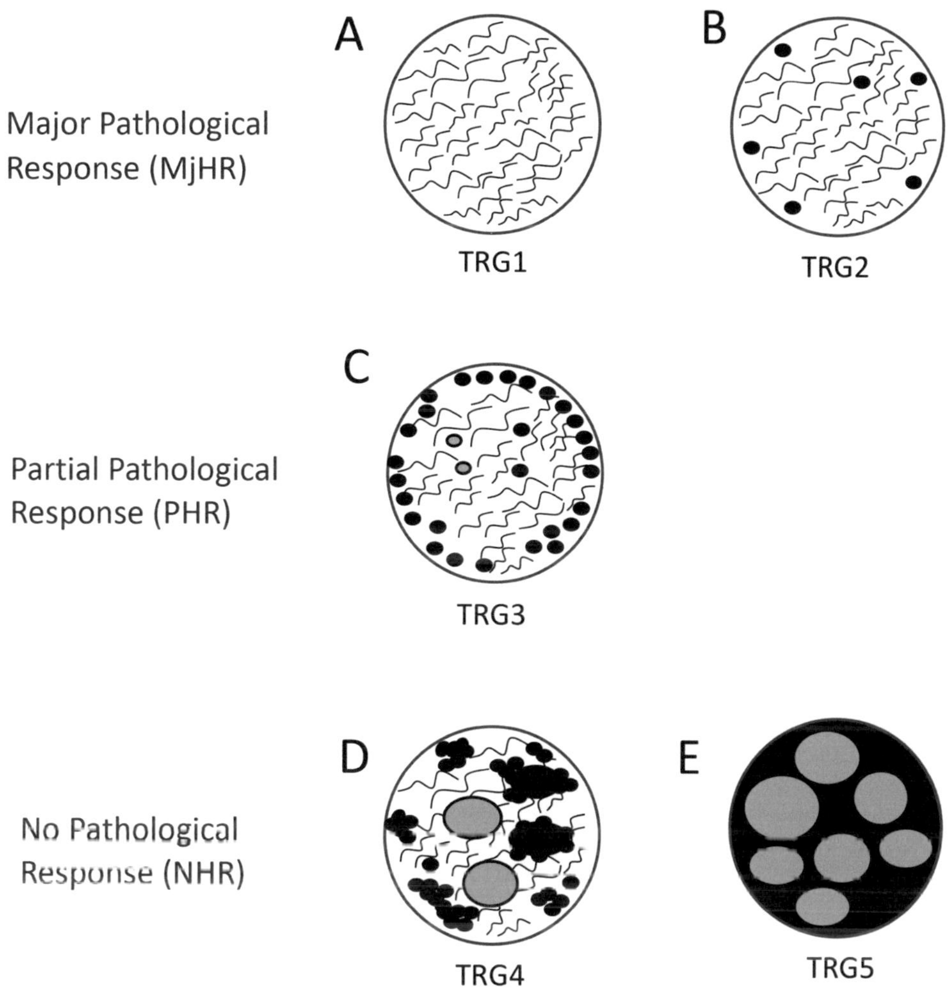

Figure 3.
Tumour regression grade (TRG) scoring system as a component of measuring pathological response in treated CRLMs. (A–E) TRG as scored on haematoxylin and eosin sections of CRLMs based on the proportion of fibrosis to viable tumour cells. The five TRGs shown in this cartoon roughly illustrate the different proportions of fibrosis (fibrils) to tumour cells (black areas). (A) TRG1. There is an absence of viable tumour cells and large amounts of fibrosis. (B) TRG2. The presence of viable tumour cells is rare and they are scattered throughout the fibrosis. (C) TRG3. There is the presence of more residual tumour cells but fibrosis predominates. (D) TRG4. Residual cancer cells predominate over fibrosis. (E) TRG5. There are no signs of tumour regression. The percentage of the CRLM surface area occupied by necrosis is also incorporated as a parameter for pathological response (grey areas). 3 main pathological response groups: TRG1-2: major response (MjHR), TRG3: partial response (PHR), TRG4-5: no histological response (NHR).

Tumour response was scored according to five tumour regression grades (TRG1-5) based on the proportion of fibrosis to viable tumour cells. Later, this TRG scoring system was modified for its application in CRLMs receiving different chemotherapy backbones prior to liver resection (**Figure 3A–E**) [116]. Correlation analyses have demonstrated a significant association of major histological responders with increased survival.

Similar retrospective studies using the TRG in CRLMs were undertaken to see whether adding bevacizumab to chemotherapy would further increase pathological response rate, without necessarily increasing radiographic response rate, after liver resection. Indeed, several retrospective analyses demonstrated that a significantly increased percentage of patients treated with bevacizumab achieved a major pathological response and a significantly higher percentage area of tumour necrosis compared to chemotherapy-only treated patients [117]. Furthermore, the extent of pathological response correlated significantly with long-term-outcomes such as 3- and 5-year overall survival.

11. Mechanisms of resistance to anti-VEGF therapy

As is the case with most cancer therapeutics, drug resistance is considered to be a major factor that limits the efficacy of anti-angiogenic agents. Two 'modes' of resistance to anti-angiogenic therapy are currently recognised: intrinsic resistance, whereby the tumour fails to respond to the therapy from the outset, and acquired resistance, whereby the tumour develops means to evade the therapy after a period of response [21, 29, 118]. It is important to realise that resistance to anti-angiogenic therapy may be attributable to either the tumour cells themselves or due to interactions with their microenvironment. In terms of specific mechanisms mediating resistance to anti-angiogenic therapy, several have been proposed.

11.1 Vessel heterogeneity

Pre-clinical work has demonstrated that although anti-angiogenic agents thwart the growth of newly established tumour vessels, they are less effective against more mature blood vessels, indicating that they may be less dependent on VEGF (**Figure 4A**) [29]. This may be due to PDGF secretion mediating pericyte recruitment, allowing young vessels to mature and survive [119]. Co-inhibition of VEGF and PDGF has been shown to generate significant anti-angiogenic and anti-tumour effects than with VEGF inhibition alone [120].

11.2 Alternative pro-angiogenic signalling pathways

Alternative pro-angiogenic signalling pathways may allow tumour vascularisation to proceed when VEGF signalling is blocked (**Figure 4B**) [29]. A large body of preclinical work has identified candidate pathways that may provide such an alternative pro-angiogenic stimulus. These include fibroblast growth factors 1 and 2 (FGF1 and FGF2) [121], hepatocyte growth factor (HGF) [122] and epidermal growth factor (EGF) [123]. Most of the above preclinical work suggests that, by inhibiting both VEGF signalling and the candidate pathway, improvements in the anti-tumour efficacy can be seen. Therefore, targeting multiple pro-angiogenic pathways may prove more beneficial than employing agents that inhibit VEGF signalling alone.

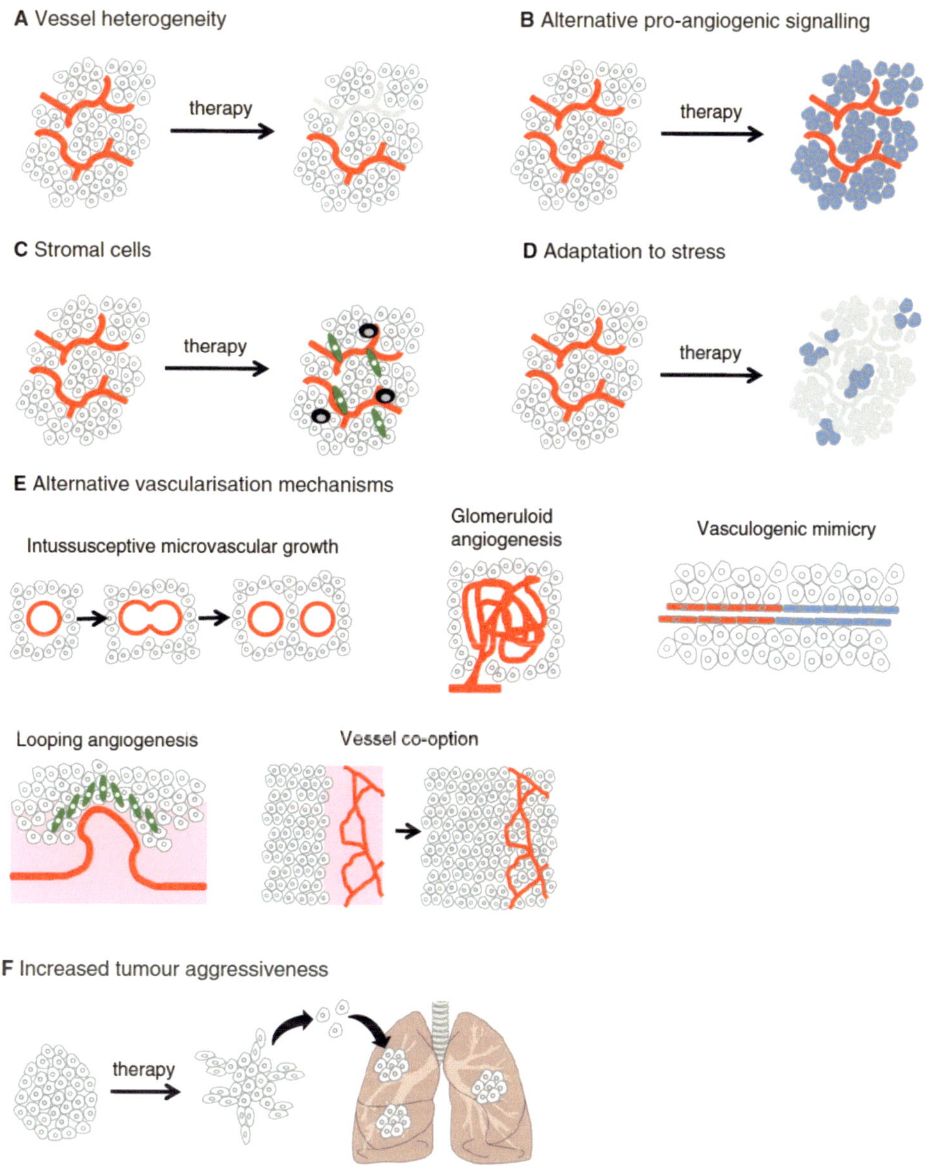

Figure 4.

Proposed mechanisms of resistance to anti-angiogenic therapy. (A–F) The potential mechanisms that tumours can utilise to evade anti-angiogenic therapy. (A) Vessel heterogeneity. Tumours can contain vessels that are at different stages of maturation making some more sensitive to therapy than others. For example, here the top vessel is immature and is abolished by therapy (grey), whilst the bottom one is mature and remains viable (red). (B) Alternative proangiogenic signalling pathway scan affect the susceptibility of vessels to therapy. Here, tumour cells (blue) have up-regulated an alternative pro-angiogenic growth factor to facilitate persistent blood vessel growth and survival despite VEGF blockade. (C) Stromal cells infiltrating into of the tumour, such as myeloid progenitors (black) or fibroblasts (green), can also mediate resistance by releasing pro-angiogenic growth factors or by physically incorporating into vessels. (D) Tumour cell adaptation to stress. Subpopulations of cancer cells in the tumour (blue) can survive the hypoxic conditions and nutrient shortage resulting from vascular destruction by employing different adaptation mechanisms. (E) Alternative tumour vascularisation mechanisms. Apart from sprouting angiogenesis, tumours may utilise alternative mechanisms to recruit a vascular supply. In intussusceptive microvascular growth, new vessels are generated by the fission of pre-existing vessels. Glomeruloid angiogenesis is where tight nests of vessels, resembling the renal glomerulus, are formed. Vasculogenic mimicry is a process whereby tumour cells can create vascular-like structures themselves (blue) which are perfused as they become continuous with the host vasculature (red). In looping angiogenesis, contractile myofibroblasts (green) pull host vessels (red) out of the surrounding parenchymal tissue (pink region). Vessel co-option is a process whereby invading tumour cells engulf pre-existing vessels (red) in the normal parenchyma (pink region). (F) Selection of aggressive cells. Therapy alters the biology of the tumour cells in that they become more invasive and/or facilitate accelerated growth of metastases.

11.3 Role of stromal cells

Preclinical data suggest that cells in the tumour stroma, including fibroblasts, neutrophils, macrophages and myeloid progenitors, mediate resistance to VEGF-targeted agents (**Figure 4C**) [124]. For example, tumour-derived granulocyte-colony stimulating factor (G-CSF) mobilises myeloid cells from bone marrow, and is believed to promote pro-angiogenic Bv8 signalling by myeloid cells, which in tumours may confer resistance to anti-VEGF treatment [125]. Immunohistochemistry studies in human tumours showed expression of Bv8 in tumour-infiltrating neutrophils, which were seen in around 15% of breast carcinomas [126].

11.4 Tumour cell adaptation to stress

It is presumed that the inhibition of tumour vascularisation by anti-angiogenic agents will lead to a reduction in oxygen and nutrients available to the tumour thus causing retardation of tumour growth. However, tumours may develop a number of survival mechanisms enabling them to adapt to such hostile conditions (**Figure 4D**).

11.4.1 Metabolism

Some studies have suggested that anti-angiogenic therapy leads to metabolic reprogramming of tumour cells, allowing them to adapt to reduced vascular supply. Preclinical studies have demonstrated that treatment with anti-VEGF antibodies can lead to tumour cells relying on anaerobic metabolism and the glycolytic pathway for ATP [127]. Furthermore, the withdrawal of anti-angiogenic therapy has been shown to cause an increase in lipid metabolism, leading to a rebound in tumour growth [127].

11.4.2 Autophagy

Tumours treated with anti-angiogenic agents may also adapt to survive by activation of autophagy. Autophagy can occur in response to treatment related stressors such as hypoxia and occurs when organelles and proteins in the cell are degraded and recycled by lysosomes [128]. Autophagy-mediating molecules such as BNIP3 have been identified in GBM tumour cells after exposure (a) to hypoxic conditions in vitro, (b) to bevacizumab therapy in vivo or (c) to bevacizumab therapy in human tumours [129]. Furthermore, a recent study has reported that when MDA-MB-231 breast cancer cells were treated with an agent that induced autophagy, they exhibited increased invasiveness [130].

11.4.3 Cancer stem cells (CSCs)

It is becoming clear that many solid tumours contain relatively rare subpopulations of cancer stem cells. These are clones of tumour cells that are able to sustain self-renewal and can tolerate hostile environments [131]. Furthermore, it has been proposed that hypoxia induced by anti-angiogenic therapy can (a) select for CSCs, and (b) maintain the niche that supports the survival of CSCs [132]. Conceivably, these persistent clones of CSCs may render the tumour more invasive and metastatic and may also lead to antiangiogenic therapy resistance [133].

11.4.4 Enhanced tumour aggressiveness

Anti-angiogenic therapy has been proposed to induce hypoxic tumour microenvironments, enhancing the aggressiveness of tumour cells (**Figure 4F**) [134]. This may help explain why the response to anti-angiogenic therapy is often transient as anti-angiogenic agents can cause initial reductions in tumour burden and a prolonged PFS, but with minimal or no improvement in OS [118]. Anti-angiogenic agents have demonstrated an ability to select for more aggressive cancer cells and enhance tumour cell invasion, growth and metastasis [135]. Moreover, it is now well accepted that some GBM patients with tumours treated with bevacizumab show an increase in tumour invasiveness [136].

11.5 Alternative vascularisation mechanisms

Despite the dogma that tumours primarily employ VEGF-dependent sprouting angiogenesis, emerging evidence now exists for alternative tumour vascularisation mechanisms, including: intussusceptive microvascular growth (IMG) (sometimes known merely as 'intussusception'), glomeruloid angiogenesis, vascular mimicry (also sometimes called 'vasculogenic mimicry'), looping angiogenesis, and vessel co-option (also sometimes called 'vascular co-option') (**Figure 4E**) [21]. These mechanisms may occur by alternative signalling pathways that may not be inhibited by VEGF-targeted therapies.

11.5.1 Intussusception

Intussusception is a mechanism whereby pre-existing vessels split into two daughter vessels without the need for endothelial cell proliferation and sprouting (**Figure 4E**). It has been observed in embryonic development and within experimental tumours recovering from anti-angiogenic therapy and radiotherapy [137]. The molecular mechanisms that control this process are still not well understood.

11.5.2 Vascular mimicry

Vascular mimicry (VM) is a process observed in clinical and preclinical studies whereby tumour cells differentiate into vascular-like structures themselves [138] (**Figure 4E**). It has been shown that basic fibroblast growth factor (bFGF) and VEGF, are incapable of inducing VM channels and networks in poorly aggressive melanoma cell lines, suggesting that VM channel formation maybe be independent of these classical pro-angiogenic growth factors [139]. However, further mechanistic detail is lacking.

11.5.3 Vessel co-option

Vessel co-option is the process whereby, when a tumour invades, existing local vessels become directly incorporated into the tumour (**Figure 4E**). Histopathological studies have indicated that colorectal and breast cancer liver metastases may utilise vessel co-option [140, 141].

Vessel co-option has been shown to mediate resistance to VEGF inhibitors in mouse models of melanoma metastasis to the brain and in mouse models of glioblastoma multiforme, and has been observed in glioblastoma patients who have progressed on anti-VEGF therapy [142–144]. Recently, it has been demonstrated that vessel co-option plays a role in mediating resistance to anti-angiogenic therapy in colorectal cancer liver metastases [145].

In tumour samples obtained from primary lung cancer patients, gene expression arrays have been utilised to identify pathways differentially expressed between angiogenic tumours and vessel co-opting tumours [146]. Stromal expression of thrombospondin-1 appeared to be up regulated in angiogenic tumours, whilst in vessel co-option tumours, there was increased expression of genes involved in oxidative phosphorylation in primary [146]. Surprisingly, no differences in classic hypoxia or angiogenesis related genes were found between angiogenic and non-angiogenic tumours.

In a glioma rat model of breast cancer brain and lung metastasis, co-opted blood vessels were seen in early-stage tumours and these vessels were found to overexpress angiopoietin-2, a natural antagonist of angiopoietin-1 [147]. As these tumours grew to become more hypoxic, VEGF was upregulated at the hypoxic tumour periphery and stimulated angiogenesis [147]. These observations suggest that a transition from vessel co-option to angiogenesis, or vice versa, may be dependent on the relative expression of pro-angiogenic growth factors (angiopoeitin-1, VEGF) and anti-angiogenic factors (angiopoeitin-2).

Cell adhesion molecules have been implicated in facilitating the process of vessel co-option. In a preclinical brain metastasis model, Carbonell et al. demonstrated that the β1 integrin subunit in breast cancer and lymphoma cells facilitates (a) tumour cell adhesion to the vascular basement membrane of existing brain vessels, (b) tumour cell invasion and (c) the process of vessel co-option [148]. When the function of the β1 integrin subunit was blocked, adhesion to vessels was attenuated and brain metastasis colonies failed to become established and grow [148].

Furthermore, the L1 cell adhesion molecule (L1CAM) has been shown to be involved in vessel co-option in the brain [149]. The ability of cancer cells to co-opt blood vessels was suppressed when L1CAM expression was depleted using shRNA. Conversely, when L1CAM was overexpressed, tumour cells demonstrated enhanced adherence to the outer surface of vessels and tumour growth alongside them. Although such mechanisms are likely to be more specific for vessel co-option in the brain, similar mechanisms may be at work during vessel co-option at other anatomical sites.

12. Conclusion

Tumour vascularisation is modulated by the complex interplay of several endogenous factors and processes that can be up-regulated or downregulated, depending on the tumour microenvironment and the treatment pressures that are imposed on it. A multitude of studies have shown that the majority of solid tumours exhibit an overexpression of VEGF, one of the key drivers of sprouting angiogenesis. As a result, various anti-angiogenic therapies targeting VEGF or VEGFR have now been developed and are used conventionally in the clinic. Compellingly, recent pre-clinical and clinical studies using anti-angiogenic agents in combination with immunotherapies (e.g. ICI's), have demonstrated a synergistic effect in reducing tumour growth. This highlights that there is promise, not only in incorporating anti-angiogenic therapy in the management of most cancers, but also in combining such agents with immunomodulatory agents.

However, as is the case with many cancer treatments, drug resistance can limit the efficacy of these agents. Trials of VEGF-targeted therapies in advanced malignancies have not consistently demonstrated beneficial outcomes in terms of tumour response and survival. Importantly, only a proportion of patients benefit from anti-angiogenic therapy, control of tumour growth is generally transient, there remains significant risk for therapeutic toxicity and we are still challenged by the burden of health costs.

Limited clinical outcomes with anti-angiogenic therapies are felt to be driven by either intrinsic or acquired resistance mechanisms, and several of these have now been proposed. In this chapter, we have reviewed the most commonly used anti-angiogenic agents in the clinic and have highlighted the spectrum of mechanisms that may be involved in therapeutic resistance. However, despite the plethora of pre-clinical and clinical studies that have been undertaken, these mechanisms are yet to be entirely elucidated. Importantly, the clinically relevant mechanisms that mediate such resistance to anti-angiogenic therapy are poorly understood and we still do not have means to select patients who will benefit from these agents. Furthermore, there has been a rapid expansion in the development of multiple next generation anti-vascular agents, but there is still little clarity regarding important biological pathways that may affect their efficacy.

The data supporting the role of candidate biomarkers for response and resistance to anti-angiogenic therapies thus far have been generated from basic research, retrospective studies and limited prospective correlative studies. As such there remains a crucial need for substantial research of clinically relevant predictive biomarkers with the use of large, prospective randomised trials. This could also provide a platform for longitudinal and frequent biospecimen collection in order to further interrogate the mechanisms involved in tumour vascularisation and therapeutic resistance over time.

Author details

Sophia Frentzas[1,2]*, Caroline Lum[1] and Ting-Yu Chen[3]

1 Department of Medical Oncology, Monash Health, Clayton, Victoria, Australia

2 Department of Oncology, Monash University, Clayton, Victoria, Australia

3 Faculty of Medicine, Nursing and Health Sciences, Monash University, Clayton, Victoria, Australia

*Address all correspondence to: sophia.frentzas@monash.edu

IntechOpen

© 2019 The Author(s). Licensee IntechOpen. This chapter is distributed under the terms of the Creative Commons Attribution License (http://creativecommons.org/licenses/by/3.0), which permits unrestricted use, distribution, and reproduction in any medium, provided the original work is properly cited.

References

[1] Pang RWC, Poon RTP. Clinical implications of angiogenesis in cancers. Vascular Health and Risk Management. 2006;**2**(2):97-108

[2] Folkman J. Tumor angiogenesis: Therapeutic implications. The New England Journal of Medicine. 1971;**285**(21):1182-1186

[3] Hanahan D, Folkman J. Patterns and emerging mechanisms of the angiogenic switch during tumorigenesis. Cell. 1996;**86**(3):353-364

[4] Yang EV, Sood AK, Chen M, Li Y, Eubank TD, Marsh CB, et al. Norepinephrine up-regulates the expression of vascular endothelial growth factor, matrix metalloproteinase (MMP)-2, and MMP-9 in nasopharyngeal carcinoma tumor cells. Cancer Research. 2006;**66**(21):10357-10364

[5] Tugues S, Koch S, Gualandi L, Li X, Claesson-Welsh L. Vascular endothelial growth factors and receptors: Anti-angiogenic therapy in the treatment of cancer. Molecular Aspects of Medicine. 2011;**32**(2):88-111

[6] Carmeliet P. VEGF as a key mediator of angiogenesis in cancer. Oncology. 2005;**69**(Suppl 3):4-10

[7] Brahimi-Horn C, Pouyssegur J. The role of the hypoxia-inducible factor in tumor metabolism growth and invasion. Bulletin du Cancer. 2006;**93**(8):E73-E80

[8] Takahashi H, Shibuya M. The vascular endothelial growth factor (VEGF)/VEGF receptor system and its role under physiological and pathological conditions. Clinical Science (London, England). 2005;**109**(3):227-241

[9] Carmeliet P, Jain RK. Molecular mechanisms and clinical applications of angiogenesis. Nature. 2011;**473**(7347):298-307

[10] Gerber HP, Ferrara N. Pharmacology and pharmacodynamics of bevacizumab as monotherapy or in combination with cytotoxic therapy in preclinical studies. Cancer Research. 2005;**65**(3):671-680

[11] Olsson AK, Dimberg A, Kreuger J, Claesson-Welsh L. VEGF receptor signalling—In control of vascular function. Nature Reviews. Molecular Cell Biology. 2006;**7**(5):359-371

[12] Dougher M, Terman BI. Autophosphorylation of KDR in the kinase domain is required for maximal VEGF-stimulated kinase activity and receptor internalization. Oncogene. 1999;**18**(8):1619-1627

[13] Lamalice L, Houle F, Huot J. Phosphorylation of Tyr1214 within VEGFR-2 triggers the recruitment of Nck and activation of Fyn leading to SAPK2/p38 activation and endothelial cell migration in response to VEGF. The Journal of Biological Chemistry. 2006;**281**(45):34009-34020

[14] Wong C, Jin ZG. Protein kinase C-dependent protein kinase D activation modulates ERK signal pathway and endothelial cell proliferation by vascular endothelial growth factor. The Journal of Biological Chemistry. 2005;**280**(39):33262-33269

[15] Lee SJ, Tsang PS, Diaz TM, Wei BY, Stetler-Stevenson WG. TIMP-2 modulates VEGFR-2 phosphorylation and enhances phosphodiesterase activity in endothelial cells. Laboratory Investigation. 2010;**90**(3):374-382

[16] Nelson AR, Fingleton B, Rothenberg ML, Matrisian LM. Matrix metalloproteinases: Biologic activity and clinical implications. Journal of Clinical Oncology: Official Journal of the

American Society of Clinical Oncology. 2000;**18**(5):1135-1149

[17] Abramsson A, Lindblom P, Betsholtz C. Endothelial and nonendothelial sources of PDGF-B regulate pericyte recruitment and influence vascular pattern formation in tumors. The Journal of Clinical Investigation. 2003;**112**(8):1142-1151

[18] Yang D-H, Park J-S, Jin C-J, Kang H-K, Nam J-H, Rhee J-H, et al. The dysfunction and abnormal signaling pathway of dendritic cells loaded by tumor antigen can be overcome by neutralizing VEGF in multiple myeloma. Leukemia Research. 2009;**33**(5):665-670

[19] Yang J, Yan J, Liu B. Targeting VEGF/VEGFR to modulate antitumor immunity. Frontiers in Immunology. 2018;**9**(978):1-9

[20] Martino EC, Misso G, Pastina P, Costantini S, Vanni F, Gandolfo C, et al. Immune-modulating effects of bevacizumab in metastatic non-small-cell lung cancer patients. Cell Death Discovery. 2016;**2**(16026):1-8

[21] Vasudev NS, Reynolds AR. Anti-angiogenic therapy for cancer: Current progress, unresolved questions and future directions. Angiogenesis. 2014;**17**(3):471-494

[22] Eichholz A, Merchant S, Gaya AM. Anti-angiogenesis therapies: Their potential in cancer management. OncoTargets and Therapy. 2010;**3**:69-82

[23] Ferrara N, Hillan KJ, Gerber HP, Novotny W. Discovery and development of bevacizumab, an anti-VEGF antibody for treating cancer. Nature Reviews. Drug Discovery. 2004;**3**(5):391-400

[24] Margolin K, Gordon MS, Holmgren E, Gaudreault J, Novotny W, Fyfe G, et al. Phase Ib trial of intravenous recombinant humanized monoclonal antibody to vascular endothelial growth factor in combination with chemotherapy in patients with advanced cancer: Pharmacologic and long-term safety data. Journal of Clinical Oncology: Official Journal of the American Society of Clinical Oncology. 2001;**19**(3):851-856

[25] Hurwitz H, Fehrenbacher L, Novotny W, Cartwright T, Hainsworth J, Heim W, et al. Bevacizumab plus irinotecan, fluorouracil, and leucovorin for metastatic colorectal cancer. The New England Journal of Medicine. 2004;**350**(23):2335-2342

[26] Cunningham D, Lang I, Marcuello E, Lorusso V, Ocvirk J, Shin DB, et al. Bevacizumab plus capecitabine versus capecitabine alone in elderly patients with previously untreated metastatic colorectal cancer (AVEX): An open-label, randomised phase 3 trial. The Lancet Oncology. 2013;**14**(11):1077-1085

[27] Giantonio BJ, Catalano PJ, Meropol NJ, O'Dwyer PJ, Mitchell EP, Alberts SR, et al. Bevacizumab in combination with oxaliplatin, fluorouracil, and leucovorin (FOLFOX4) for previously treated metastatic colorectal cancer: Results from the Eastern Cooperative Oncology Group Study E3200. Journal of Clinical Oncology. 2007;**25**(12):1539-1544

[28] Saltz LB, Clarke S, Diaz-Rubio E, Scheithauer W, Figer A, Wong R, et al. Bevacizumab in combination with oxaliplatin-based chemotherapy as first-line therapy in metastatic colorectal cancer: A randomized phase III study. Journal of Clinical Oncology. 2008;**26**(12):2013-2019

[29] Bergers G, Hanahan D. Modes of resistance to anti-angiogenic therapy. Nature Reviews. Cancer. 2008;**8**(8):592-603

[30] Nordlinger B, Van Cutsem E, Gruenberger T, Glimelius B, Poston G, Rougier P, et al. Combination of surgery and chemotherapy and the role of targeted agents in the treatment of patients with colorectal liver metastases: Recommendations from an expert panel. Annals of Oncology. 2009;**20**(6):985-992

[31] Wong R, Cunningham D, Barbachano Y, Saffery C, Valle J, Hickish T, et al. A multicentre study of capecitabine, oxaliplatin plus bevacizumab as perioperative treatment of patients with poor-risk colorectal liver-only metastases not selected for upfront resection. Annals of Oncology. 2011;**22**(9):2042-2048

[32] Gruenberger T, Arnold D, Rubbia-Brandt L. Pathologic response to bevacizumab-containing chemotherapy in patients with colorectal liver metastases and its correlation with survival. Surgical Oncology. 2012;**21**(4):309-315

[33] Okines A, Puerto OD, Cunningham D, Chau I, Van Cutsem E, Saltz L, et al. Surgery with curative-intent in patients treated with first-line chemotherapy plus bevacizumab for metastatic colorectal cancer first BEAT and the randomised phase-III NO16966 trial. British Journal of Cancer. 2009;**101**(7):1033-1038

[34] Grothey A, Sugrue MM, Purdie DM, Dong W, Sargent D, Hedrick E, et al. Bevacizumab beyond first progression is associated with prolonged overall survival in metastatic colorectal cancer: Results from a large observational cohort study (BRiTE). Journal of Clinical Oncology. 2008;**26**(33):5326-5334

[35] Grothey A, Flick ED, Cohn AL, Bekaii-Saab TS, Bendell JC, Kozloff M, et al. Bevacizumab exposure beyond first disease progression in patients with metastatic colorectal cancer: Analyses of the ARIES observational cohort study. Pharmacoepidemiology and Drug Safety. 2014;**23**(7):726-734

[36] Bennouna J, Sastre J, Arnold D, Osterlund P, Greil R, Van Cutsem E, et al. Continuation of bevacizumab after first progression in metastatic colorectal cancer (ML18147): A randomised phase 3 trial. The Lancet Oncology. 2013;**14**(1):29-37

[37] de Gramont A, Van Cutsem E, Schmoll HJ, Tabernero J, Clarke S, Moore MJ, et al. Bevacizumab plus oxaliplatin-based chemotherapy as adjuvant treatment for colon cancer (AVANT): A phase 3 randomised controlled trial. The Lancet Oncology. 2012;**13**(12):1225-1233

[38] Allegra CJ, Yothers G, O'Connell MJ, Sharif S, Petrelli NJ, Lopa SH, et al. Bevacizumab in stage II-III colon cancer: 5-year update of the National Surgical Adjuvant Breast and Bowel Project C-08 trial. Journal of Clinical Oncology. 2013;**31**(3):359-364

[39] Reck M, von Pawel J, Zatloukal P, Ramlau R, Gorbounova V, Hirsh V, et al. Phase III trial of cisplatin plus gemcitabine with either placebo or bevacizumab as first-line therapy for nonsquamous non-small-cell lung cancer: AVAil. Journal of Clinical Oncology. 2009;**27**(8):1227-1234

[40] Sandler A, Gray R, Perry MC, Brahmer J, Schiller JH, Dowlati A, et al. Paclitaxel-carboplatin alone or with bevacizumab for non-small-cell lung cancer. The New England Journal of Medicine. 2006;**355**(24):2542-2550

[41] Soria JC, Mauguen A, Reck M, Sandler AB, Saijo N, Johnson DH, et al. Systematic review and meta-analysis of randomised, phase II/III trials adding bevacizumab to platinum-based chemotherapy as first-line treatment in patients with advanced non-small-cell

lung cancer. Annals of Oncology. 2013;**24**(1):20-30

[42] Socinski MA, Jotte RM, Cappuzzo F, Orlandi F, Stroyakovskiy D, Nogami N, et al. Atezolizumab for first-line treatment of metastatic nonsquamous NSCLC. The New England Journal of Medicine. 2018;**378**(24):2288-2301

[43] Burger RA, Brady MF, Bookman MA, Fleming GF, Monk BJ, Huang H, et al. Incorporation of bevacizumab in the primary treatment of ovarian cancer. The New England Journal of Medicine. 2011;**365**(26):2473-2483

[44] Taal W, Oosterkamp HM, Walenkamp AM, Dubbink HJ, Beerepoot LV, Hanse MC, et al. Single-agent bevacizumab or lomustine versus a combination of bevacizumab plus lomustine in patients with recurrent glioblastoma (BELOB trial): A randomised controlled phase 2 trial. The Lancet Oncology. 2014;**15**(9):943-953

[45] Gilbert MR, Dignam JJ, Armstrong TS, Wefel JS, Blumenthal DT, Vogelbaum MA, et al. A randomized trial of bevacizumab for newly diagnosed glioblastoma. New England Journal of Medicine. 2014;**370**(8):699-708

[46] Rini BI, Powles T, Atkins MB, Escudier B, McDermott DF, Suarez C, et al. Atezolizumab plus bevacizumab versus sunitinib in patients with previously untreated metastatic renal cell carcinoma (IMmotion151): A multicentre, open-label, phase 3, randomised controlled trial. The Lancet. 2019;**15**;393(10189):2362-2364

[47] Rossari JR, Metzger-Filho O, Paesmans M, Saini KS, Gennari A, de Azambuja E, et al. Bevacizumab and breast cancer: A meta-analysis of first-line phase III studies and a critical reappraisal of available evidence. Journal of Oncology. 2012;**2012**:417673

[48] Spratlin JL, Cohen RB, Eadens M, Gore L, Camidge DR, Diab S, et al. Phase I pharmacologic and biologic study of ramucirumab (IMC-1121B), a fully human immunoglobulin G1 monoclonal antibody targeting the vascular endothelial growth factor receptor-2. Journal of Clinical Oncology. 2010;**28**(5):780-787

[49] Fuchs CS, Tomasek J, Yong CJ, Dumitru F, Passalacqua R, Goswami C, et al. Ramucirumab monotherapy for previously treated advanced gastric or gastro-oesophageal junction adenocarcinoma (REGARD): An international, randomised, multicentre, placebo-controlled, phase 3 trial. The Lancet. 2014;**383**(9911):31-39

[50] Wilke H, Muro K, Van Cutsem E, Oh S-C, Bodoky G, Shimada Y, et al. Ramucirumab plus paclitaxel versus placebo plus paclitaxel in patients with previously treated advanced gastric or gastro-oesophageal junction adenocarcinoma (RAINBOW): A double-blind, randomised phase 3 trial. The Lancet Oncology. 2014;**15**(11):1224-1235

[51] Fuchs CS, Shitara K, Bartololmeo MD, Lonardi S, Al-Batran SE, Van Cutsem E, et al. Ramucirumab with cisplatin and fluoropyrimidine as first-line therapy in patients with metastatic gastric or junctional adenocarcinoma (RAINFALL): A double-blind, randomised, placebo-controlled, phase 3 trial. The Lancet Oncology. 2019;**20**(3):420-435

[52] Garon EB, Ciuleanu T-E, Arrieta O, Prabhash K, Syrigos KN, Goksel T, et al. Ramucirumab plus docetaxel versus placebo plus docetaxel for second-line treatment of stage IV non-small-cell lung cancer after disease

progression on platinum-based therapy (REVEL): A multicentre, double-blind, randomised phase 3 trial. The Lancet. 2014;**384**(9944):665-673

[53] Petrylak DP, de Wit R, Chi KN, Drakaki A, Sternberg CN, Nishiyama H, et al. Ramucirumab plus docetaxel versus placebo plus docetaxel in patients with locally advanced or metastatic urothelial carcinoma after platinum-based therapy (RANGE): A randomised, double-blind, phase 3 trial. The Lancet. 2017;**390**(10109):2266-2277

[54] Fischer C, Jonckx B, Mazzone M, Zacchigna S, Loges S, Pattarini L, et al. Anti-PlGF inhibits growth of VEGF(R)-inhibitor-resistant tumors without affecting healthy vessels. Cell. 2007;**131**(3):463-475

[55] Byrne AT, Ross L, Holash J, Nakanishi M, Hu L, Hofmann JI, et al. Vascular endothelial growth factor-trap decreases tumor burden, inhibits ascites, and causes dramatic vascular remodeling in an ovarian cancer model. Clinical Cancer Research. 2003;**9**(15):5721-5728

[56] Van Cutsem E, Tabernero J, Lakomy R, Prenen H, Prausova J, Macarulla T, et al. Addition of aflibercept to fluorouracil, leucovorin, and irinotecan improves survival in a phase III randomized trial in patients with metastatic colorectal cancer previously treated with an oxaliplatin-based regimen. Journal of Clinical Oncology. 2012;**30**(28):3499-3506

[57] Tabernero J, Van Cutsem E, Lakomy R, Prausova J, Ruff P, van Hazel GA, et al. Aflibercept versus placebo in combination with fluorouracil, leucovorin and irinotecan in the treatment of previously treated metastatic colorectal cancer: Prespecified subgroup analyses from the VELOUR trial. European Journal of Cancer. 2014;**50**(2):320-331

[58] Faivre S, Demetri G, Sargent W, Raymond E. Molecular basis for sunitinib efficacy and future clinical development. Nature Reviews. Drug Discovery. 2007;**6**(9):734-745

[59] Mendel DB, Laird AD, Xin X, Louie SG, Christensen JG, Li G, et al. In vivo antitumor activity of SU11248, a novel tyrosine kinase inhibitor targeting vascular endothelial growth factor and platelet-derived growth factor receptors: Determination of a pharmacokinetic/pharmacodynamic relationship. Clinical Cancer Research. 2003;**9**(1):327-337

[60] Griffioen AW, Mans LA, de Graaf AM, Nowak-Sliwinska P, de Hoog CL, de Jong TA, et al. Rapid angiogenesis onset after discontinuation of sunitinib treatment of renal cell carcinoma patients. Clinical Cancer Research. 2012;**18**(14):3961-3971

[61] Escudier B, Roigas J, Gillessen S, Harmenberg U, Srinivas S, Mulder SF, et al. Phase II study of sunitinib administered in a continuous once-daily dosing regimen in patients with cytokine-refractory metastatic renal cell carcinoma. Journal of Clinical Oncology. 2009;**27**(25):4068-4075

[62] Motzer RJ, Hutson TE, Tomczak P, Michaelson MD, Bukowski RM, Oudard S, et al. Overall survival and updated results for sunitinib compared with interferon alfa in patients with metastatic renal cell carcinoma. Journal of Clinical Oncology. 2009;**27**(22):3584-3590

[63] Rini BI, Plimack ER, Stus V, Gafanov R, Hawkins R, Nosov D, et al. Pembrolizumab plus axitinib versus sunitinib for advanced renal-cell carcinoma. New England Journal of Medicine. 2019;**380**(12):1116-1127

[64] Christensen JG. A preclinical review of sunitinib, a multitargeted receptor tyrosine kinase inhibitor

with anti-angiogenic and antitumour activities. Annals of Oncology. 2007;**18**(Suppl 10):x3-x10

[65] Carrato A, Swieboda-Sadlej A, Staszewska-Skurczynska M, Lim R, Roman L, Shparyk Y, et al. Fluorouracil, leucovorin, and irinotecan plus either sunitinib or placebo in metastatic colorectal cancer: A randomized, phase III trial. Journal of Clinical Oncology. 2013;**31**(10):1341-1347

[66] Wilhelm SM, Carter C, Tang L, Wilkie D, McNabola A, Rong H, et al. BAY 43-9006 exhibits broad spectrum oral antitumor activity and targets the RAF/MEK/ERK pathway and receptor tyrosine kinases involved in tumor progression and angiogenesis. Cancer Research. 2004;**64**(19):7099-7109

[67] Wilhelm SM, Dumas J, Adnane L, Lynch M, Carter CA, Schutz G, et al. Regorafenib (BAY 73-4506): A new oral multikinase inhibitor of angiogenic, stromal and oncogenic receptor tyrosine kinases with potent preclinical antitumor activity. International Journal of Cancer. 2011;**129**(1):245-255

[68] Grothey A, Van Cutsem E, Sobrero A, Siena S, Falcone A, Ychou M, et al. Regorafenib monotherapy for previously treated metastatic colorectal cancer (CORRECT): An international, multicentre, randomised, placebo-controlled, phase 3 trial. Lancet. 2013;**381**(9863):303-312

[69] Demetri GD, Reichardt P, Kang Y-K, Blay J-Y, Rutkowski P, Gelderblom H, et al. Efficacy and safety of regorafenib for advanced gastrointestinal stromal tumours after failure of imatinib and sunitinib (GRID): An international, multicentre, randomised, placebo-controlled, phase 3 trial. The Lancet. 2013;**381**(9863):295-302

[70] Bruix J, Qin S, Merle P, Granito A, Huang YH, Bodoky G, et al. Regorafenib for patients with hepatocellular carcinoma who progressed on sorafenib treatment (RESORCE): A randomised, double-bind, placebo-controlled, phase 3 trial. The Lancet. 2017;**389**(10064):56-66

[71] Jain RK. Molecular regulation of vessel maturation. Nature Medicine. 2003;**9**(6):685-693

[72] Kaye SB. Bevacizumab for the treatment of epithelial ovarian cancer: Will this be its finest hour? Journal of Clinical Oncology. 2007;**25**(33):5150-5152

[73] Jain RK. Normalization of tumor vasculature: An emerging concept in antiangiogenic therapy. Science. 2005;**307**(5706):58-62

[74] Van der Veldt AA, Lubberink M, Bahce I, Walraven M, de Boer MP, Greuter HN, et al. Rapid decrease in delivery of chemotherapy to tumors after anti-VEGF therapy: Implications for scheduling of anti-angiogenic drugs. Cancer Cell. 2012;**21**(1):82-91

[75] Kerbel RS. Antiangiogenic therapy: A universal chemosensitization strategy for cancer? Science. 2006;**312**(5777):1171-1175

[76] Shaked Y, Henke E, Roodhart JM, Mancuso P, Langenberg MH, Colleoni M, et al. Rapid chemotherapy-induced acute endothelial progenitor cell mobilization: Implications for antiangiogenic drugs as chemosensitizing agents. Cancer Cell. 2008;**14**(3):263-273

[77] Kamoun WS, Ley CD, Farrar CT, Duyverman AM, Lahdenranta J, Lacorre DA, et al. Edema control by cediranib, a vascular endothelial growth factor receptor-targeted kinase inhibitor, prolongs survival despite persistent brain tumor growth in

mice. Journal of Clinical Oncology. 2009;**27**(15):2542-2552

[78] Gianni L, Romieu GH, Lichinitser M, Serrano SV, Mansutti M, Pivot X, et al. AVEREL: A randomized phase III trial evaluating bevacizumab in combination with docetaxel and trastuzumab as first-line therapy for HER2-positive locally recurrent/metastatic breast cancer. Journal of Clinical Oncology. 2013;**31**(14):1719-1725

[79] Smith NR, Baker D, Farren M, Pommier A, Swann R, Wang X, et al. Tumor stromal architecture can define the intrinsic tumor response to VEGF-targeted therapy. Clinical Cancer Research. 2013;**19**(24):6943-6956

[80] Yasuda S, Sho M, Yamato I, Yoshiji H, Wakatsuki K, Nishiwada S, et al. Simultaneous blockade of programmed death 1 and vascular endothelial growth factor receptor 2 (VEGFR2) induces synergistic anti-tumour effect in vivo. Clinical and Experimental Immunology. 2013;**172**(3):500-506

[81] Malo CS, Khadka RH, Ayasoufi K, Jin F, AbouChehade JE, Hansen MJ, et al. Immunomodulation mediated by anti-angiogenic therapy improves CD8 T cell immunity against experimental glioma. Frontiers in Oncology. 2018;**8**(320):1-6

[82] Hodi FS, Lawrence D, Lezcano C, Wu X, Zhou J, Sasada T, et al. Bevacizumab plus ipilimumab in patients with metastatic melanoma. Cancer Immunology Research. 2014;**2**(7):632-642

[83] Wallin JJ, Bendell JC, Funke R, Sznol M, Korski K, Jones S, et al. Atezolizumab in combination with bevacizumab enhances migration of antigen-specific T-cells in metastatic renal cell carcinoma. Nature Communications. 2016;7:12624

[84] McDermott DF, Huseni MA, Atkins MB, Motzer RJ, Rini BI, Escudier B, et al. Clinical activity and molecular correlates of response to atezolizumab alone or in combination with bevacizumab versus sunitinib in renal cell carcinoma. Nature Medicine. 2018;**24**(6):749-757

[85] Zhu AX, Duda DG, Sahani DV, Jain RK. HCC and angiogenesis: Possible targets and future directions. Nature Reviews. Clinical Oncology. 2011;**8**(5):292-301

[86] Bernaards C, Hegde P, Chen D, Holmgren E, Zheng M, Jubb AM, et al. Circulating vascular endothelial growth factor (VEGF) as a biomarker for bevacizumab-based therapy in metastatic colorectal, non-small cell lung, and renal cell cancers: Analysis of phase III studies. Journal of Clinical Oncology. 2010;**28**(15_suppl):10519

[87] Duda DG, Willett CG, Ancukiewicz M, di Tomaso E, Shah M, Czito BG, et al. Plasma soluble VEGFR-1 is a potential dual biomarker of response and toxicity for bevacizumab with chemoradiation in locally advanced rectal cancer. The Oncologist. 2010;**15**(6):577-583

[88] Kopetz S, Hoff PM, Morris JS, Wolff RA, Eng C, Glover KY, et al. Phase II trial of infusional fluorouracil, irinotecan, and bevacizumab for metastatic colorectal cancer: Efficacy and circulating angiogenic biomarkers associated with therapeutic resistance. Journal of Clinical Oncology. 2010;**28**(3):453-459

[89] Cetin B, Kaplan MA, Berk V, Ozturk SC, Benekli M, Isikdogan A, et al. Prognostic factors for overall survival in patients with metastatic colorectal carcinoma treated with vascular endothelial growth factor-targeting agents. Asian Pacific

Journal of Cancer Prevention. 2012;**13**(3):1059-1063

[90] Manzoni M, Mariucci S, Delfanti S, et al. Circulating endothelial cells and their apoptotic fraction are mutually independent predictive biomarkers in Bevacizumab-based treatment for advanced colorectal cancer. Journal of Cancer Research and Clinical Oncology. 2012;**138**(7):1187-1196

[91] Jubb AM, Miller KD, Rugo HS, Harris AL, Chen D, Reimann JD, et al. Impact of exploratory biomarkers on the treatment effect of bevacizumab in metastatic breast cancer. Clinical Cancer Research. 2011;**17**(2):372-381

[92] Jubb AM, Hurwitz HI, Bai W, Holmgren EB, Tobin P, Guerrero AS, et al. Impact of vascular endothelial growth factor-a expression, thrombospondin-2 expression, and microvessel density on the treatment effect of Bevacizumab in metastatic colorectal. Cancer. 2006;**24**(2):217-227

[93] Relf M, LeJeune S, Scott PA, Fox S, Smith K, Leek R, et al. Expression of the angiogenic factors vascular endothelial cell growth factor, acidic and basic fibroblast growth factor, tumor growth factor beta-1, platelet-derived endothelial cell growth factor, placenta growth factor, and pleiotrophin in human primary breast cancer and its relation to angiogenesis. Cancer Research. 1997;**57**(5):963-969

[94] Ebos JM, Lee CR, Christensen JG, Mutsaers AJ, Kerbel RS. Multiple circulating proangiogenic factors induced by sunitinib malate are tumor-independent and correlate with antitumor efficacy. Proceedings of the National Academy of Sciences of the United States of America. 2007;**104**(43):17069-17074

[95] Maru D, Venook AP, Ellis LM. Predictive biomarkers for bevacizumab: Are we there yet? Clinical Cancer Research. 2013;**19**(11):2824-2827

[96] Jain RK, Duda DG, Willett CG, Sahani DV, Zhu AX, Loeffler JS, et al. Biomarkers of response and resistance to antiangiogenic therapy. Nature Reviews Clinical Oncology. 2009;**6**(6):327-338

[97] Tran HT, Liu Y, Zurita AJ, Lin Y, Baker-Neblett KL, Martin AM, et al. Prognostic or predictive plasma cytokines and angiogenic factors for patients treated with pazopanib for metastatic renal-cell cancer: A retrospective analysis of phase 2 and phase 3 trials. The Lancet Oncology. 2012;**13**(8):827-837

[98] Schneider BP, Wang M, Radovich M, Sledge GW, Badve S, Thor A, et al. Association of vascular endothelial growth factor and vascular endothelial growth factor receptor-2 genetic polymorphisms with outcome in a trial of paclitaxel compared with paclitaxel plus bevacizumab in advanced breast cancer: ECOG 2100. Journal of Clinical Oncology. 2008;**26**(28):4672-4678

[99] Koutras AK, Antonacopoulou AG, Eleftheraki AG, Dimitrakopoulos FI, Koumarianou A, Varthalitis I, et al. Vascular endothelial growth factor polymorphisms and clinical outcome in colorectal cancer patients treated with irinotecan-based chemotherapy and bevacizumab. The Pharmacogenomics Journal. 2012;**12**(6):468-475

[100] Lambrechts D, Claes B, Delmar P, Reumers J, Mazzone M, Yesilyurt BT, et al. VEGF pathway genetic variants as biomarkers of treatment outcome with bevacizumab: An analysis of data from the AViTA and AVOREN randomised trials. The Lancet Oncology. 2012;**13**(7):724-733

[101] Beuselinck B, Karadimou A, Lambrechts D, Claes B, Wolter P, Couchy G, et al. VEGFR1 single

nucleotide polymorphisms associated with outcome in patients with metastatic renal cell carcinoma treated with sunitinib—A multicentric retrospective analysis. Acta Oncologica. 2014;**53**(1):103-112

[102] O'Connor JP, Jayson GC. Do imaging biomarkers relate to outcome in patients treated with VEGF inhibitors? Clinical Cancer Research. 2012;**18**(24):6588-6598

[103] Fournier LS, Oudard S, Thiam R, Trinquart L, Banu E, Medioni J, et al. Metastatic renal carcinoma: Evaluation of antiangiogenic therapy with dynamic contrast-enhanced CT. Radiology. 2010;**256**(2):511-518

[104] Vasudev NS, Goh V, Juttla JK, Thompson VL, Larkin JM, Gore M, et al. Changes in tumour vessel density upon treatment with anti-angiogenic agents: Relationship with response and resistance to therapy. British Journal of Cancer. 2013;**109**(5):1230-1242

[105] Grothey A, Hedrick EE, Mass RD, Sarkar S, Suzuki S, Ramanathan RK, et al. Response-independent survival benefit in metastatic colorectal cancer: A comparative analysis of N9741 and AVF2107. Journal of Clinical Oncology. 2008;**26**(2):183-189

[106] Kerbel RS. Clinical trials of antiangiogenic drugs: Opportunities, problems, and assessment of initial results. Journal of Clinical Oncology. 2001;**19**(18 Suppl):45S-51S

[107] Kim KJ, Li B, Winer J, Armanini M, Gillett N, Phillips HS, et al. Inhibition of vascular endothelial growth factor-induced angiogenesis suppresses tumour growth in vivo. Nature. 1993;**362**(6423):841-844

[108] Chun YS, Vauthey JN, Boonsirikamchai P, Maru DM, Kopetz S, Palavecino M, et al. Association of computed tomography morphologic criteria with pathologic response and survival in patients treated with bevacizumab for colorectal liver metastases. JAMA: The Journal of the American Medical Association. 2009;**302**(21):2338-2344

[109] Shindoh J, Loyer EM, Kopetz S, Boonsirikamchai P, Maru DM, Chun YS, et al. Optimal morphologic response to preoperative chemotherapy: An alternate outcome end point before resection of hepatic colorectal metastases. Journal of Clinical Oncology. 2012;**30**(36):4566-4572

[110] Lee HY, Lee KS, Hwang HS, Lee JW, Ahn MJ, Park K, et al. Molecularly targeted therapy using bevacizumab for non-small cell lung cancer: A pilot study for the new CT response criteria. Korean Journal of Radiology. 2010;**11**(6):618-626

[111] Schott AF, Roubidoux MA, Helvie MA, Hayes DF, Kleer CG, Newman LA, et al. Clinical and radiologic assessments to predict breast cancer pathologic complete response to neoadjuvant chemotherapy. Breast Cancer Research and Treatment. 2005;**92**(3):231-238

[112] Bouzourene H, Bosman FT, Seelentag W, Matter M, Coucke P. Importance of tumor regression assessment in predicting the outcome in patients with locally advanced rectal carcinoma who are treated with preoperative radiotherapy. Cancer. 2002;**94**(4):1121-1130

[113] Ajani JA, Mansfield PF, Crane CH, Wu TT, Lunagomez S, Lynch PM, et al. Paclitaxel-based chemoradiotherapy in localized gastric carcinoma: Degree of pathologic response and not clinical parameters dictated patient outcome. Journal of Clinical Oncology. 2005;**23**(6):1237-1244

[114] Ribero D, Wang H, Donadon M, Zorzi D, Thomas MB, Eng C, et al. Bevacizumab improves pathologic

response and protects against hepatic injury in patients treated with oxaliplatin-based chemotherapy for colorectal liver metastases. Cancer. 2007;**110**(12):2761-2767

[115] Mandard AM, Dalibard F, Mandard JC, Marnay J, Henry-Amar M, Petiot JF, et al. Pathologic assessment of tumor regression after preoperative chemoradiotherapy of esophageal carcinoma. Clinicopathologic Correlations. Cancer. 1994;**73**(11):2680-2686

[116] Rubbia-Brandt L, Giostra E, Brezault C, Roth AD, Andres A, Audard V, et al. Importance of histological tumor response assessment in predicting the outcome in patients with colorectal liver metastases treated with neo-adjuvant chemotherapy followed by liver surgery. Annals of Oncology. 2007;**18**(2):299-304

[117] Klinger M, Tamandl D, Eipeldauer S, Hacker S, Herberger B, Kaczirek K, et al. Bevacizumab improves pathological response of colorectal cancer liver metastases treated with XELOX/FOLFOX. Annals of Surgical Oncology. 2010;**17**(8):2059-2065

[118] Ebos JM, Kerbel RS. Antiangiogenic therapy: Impact on invasion, disease progression, and metastasis. Nature Reviews Clinical Oncology. 2011;**8**(4):210-221

[119] Franco M, Roswall P, Cortez E, Hanahan D, Pietras K. Pericytes promote endothelial cell survival through induction of autocrine VEGF-A signaling and Bcl-w expression. Blood. 2011;**118**(10):2906-2917

[120] Erber R, Thurnher A, Katsen AD, Groth G, Kerger H, Hammes HP, et al. Combined inhibition of VEGF and PDGF signaling enforces tumor vessel regression by interfering with pericyte-mediated endothelial cell survival mechanisms. FASEB Journal: Official Publication of the Federation of American Societies for Experimental Biology. 2004;**18**(2):338-340

[121] Welti JC, Gourlaouen M, Powles T, Kudahetti SC, Wilson P, Berney DM, et al. Fibroblast growth factor 2 regulates endothelial cell sensitivity to sunitinib. Oncogene. 2011;**30**(10):1183-1193

[122] Shojaei F, Lee JH, Simmons BH, Wong A, Esparza CO, Plumlee PA, et al. HGF/c-Met acts as an alternative angiogenic pathway in sunitinib-resistant tumors. Cancer Research. 2010;**70**(24):10090-10100

[123] Cascone T, Herynk MH, Xu L, Du Z, Kadara H, Nilsson MB, et al. Upregulated stromal EGFR and vascular remodeling in mouse xenograft models of angiogenesis inhibitor-resistant human lung adenocarcinoma. The Journal of Clinical Investigation. 2011;**121**(4):1313-1328

[124] Shojaei F, Wu X, Qu X, Kowanetz M, Yu L, Tan M, et al. G-CSF-initiated myeloid cell mobilization and angiogenesis mediate tumor refractoriness to anti-VEGF therapy in mouse models. Proceedings of the National Academy of Sciences of the United States of America. 2009;**106**(16):6742-6747

[125] Shojaei F, Wu X, Malik AK, Zhong C, Baldwin ME, Schanz S, et al. Tumor refractoriness to anti-VEGF treatment is mediated by CD11b+Gr1+ myeloid cells. Nature Biotechnology. 2007;**25**(8):911-920

[126] Jubb AM, Soilleux EJ, Turley H, Steers G, Parker A, Low I, et al. Expression of vascular notch ligand delta-like 4 and inflammatory markers in breast cancer. The American Journal of Pathology. 2010;**176**(4):2019-2028

[127] Xu J, Wang J, Xu B, Ge H, Zhou X, Fang JY. Colorectal cancer cells refractory to anti-VEGF treatment are vulnerable to glycolytic blockade due to persistent impairment of mitochondria. Molecular Cancer Therapeutics. 2013;**12**(5):717-724

[128] Viry E, Paggetti J, Baginska J, Mgrditchian T, Berchem G, Moussay E, et al. Autophagy: An adaptive metabolic response to stress shaping the antitumor immunity. Biochemical Pharmacology. 2014

[129] Hu YL, DeLay M, Jahangiri A, Molinaro AM, Rose SD, Carbonell WS, et al. Hypoxia-induced autophagy promotes tumor cell survival and adaptation to antiangiogenic treatment in glioblastoma. Cancer Research. 2012;**72**(7):1773-1783

[130] Indelicato M, Pucci B, Schito L, Reali V, Aventaggiato M, Mazzarino MC, et al. Role of hypoxia and autophagy in MDA-MB-231 invasiveness. Journal of Cellular Physiology. 2010;**223**(2):359-368

[131] Kasai T, Chen L, Mizutani A, Kudoh T, Murakami H, Fu L, et al. Cancer stem cells converted from pluripotent stem cells and the cancerous niche. Journal of Stem Cells and Regenerative Medicine. 2014;**10**(1):2-7

[132] Conley SJ, Gheordunescu E, Kakarala P, Newman B, Korkaya H, Heath AN, et al. Antiangiogenic agents increase breast cancer stem cells via the generation of tumor hypoxia. Proceedings of the National Academy of Sciences of the United States of America. 2012;**109**(8):2784-2789

[133] Ebos JM, Lee CR, Cruz-Munoz W, Bjarnason GA, Christensen JG, Kerbel RS. Accelerated metastasis after short-term treatment with a potent inhibitor of tumor angiogenesis. Cancer Cell. 2009;**15**(3):232-239

[134] Sullivan R, Graham CH. Hypoxia-driven selection of the metastatic phenotype. Cancer Metastasis Reviews. 2007;**26**(2):319-331

[135] Paez-Ribes M, Allen E, Hudock J, Takeda T, Okuyama H, Vinals F, et al. Antiangiogenic therapy elicits malignant progression of tumors to increased local invasion and distant metastasis. Cancer Cell. 2009;**15**(3):220-231

[136] Zuniga RM, Torcuator R, Jain R, Anderson J, Doyle T, Ellika S, et al. Efficacy, safety and patterns of response and recurrence in patients with recurrent high-grade gliomas treated with bevacizumab plus irinotecan. Journal of Neuro-oncology. 2009;**91**(3):329-336

[137] Gianni-Barrera R, Trani M, Reginato S, Banfi A. To sprout or to split? VEGF, Notch and vascular morphogenesis. Biochemical Society Transactions. 2011;**39**(6):1644-1648

[138] Folberg R, Hendrix MJ, Maniotis AJ. Vasculogenic mimicry and tumor angiogenesis. The American Journal of Pathology. 2000;**156**(2):361-381

[139] Paulis YW, Soetekouw PM, Verheul HM, Tjan-Heijnen VC, Griffioen AW. Signalling pathways in vasculogenic mimicry. Biochimica et Biophysica Acta. 2010;**1806**(1):18-28

[140] Vermeulen PB, Colpaert C, Salgado R, Royers R, Hellemans H, Van Den Heuvel E, et al. Liver metastases from colorectal adenocarcinomas grow in three patterns with different angiogenesis and desmoplasia. The Journal of Pathology. 2001;**195**(3):336-342

[141] Stessels F, Van den Eynden G, Van der Auwera I, Salgado R, Van den Heuvel E, Harris AL, et al. Breast adenocarcinoma liver metastases, in contrast to colorectal cancer

liver metastases, display a non-angiogenic growth pattern that preserves the stroma and lacks hypoxia. British Journal of Cancer. 2004;**90**(7):1429-1436

[142] Kienast Y, von Baumgarten L, Fuhrmann M, Klinkert WE, Goldbrunner R, Herms J, et al. Real-time imaging reveals the single steps of brain metastasis formation. Nature Medicine. 2010;**16**(1):116-122

[143] Leenders WP, Kusters B, Verrijp K, Maass C, Wesseling P, Heerschap A, et al. Antiangiogenic therapy of cerebral melanoma metastases results in sustained tumor progression via vessel co-option. Clinical Cancer Research. 2004;**10**(18 Pt 1):6222-6230

[144] di Tomaso E, Snuderl M, Kamoun WS, Duda DG, Auluck PK, Fazlollahi L, et al. Glioblastoma recurrence after cediranib therapy in patients: Lack of "rebound" revascularization as mode of escape. Cancer Research. 2011;**71**(1):19-28

[145] Frentzas S, Simoneau E, Bridgeman VL, Vermeulen PB, Foo S, Kostaras E, et al. Vessel co-option mediates resistance to anti-angiogenic therapy in liver metastases. Nature Medicine. 2016;**22**(11):1294-1302

[146] Hu J, Bianchi F, Ferguson M, Cesario A, Margaritora S, Granone P, et al. Gene expression signature for angiogenic and nonangiogenic non-small-cell lung cancer. Oncogene. 2005;**24**(7):1212-1219

[147] Holash J, Maisonpierre PC, Compton D, Boland P, Alexander CR, Zagzag D, et al. Vessel cooption, regression, and growth in tumors mediated by angiopoietins and VEGF. Science. 1999;**284**(5422):1994-1998

[148] Carbonell WS, Ansorge O, Sibson N, Muschel R. The vascular basement membrane as "soil" in brain metastasis. PLoS One. 2009;**4**(6):e5857

[149] Valiente M, Obenauf AC, Jin X, Chen Q, Zhang XH, Lee DJ, et al. Serpins promote cancer cell survival and vascular co-option in brain metastasis. Cell. 2014;**156**(5):1002-1016

Chapter 3

The Influence of Microbial Metabolites in the Gastrointestinal Microenvironment on Anticancer Immunity

Silke Neumann, Estelle M. Peyroux, Matt J. Woodall, Nick J. Shields, Sarah L. Young and Sharon T. Pattison

Abstract

The gastrointestinal (GI) tumour microenvironment is characterised by its unique colonisation with bacteria that are estimated to match the total number of cells in our body. It is becoming increasingly clear that the microbiome and its metabolites are important orchestrators of local and systemic immune responses, anticancer immunity and the host response to cancer therapy. Apart from their role as an energy source, metabolites have been shown to modulate inflammation, immune cell function and cancer cell survival. The polarisation of immune cell subsets by microbial metabolites towards either pro- or antitumorigenic functions strongly affects cancer progression and outcomes. In this chapter, we will discuss the link between microbial metabolites in the GI tumour microenvironment, anticancer immune responses and cancer progression.

Keywords: gastrointestinal tumour environment, host immune response, innate immunity, microbial metabolites, metabolism

1. Introduction

The GI tract is a complex ecosystem, populated by a large variety of bacteria, fungi and viruses that together form the intestinal microbiome. A surprising amount of local and systemic bodily functions are affected by the composition of the microbiome and its produced metabolites. This includes the generation of energy, metabolism of dietary components and synthesis of vitamins as well as regulation of immune responses, behaviour and mood. Perturbations of microbial populations, commonly referred to as dysbiosis, have been associated with a large number of diseases, such as inflammatory bowel disease [1], diabetes [2], obesity [3], autism [4], depression [5] and colorectal cancer [6, 7]. Understanding the reciprocal relationship between the microbiota and immunity has received great attention as it is becoming increasingly clear that inflammatory processes underlie many pathologies. The complexity of microbiome-immune interactions is staggering as not only the presence or absence of bacterial species shape immunity, but metabolites produced and modified by bacteria have a direct effect on the immune system's ability to react to infectious and non-communicable diseases [8].

Microbial metabolites, as the sum of products modified and synthesised by microbiota, can be a useful tool to understand microbiota-driven immune modulation when analysis of bacterial lineages proves difficult. Diversity and abundance of microbial communities varies greatly amongst healthy individuals, whereas metabolic pathways are conserved and stable [9, 10]. Therefore, assessing changes of metabolic pathways and how they affect immunity may provide crucial insights into the role of the GI microenvironment in health and disease. Microbial metabolites are commonly divided into three categories, (1) metabolites produced by bacteria, derived from host products; (2) metabolites modified by bacteria, derived from host products; and (3) metabolites synthesised by bacteria directly.

In the following sections, we will briefly describe GI cancers and components of the GI tract that shape the tumour microenvironment. Furthermore, we will discuss the evidence for connecting changes in the microbiome and its metabolites with carcinogenesis and the role of bacterial metabolites in shaping immunity and in particular anticancer immunity.

2. The GI cancer microenvironment

2.1 The gastrointestinal tract

The gastrointestinal tract starts at the mouth, extends to the anus and includes the oesophagus, stomach, small intestine, large intestine, liver and pancreas. Its main functions are primarily the disruption and digestion of food, absorption of nutrients and elimination of waste products. With the diverse functions of the GI tract, it is not unsurprising that it has a number of diverse environments which are contributed to by various types of immune cells and the multiple bacteria that reside in the GI tract.

Movement of food down the GI tract is facilitated by muscular contractions. Much of the tube that makes up the GI tract is muscle lined to enable this to occur, with sphincters at particular junctures to enable control of food passage. The muscle layers are coated by a mucous membrane which varies depending on the function of that section of the GI tract.

The epithelium that lines the GI tract can be broadly divided into three subtypes, primarily based on their function. Squamous epithelium is found at the start (mouth and oesophagus) and end (anus) of the GI tract providing a protective covering. Secretory epithelium is found in the stomach. Absorptive epithelium is found in both the small and large intestines. The small intestine has numerous fingerlike projections, called villi, that increase the surface area to facilitate absorption of nutrients with interspersed crypts, or glands, which contain the stem cells that give rise to the epithelial cells. The absorptive epithelium of the large intestine is more closely packed with glands specialised for water absorption and mucus-secreting cells to lubricate the passage of faecal material down the GI tract.

The tube that forms the GI tract has a number of layers that lie between the outer muscular wall (the muscularis propria) and the innermost epithelium. The epithelium forms the innermost layer of the mucosa, which has two additional components, the lamina propria (composed of supportive connective tissue) and a thin layer of smooth muscle, the muscularis mucosae. Underneath the mucosa is the submucosa, which contains connective tissue, nerves and lymphatic and blood vessels. The submucosa is surrounded by the outer muscularis propria, the muscle layer whose contractions facilitate passage of material down the GI tract. The supporting tissue surrounding the GI tract is called the adventitia or serosa and contains major nerves and blood vessels.

The GI tract includes two large glands, the liver and pancreas. Both develop from the primitive foregut embryonically and have functions that contribute to digestion by generating digestive fluids. The liver produces bile, which can be stored and concentrated in the gallbladder. When lipids enter the duodenum, neuroendocrine cells of the duodenal mucosa are stimulated to release cholecystokinin-pancreozymin (CCK) causing contraction of the gallbladder releasing bile into the duodenum. Bile acids are emulsifying agents which aid in lipid digestion. Pancreatic secretions reach the duodenum via the pancreatic duct and contain a high content of alkaline bicarbonate ions which assist in neutralising the acidic fluid that has come from the stomach. The pancreas also produces a number of enzymes including trypsin, chymotrypsin, amylase, lipase and carboxypeptidases which are involved in the breakdown of proteins, carbohydrates and lipids.

2.2 Microbiota in the GI tract

Our lifestyle, including diet, exercise, childhood microbial exposure and the use of antibiotics strongly, influences the composition of our microbiota [9, 11–14]. Two phyla of bacteria dominate the human gut *Bacteroidetes* and *Firmicutes*. Over decades the ability to classify bacteria into their genus and species has evolved with technology resulting in numerous reclassifications. Bacteria can be additionally classified into subspecies on the basis of small but relevant differences within a species. Further classifications into strains or serovars, indicating variable immune antigens present on their surface, can be allocated outside nomenclature rules. This level of complexity demonstrates the purpose of studying microbial metabolites in the context of gut immunity, thereby avoiding the complexities of bacterial species, focusing instead on their metabolic output.

Epidemiological data initially made links between bacteria and cancer development. However, identifying the role of bacteria in cancer development has been challenging due to the importance of host factors in cancer susceptibility combined with the ubiquitous nature of bacteria and the prolonged period between introduction of a bacterium and development of overt cancer [15]. This is further complicated by environmental factors which are thought to play a much larger role than genetic makeup in determining the makeup of an individual's microbiota [16].

While the knowledge of outcomes from bacterial interactions with human cells is growing, there is enormous potential for further discovery when accommodating other microbes that populate different levels of the gastrointestinal tract such as fungi and viruses [17].

2.3 Gastrointestinal cancers

Gastrointestinal (GI) cancers are as diverse as the environments of the GI tract and the various cell types found in the GI tract. Squamous cell carcinomas arise in the squamous epithelium of the oral cavity, oesophagus and anus. Those that arise in the oral cavity are considered head and neck cancers rather than GI cancers. Adenocarcinomas are cancers that arise from glandular epithelium and can arise in the oesophagus, stomach, small intestine, pancreas and large intestine. Other cancers that can arise from the GI tract include cholangiocarcinoma, with origin from bile duct cells; hepatocellular carcinoma (HCC), originating from hepatocytes (liver cells); gastrointestinal stromal tumours, originating from the interstitial cells of Cajal which have a role in the control of peristaltic contractions [18]; and neuroendocrine cancers which can arise from neuroendocrine cells throughout the GI tract. Multiple studies examining these GI cancers have demonstrated diverse molecular alterations within cancers that arise from the same cell type in the same organ of the GI tract, highlighting the multitude of malignancies that can arise in the GI tract [19–27].

Chronic inflammation and infection are intimately associated with the development of cancer, with 15% of global cancer cases in 2012 being attributed to a carcinogenic infection [28]. Examples from the GI tract include HCC with hepatitis B and C virus infections contributing to more than 70% of global HCC diagnoses in 2012 [28]. In gastric adenocarcinoma four molecular subtypes were described by The Cancer Genome Atlas (TCGA) in 2014, one is characterised by Epstein-Barr virus positivity and shows extreme DNA hypermethylation [29]. *Helicobacter pylori* (*H. pylori*) is considered a class I carcinogen by the World Health Organization due to the association of chronic infection with the development of gastric adenocarcinoma and mucosa-associated lymphoid tissue (MALT) lymphoma, a form of B cell lymphoma in the stomach [30, 31]. The risk of developing gastric cancer with *H. pylori* is dependent on the virulence factors of the strain causing infection, other environmental factors and host genetics [32–34].

In colorectal cancer studies, *Fusobacterium* subspecies were consistently identified as being differentially present in tumour samples; however, these findings are still limited by small sample sizes [35]. A study of the microbiome in a hereditary form of CRC has implicated oncotoxins produced by co-colonisation with *Bacteroides fragilis* (*B. fragilis*) and *Escherichia coli* (*E. coli*) subspecies in mucosal biofilms. Further animal studies have revealed the bacterial synergy involved in carcinogenesis whereby the *B. fragilis* toxin increases expression of the pro-inflammatory cytokine interleukin (IL)-17 enabling the oncotoxin-producing *E. coli* to invade the mucosa inducing DNA damage in epithelial cells [36].

In addition to bacteria and viruses being implicated in carcinogenesis, parasitic infections have also been implicated in cancer development in the GI tract, with liver fluke infection, particularly *Opisthorchis viverrini,* being associated with the development of cholangiocarcinoma [37].

2.4 Inflammation in the GI tract

Acute inflammation is an integral part of the host defence against pathogens and tissue damage and is also required for the initiation of beneficial antitumour immunity [38, 39]. In contrast, it is ongoing 'smouldering' inflammation that contributes to tumour development, progression, invasion and metastasis [40]. Low-grade inflammation affects the function of immune cells and promotes an immune-suppressive, tumour-promoting phenotype [41, 42]. This in turn is associated with reduced immune surveillance and clearance of tumour cells by the immune system.

Chronic inflammation can be induced through a variety of mechanisms, including chronic infections [43], autoimmunity [44], metabolic disorders [45] and altered microbiota [46, 47]. In the GI tract in particular, the host immune system has to maintain a delicate balance, and pathogens and malignant cells need to be cleared, whereas normal flora has to be tolerated. Disruption of immune tolerance or dysbiosis may result in loss of epithelial barrier function and overstimulation of immune cells, leading to tissue damage and chronic inflammation.

Conditions associated with recurrent or chronic inflammation, such as inflammatory bowel disease (IBD), have been shown to contribute to the risk of developing small and large intestine cancers [48, 49]. Mechanistically, this has been related to increased stimulation of inflammation-promoting immune cells by altered microbiota [46]. As a result, pro-inflammatory cytokines and chemokines are secreted, attract further immune cells into the tissue and polarise them towards tumour-promoting functions [50–52]. Particularly the presence of pathogenic

T-cell subsets, induced by pro-inflammatory cytokines, has been shown to be a predictor of poor prognosis in colorectal cancer patients [53]. Chronic inflammation also contributes to the expansion of oncogenic bacteria thereby re-enforcing disease progression [54]. See **Box 1** for an overview of the immune cell populations involved in intestinal antitumour immune responses.

Dendritic cells
DCs are innate immune cells that develop from myeloid precursors in the bone marrow. They are capable of detecting pathogens or tissue disturbances and initiate an inflammatory response. In the tumour microenvironment, they are thought to engulf dead tumour cells and debris and present fragments thereof to T cells, thus initiating anticancer immune responses.

Macrophages
Macrophages are antigen-presenting cells that arise from either circulating monocytes or embryonic progenitors that persist into adulthood, both giving rise to tissue-specific macrophage populations that are capable of self-renewal [186, 187]. Macrophages serve important functions in immunity, cancer, metabolism and tissue repair. Macrophages play an important role in in the antitumour immune response but can also adopt a pro-tumour phenotype in the tumour environment [188, 189].

Cytotoxic T cells (CD8+ T cells)
CTLs express the CD8 receptor and recognise antigens presented on the surface of antigen-presenting cells. Once primed by this encounter, CTLs are capable of recognising the same antigens and kill target cells expressing the antigen. Tumour-specific CTL responses are crucial for controlling tumour growth.

Helper T cells (CD4+ T cells)
Th cells express the CD4 receptor and support functions of innate and adaptive immune cells by secreting cytokines. Depending on the environment they encounter, Th cells develop into subsets with a wide range of functions [190]. Cytokines, such as IL-12, promote the development of Th1 cells, which are efficient at secreting IFN-γ and TNF-α, important cytokines for antitumour immunity. When naïve $CD4^+$ T cells reside an environment high in IL-6 and TGF-β, they develop into Th17 cells, which promote autoimmunity and are a negative prognostic marker for colorectal cancer [49]. Th cells can develop into immune-suppressive Tregs in the presence of TGF-β when expressing the transcription factor *FOXP3*.

Mucosa-activated invariant T cells (MAIT cells)
MAIT cells reside at mucosal surfaces in the lung and the intestine [163] and are widely distributed in tissue and the systemic blood circulation [164, 165]. They have innate immune cell features but also express a semi-invariant T-cell receptor, which can recognise antigens presented on a monomorphic MHC class 1-related protein (MR1) expressed by antigen-presenting cells [166]. MAIT cells are first responders to a variety of infections caused by bacteria, fungi and viruses through detection of microbial B vitamin antigens.

Innate lymphoid cells (ILCs)
ILCs stem from the lymphoid lineage but have innate immune cell characteristics [109]. They are quick responders and contribute to elimination of pathogens and tissue homeostasis by producing a variety of cytokines. Based on their specific cytokine secretion, ILCs are grouped into different classes that resemble their T-cell counterparts, for example, group 3 ILCs (ILC3s) resemble Th17 cells and produce IL-17 and IL-22 [109].

Box 1. *Overview of immune cell populations involved in intestinal antitumour immune responses.*

3. Microbial metabolites that shape antitumour immunity

Metabolites produced or modified by bacteria significantly impact health and disease by acting locally on GI tract cells but can also have systemic effects by influencing the function and activation states of immune cells. The 'metabolome' constitutes the sum of small molecules produced by a biological system and is a powerful approach to explore the current condition of that system [55]. Metabolomics refers to the analysis of metabolites using techniques, such as mass spectrometry, nuclear magnetic resonance analysis, high-performance liquid chromatography and gas chromatography coupled with mass spectrometry. Obtained peak patterns can be compared against spectral databases for identification of metabolites. Metabolomics can be combined with metagenomics, investigating the genetic material of the entire community, and metatranscriptomics, exploring which genes are expressed, to increase our understanding of microbiomes. The benefits, disadvantages and technical challenges of these omics techniques are reviewed extensively elsewhere [56–59].

In the following sections, we will discuss the impact of microbial metabolites on immune cell function, focusing on how these metabolites shape the immune response. The anatomical components of the intestinal immune system including immune and epithelial cell populations and the mechanisms employed by these cell populations to discriminate between commensal and pathogenic bacteria have been reviewed extensively recently [60–66].

3.1 Metabolites produced by bacteria from dietary components

3.1.1 Short-chain fatty acids

Short-chain fatty acids (SCFAs) are 1–6 carbon volatile fatty acids which can either be in straight or branched chain conformation [67]. They are end products of fermentation of indigestible carbohydrates such as starch and fibre, by anaerobic microbiota in the caecum and large intestine [68]. SCFAs are the most abundant metabolite in the colon and consist almost entirely of acetate (C2), propionate (C3) and butyrate (C4) [69]. Acetate is the most common SCFA (60% of total SCFAs) in the colon and can also reach the systemic circulation after absorption from the GI tract. Propionate and butyrate make up roughly 20% of the SCFAs in faeces each [68, 70]. Propionate is mainly metabolised in the liver after draining into the portal vein after absorption from the gut mucosa, while butyrate is the preferred energy source of colonocytes and is digested locally [71].

SCFAs affect host physiology and pathology through a multitude of local and systemic mechanisms of action (**Figure 1**). In the GI tract, they act through binding to transmembrane G protein-coupled receptors (GPRs) and diffusion into epithelial and immune cells where they modify post-translational gene expression and function as energy source.

GPRs implicated in SCFA signalling are free fatty acid receptors GPR41, GPR43 and GPR109a. The SCFAs acetate, propionate and butyrate have differing selectivity for these receptors with all three binding to GPR43, expressed on the GI epithelium and immune cells [72, 73]. Propionate and butyrate bind to GPR41, expressed by lamina propria cells in the large intestine, immune cells and cells of the peripheral nervous system [72]. Butyrate has also been found to ligate GPR109a expressed by large intestinal epithelium and certain subsets of immune cells [73].

Activation of the GPRs leads to changes in intracellular potassium concentrations [K^+], which directly activate intracellular danger-sensing molecular complexes, called inflammasomes. Integral components of inflammasomes are Nod-like receptors, which are cytosolic pattern recognition receptors (PRRs). Particularly changes in the NLRP3 and NLRP6 inflammasomes (containing Nod-like receptors 3 and 6, respectively) have been implicated in exacerbating intestinal inflammation [74–76]. Inflammasome complexes can be activated through a two-step process. The first signal is considered the 'priming signal', which induces nuclear factor (NF)-kB-mediated transcription of inflammasome components and pro-IL-1β and IL-18 in epithelial and immune cells [77]. The second signal leads to the assembly of the inflammasome complex and caspase-1-dependent processing of pro-IL-1β and IL-18 into their biologically active forms.

IL-1β and IL-18 are important signalling molecules for gut homeostasis and immune effector function. IL-1β can have pro- and anti-homeostatic functions, whereas IL-18 is generally regarded as a crucial cytokine for maintaining gut barrier integrity and a healthy microbiome composition. A reduction in IL-18 secretion has been found to be associated with a shift in microbiota towards the expansion of *Bacteroidetes*, which promote colonic inflammation and carcinogenesis in mouse models [46, 76]. This aligns with findings that describe a decreased

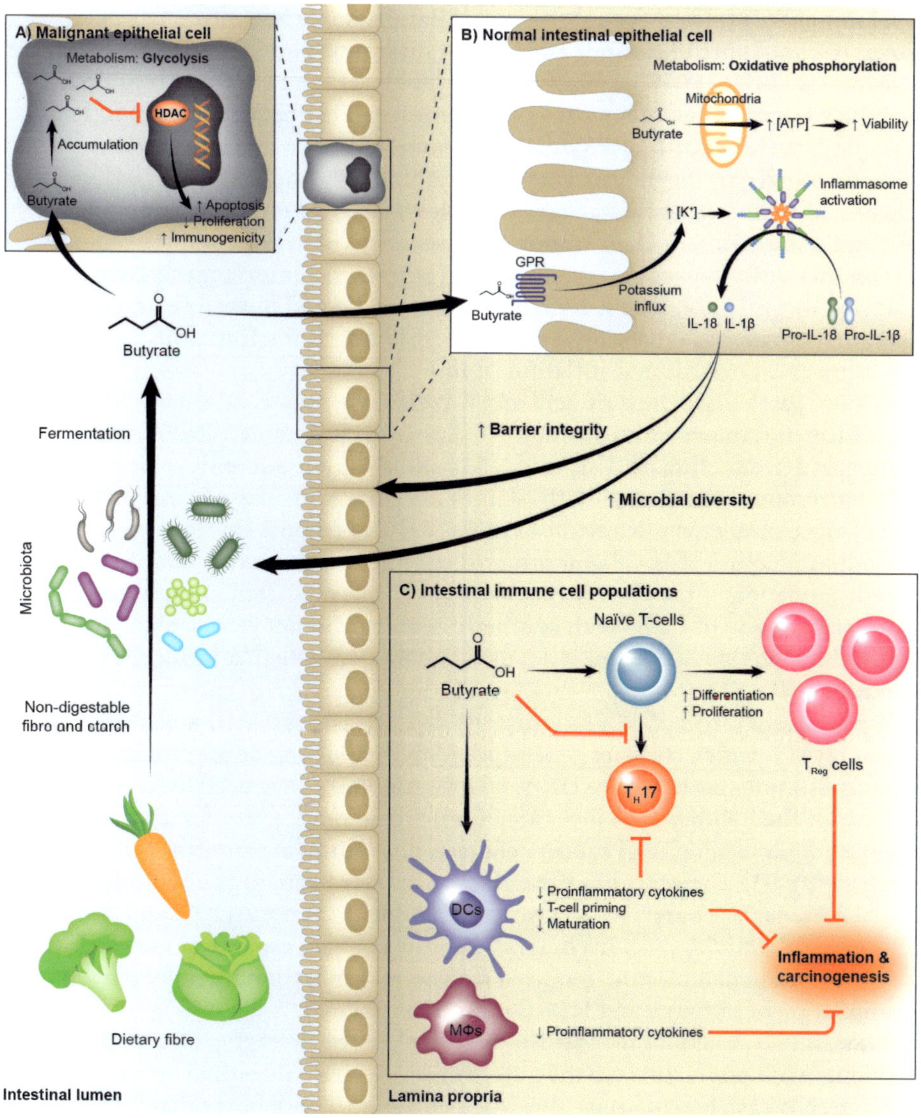

Figure 1.
Effects of the SCFA butyrate on epithelial and immune cell function. SCFAs are produced through fermentation of non-digestible fibre and starch by microbiota. (a) Cancer cells switch their metabolism to glycolysis and are less efficient at metabolising SCFAs such as butyrate, leading to accumulation of butyrate in the cell. Increased concentrations of butyrate inhibit HDAC activity and induce apoptosis, reduce proliferation and increase immunogenicity of cancer cells. (b) In healthy epithelial cells, butyrate is metabolised through oxidative phosphorylation and used as energy source by the cell. Butyrate also activates NLRP3 and NLRP6 inflammasomes through binding to GPRs, resulting in secretion of cytokines IL-1β and IL-18. In turn, IL-18 strengthens intestinal barrier integrity and promotes diversity of intestinal microbiota. (c) The effects of butyrate on immune cells in the lamina propria can be described as promoting the development and activity of anti-inflammatory populations, such as Tregs, while suppressing immune cell functions contributing to inflammation. Butyrate suppresses the maturation of DCs, limits their ability to prime CTLs and reduces the production of pro-inflammatory cytokines in DCs and macrophages. Together this reduces inflammation and the development of inflammatory Th subsets, such as Th17, which contribute to intestinal carcinogenesis.

expression of NLRP6 in gastric cancer, correlated with a reduced survival time in patients [78]. When the NLRP6 inflammasome was overexpressed, gastric cancer cell proliferation and development were inhibited, and migration and invasion of cancer cells were decreased. Furthermore, NLRP6 activity has been linked with intact epithelial barrier function and prevention of colorectal cancer development [79]. Even though NLRP3 inflammasome activation has been shown to contribute to tumour-promoting inflammation and immune infiltrate in several ways [11, 80–83], many reports highlight the beneficial functions of the NLRP3 inflammasome in preventing intestinal cancer development. For example, activation of NLRP3 inflammasomes has been demonstrated to protect from intestinal carcinogenesis via IL-18-mediated epithelial repair [84] and suppression of metastatic colon cancer growth via maturation of natural killer (NK) cells and stimulation of their tumoricidal activity [85]. The complex biology of intestinal inflammasome signalling and its role in tumorigenesis have been reviewed recently [74, 86]. It remains to be investigated how the often overlapping and controversial findings regarding inflammasome functions orchestrate induction and resolution of inflammation.

SCFAs, particularly butyric acid and β-hydroxybutyrate, stimulate NLRP3 and NLRP6 inflammasomes through binding to GPR43 and GPR109a, leading to increased production of IL-1β and IL-18 [87, 88]. Subsequently it was shown that dietary supplementation with sodium butyrate or increased consumption of dietary fibre protected mice against colitis [87] and colonic carcinogenesis [89] through production of IL-18 and promotion of gut homeostasis. Interestingly, even though activation of the NLRP3 inflammasome was mediated via activation of GPRs, stimulation of GPRs with synthetic agonists did not recapitulate these findings, indicating that SCFAs must act on additional targets that influence cytokine secretion [90].

A prominent target of SCFAs is histone deacetylases (HDAC) and acetyltransferases (HAT), which regulate gene expression by allowing or preventing access of the transcription machinery to DNA. HDAC inhibitors have been used in cancer therapy for their ability to induce cancer cell death, reduce proliferation and increase immunogenicity of cancer cells as well as stimulate anticancer immune function [91–93]. Cancer cells utilise glucose as their primary energy source, and thus SCFAs, such as butyrate, accumulate and due to increased concentration inhibit HDAC activity [94]. In contrast, healthy cells are capable of metabolising butyrate into small molecules required for energy generation, thereby preventing accumulation of butyrate and HDAC inhibition [95, 96].

Interestingly, a similar mechanism may explain the diverging effects of butyrate on immune cell populations in the gut. In order to retain intestinal homeostasis, immune cells have to remain passive when challenged with host microbiota and food antigens yet remain responsive to fight pathogenic bacteria. This diversity of function is supported by SCFAs that induce a hypo-responsive state in immune cell populations, which are capable of promoting inflammation, such as macrophages, dendritic cells (DCs) and T cells [47], yet cells involved in containing inflammation are induced and expanded by SCFAs [97, 98].

DCs and macrophages are professional antigen-presenting cells, highly proficient at scanning the environment for invaders or tissue disturbances. Once detected, pathogens or abnormal cells are engulfed, processed and presented in small fragments to T helper (Th) cells. These cells, in turn, differentiate into populations of effector Th cells, directed by cytokines from DCs. Secretion of pro-inflammatory cytokines by DCs, such as IL-6, IL-12 and IL-23 in particular, supports the polarisation of Th cells towards effector and inflammatory subsets Th1 and Th17, respectively. This is important for removal of pathogens but can be detrimental for tissue homeostasis if not regulated tightly. Th cells also facilitate the full activation and memory development of cytotoxic T cells (CTLs), which are able to kill antigen specifically and react swiftly in the case of a second encounter. SCFAs, butyrate and propionate, but not acetate, have been shown to reduce production of pro-inflammatory cytokines, such as IL-12 and IL-23, and chemokines in DCs and also impair the maturation of DCs [90, 99, 100]. Changes in cytokine secretion are associated with impaired ability of DCs to prime CTLs [101], reduced polarisation of Th-cell subsets towards effector and inflammatory subsets and induction of regulatory T cells (Tregs) [102].

Regulatory T cells have an important role in control of inflammation. Tissue inflammation and autoimmunity are promoted if Tregs are not present or dysfunctional. In contrast to many other cancers where Tregs are thought to suppress effective antitumour immunity, GI cancer patients benefit from the presence of Tregs in the tumour microenvironment [103]. Tregs limit inflammatory processes, induce tolerance towards food and microbial antigens and promote stem cell renewal in the intestine through a variety of mechanisms. This includes production of anti-inflammatory cytokines, such as IL-10 and transforming growth factor beta (TGF-β)1, expression of inhibitory molecules and restriction of nutrients required by effector T cells, particularly Th1 and Th17 cells [64, 104–106].

Interestingly, due to the high rates of glycolysis in effector and pro-inflammatory cells, such as CTLs, Th1 and Th17 subsets, butyrate accumulates in these cells, leading to an inhibitory effect mediated by both HDAC inhibition and binding to GPR109a [90, 93, 102]. In contrast, anti-inflammatory cells, such as Tregs, which rely on oxidative phosphorylation can process butyrate for energy consumption, circumventing these effects [107]. It has been demonstrated comprehensively that SCFAs drive Treg development via HDAC inhibition and GPR activation in the intestine and periphery, thereby protecting mice against colonic inflammation, colitis and colorectal cancer [97, 98, 106, 108].

3.1.2 Indole derivatives

Indoles are aromatic heterocyclic compounds, produced by gut bacteria from the degradation of tryptophan via several enzymes [109]. Tryptophan is an essential amino acid, which cannot be produced by the host and is taken up in the diet. Dietary tryptophan can be metabolised by microbiota and host cells to indole derivatives that have important immune modulatory functions in the gut [110]. Indole derivatives, such as kynurenines, are ligands for the aryl hydrocarbon receptor (AHR), an intracellular ligand-activated transcription factor with important roles in detecting environmental changes and alerting cells to them. Microbial AHR ligands are thought to play an important role in maintaining intestinal homeostasis and limiting inflammation [111]. The importance of AHR signalling has been demonstrated in $AHR^{-/-}$ mice where clearance of pathogenic bacteria was impaired while intestinal inflammation was elevated and associated with an increased risk of developing colitis [112–114].

Mechanistically, bacterial AHR ligands have been shown to induce the production of IL-22 in innate lymphoid cells (ILC3), which promotes diversity of gut microbiota and protects mucosal barrier functions [115, 116]. ILCs stem from the lymphoid lineage but have innate immune cell characteristics [117]. They are quick responders and contribute to elimination of pathogens and tissue homeostasis by producing a variety of cytokines. Based on their specific cytokine secretion, ILCs are grouped into different classes that resemble their T-cell counterparts, for example, group 3 ILCs (ILC3s) resemble Th17 cells and produce IL-17 and IL-22 [117]. Even though production of IL-22 by ILC3s is vital for mucosal homeostasis, elevated levels of ILC3s and increased production of IL-17 have been associated with IBD pathology [118, 119]. Furthermore, it has been found that IL-22 contributes to tumorigenesis in the colon when elevated chronically. This was mediated via an inflammasome-dependent reduction of IL-22 binding protein and chronic elevated IL-22 levels [50, 51].

Genetic induction of constitutively active AHR signalling in mouse models has been found to be associated with stomach and liver cancer development [120, 121], whereas the absence of AHR in $AHR^{-/-}$ mice protected from prostate cancer [122]. As AHR is crucially involved in early development, maintenance of stem cells and cell differentiation, it is difficult to discern if stable genetic induction or ablation of these signalling pathways may promote carcinogenesis directly or through disturbances in early development.

3.1.3 Polyamines

Polyamines are small polycationic molecules, derived either from the diet or synthesised by gut bacteria or host cells [123]. While they are found in almost all living cells, the method of production in mammalian and bacterial cells differs. Intestinal bacteria use inducible or constitutive forms of amino acid decarboxylase enzymes in order to produce polyamines with arginine as a precursor. Mammalian synthesis involves a series of steps to convert arginine to polyamines, with ornithine decarboxylase being the rate-limiting enzyme. Putrescine, spermidine and spermine are the major polyamines secreted by both the gut microbiota and mammalian cells and have important immune modulatory functions [124].

Along with other polyamines, spermine directly regulates cells in the innate arm of the immune system and has an anti-inflammatory effect. Spermine inhibits lipopolysaccharide-induced expression of pro-inflammatory cytokines in monocytes and macrophages [125]. In macrophages, spermine is able to increase the expression of IL-10 and suppress production of inflammatory cytokines such as IFN-γ [126]. These functions were shown to have anti-inflammatory and protective effects in animal models of local and systemic inflammation [127].

Conversely, spermine inhibits the activation of the NLRP6 inflammasome and reduces the amount of IL-1β and IL-18 released. This is counteracted by taurine, another microbial metabolite, which is discussed below. The inhibitory effect of spermine on NLRP6 activity may be counteracted by the role polyamines play in maintenance of the gut epithelial lining. Many studies have found that intestinal mucosal repair is associated with an increase in levels of spermine, spermidine and putrescine [128]. Furthermore, when the synthesis of polyamines is blocked, migration and proliferation of intestinal epithelial cells to the site of injury as well as in regular turnover of mucosal cells are significantly reduced. Polyamines promote the transcription of E-cadherin, which is important for the formation of tight junctions. In this regard, they play a role in stabilising the gut epithelium, so it is able to act as a barrier between the external and internal environment [128].

3.2 Metabolites modified by bacteria, derived from host products

3.2.1 Bile acids and derivatives

Bile acids are physiological surfactants, produced in the liver and secreted into the duodenum or stored in the gall bladder. Bile acid molecules contain a hydrophobic hemisphere and a hydrophilic one, enabling them to associate around dietary fats and fat-soluble vitamins into micelles [129]. This promotes the breakdown and absorption of these molecules in the hydrophilic environment of the GI tract [130]. Approximately 95% of bile acids are reabsorbed via active transport by the apical sodium-dependent bile acid transporter in the ileum of the small intestine [131]. Microbial bile salt hydrolases catalyse the hydrolysis of amide bond linkage in bile acids, releasing an unconjugated bile acid. The de-conjugation of bile acids causes the release of glycine and taurine, which can then be used for further metabolism and growth.

Bile acids modulate innate immune cell function by inhibiting NF-kB activity, resulting in reduced production of pro-inflammatory cytokines and molecules (TNF-α, IL-1β, IL-6, IL-12, cyclooxygenase-1 and cyclooxygenase-2, and inducible nitric oxide synthase) in stimulated monocytes, macrophages, DCs and intestinal epithelial cells [132–135]. In human macrophages, administration of bile acids leads to increased production of IL-10 and a decrease in phagocytosis [136]. The reduction in pro-inflammatory cytokines combined with the increase in anti-inflammatory cytokine production induces the development, recruitment and expansion of Tregs in the colon. Together, the properties of bile acids improve barrier integrity and outcomes in mouse models of experimental colitis, which lead to the development of inflammatory bowel disease and colorectal cancer [133]. The effects occur via bile acid-mediated activation of the farnesoid X receptor (FXR), a ligand-activated nuclear receptor, and the G protein-coupled bile acid receptor 1 (GPBAR1). These receptors also play a crucial role in bile acid-induced inhibition of the NLRP3 inflammasome, which is associated with reduced levels of secreted IL-1β and IL-18 [137, 138].

In contrast to primary bile acids, the bile acid-derivative taurine stimulates NLRP6 inflammasome activity, leading to increased production of IL-18 [139]. Levy et al. found high taurine and associated IL-18 concentrations maintained and restored functional microbiota typically present in healthy flora.

3.3 Metabolites synthesised by bacteria directly

Microbiota are able to synthesise metabolites that are either unique to prokaryotic organisms, such as capsule polysaccharides and certain vitamins, or that can also be produced by host cells, for example, adenosine triphosphate (ATP).

3.3.1 ATP

In addition to its role as universal energy source, ATP is an important signalling molecule that directly impacts immune cell function when released into the extracellular space. ATP is not only produced by living organisms but has been found to be secreted by a variety of commensal and pathogenic bacteria [140, 141]. Generally, increased levels of ATP are produced and secreted by host cells under inflammatory stress conditions and injury, often associated with inflammatory cell death [142]. Furthermore, the tumour microenvironment has high concentrations of extracellular ATP, at least partly induced by hypoxia, an activator of ATP secretion, and necrotic cell death [143, 144]. The chronic presence of ATP in the tumour microenvironment supports cancer cell proliferation, survival and metastasis as reviewed elsewhere [144]. In the immune context, most of the actions of ATP have been described to be pro-inflammatory; however, its hydrolysis product adenosine has immune-suppressive functions.

Host-, tumour- and microbial-derived ATP binds to purinergic-type receptor P2, while adenosine, the downstream product of hydrolysed ATP, binds to P1 receptors [144]. Purinergic P2 receptors are expressed highly by immune cells, and ATP exerts most of its pro-inflammatory effects through binding to P2X(1–7) ion channels and P2Y(1, 4, 6, 11–14) metabotropic purinergic receptors [145]. Activation of purinergic receptor P2X7 by ATP increases intracellular potassium and calcium concentrations [146]. Together with a priming signal, ATP is an important inducer of NLRP3 inflammasome activity [147]. As discussed previously, activation of the NLRP3 inflammasome and the subsequent secretion of IL-1β and IL-18 have important roles in shaping the magnitude of inflammatory responses, gut homeostasis and barrier function and have a controversial role in tumour progression [86].

Besides its role as inflammasome activator, ATP modulates migration of innate and adaptive immune cell subsets [148]. After release of ATP into the extracellular space, innate immune cells such as monocytes, mature DCs, neutrophils, macrophages and microglia are mobilised via activation of P2X and P2Y receptors and migrate to the source of the high ATP concentration. This migratory response is further amplified through autocrine activation of pannexin 1 channels in the membrane of innate immune cells [149–153]. Interestingly, ATP has been shown to affect migration of $CD4^+$ T-cell subsets differently, depending on their function and activation status. While activated $CD4^+$ T cells respond to high ATP concentrations and stimulation of P2X7 and P2X4 receptors with induction of apoptosis, immune-suppressive Tregs increase proliferation and migration via their P2Y2 receptor [154].

In the context of intestinal inflammation and carcinogenesis, ATP drives the polarisation of $CD4^+$ T cells towards IL-17-producing $CD4^+$ T cells, associated with a higher susceptibility to develop colitis and exacerbation of existing colitis in experimental mouse models [155, 156]. A Th17 signature in colorectal cancer patients is associated with disease progression and worse outcomes [53]. Polymorphism of the ATP-converting enzyme CD39 (hydrolysis of ATP to adenosine diphosphate (ADP)) in IBD patients and increased expression of P2X7 receptors in the inflamed epithelium of Crohn's patients have been found, suggesting another role of ATP in disease pathology [156, 157].

ATP is hydrolysed by CD39 and CD73 to adenosine, which have been widely investigated and reviewed for their immune-suppressive functions in the tumour environment [144, 151, 152, 158]. Therapeutic inhibition of ATP and adenosine receptors as well as targeting of CD39 and CD73, alone and in combination with traditional chemotherapy, has shown great promise to prevent tumour growth by overturning adenosine-induced immune suppression [159–163]. However, recent evidence demonstrates that extracellular ATP is required for the formation of long-term, antigen-specific CTL responses, which are crucial for immunological memory [164]. It remains to be determined if therapeutic targeting of purinergic receptors and conversion enzymes affects development of immunological memory in cancer, which is desirable to prevent cancer occurrence.

3.3.2 Vitamins

Humans lack the ability to produce most essential vitamins and rely on vitamins to be supplied with the diet and produced by gut bacteria. Microbiota are able to synthesise vitamin K and a large number of B vitamins, such as folate (vitamin B9), riboflavin (vitamin B2), pyridoxine (vitamin B6), cobalamin (vitamin B12) and methionine [165]. B vitamins have achieved great attention for their cancer-preventing properties, with folate being the most investigated B vitamin in the cancer context [166]. The cancer-preventing mechanisms have been attributed to the role of B vitamins as cofactors in metabolic processes related to energy generation and gene regulation [166, 167]. Folate (B9) and pyridoxine (B6) have also been found to modulate intestinal immunity by increasing $CD4^+$ T-cell proliferation, trafficking and survival of Treg subsets and NK cell cytotoxicity [168–170].

Interestingly, bacteria that synthesise vitamins B2 and B9 are recognised by mucosa-activated invariant T (MAIT) cells. MAIT cells reside at mucosal surfaces in the lung and the intestine [171] and are also widely distributed in tissue and the systemic blood circulation [172, 173]. They have innate immune cell features but also express a semi-invariant T-cell receptor, which can recognise antigens presented on a monomorphic MHC class 1-related protein (MR1) expressed by antigen-presenting cells [174]. MAIT cells are first responders to a variety of infections caused by bacteria, fungi and viruses through detection of microbial B vitamin antigens.

Upon activation, MAIT cells are able to proliferate and produce cytotoxic molecules, capable of destroying infected cells displaying microbial B vitamin antigens on their MR1 protein [175–177]. Furthermore, MAIT cells produce immune modulatory cytokines, including IFN-γ, IL-2, IL-17, IL-10 and TNF-α [178]. While IFN-γ production is highly desirable to promote antitumour immunity, an IL-17 signature has been found to be associated with worse outcomes in CRC patients [53]. Numbers of MAIT cells decrease in the peripheral circulation but accumulate in intestinal tumours [179, 180]. Several groups report a diminished ability of tumour-infiltrating MAIT cells to produce IFN-γ combined with increased secretion of IL-17 [180, 181]. Even though it appears that MAIT cells may develop a tumour-promoting phenotype in the tumour microenvironment and thus contribute to cancer progression, further studies are needed to elucidate the role of these recently discovered cells.

It is tempting to speculate that MAIT cells may impact intestinal cancer development and progression through recognition of B vitamin antigens produced by dysbiotic and carcinogenic bacteria. Since MAIT cells can be activated or inhibited depending on the B vitamin antigen presented on MR1 proteins, MAIT cells have been suggested as attractive targets for cancer immunotherapy [182]. This is in part related to their potential to be targeted in combination with chemotherapy, due the expression of drug resistance proteins that allows their survival and activation during and post-chemotherapy [172].

3.3.3 Bacterial polysaccharides

Commensal bacteria contribute to intestinal homeostasis through production of capsular polysaccharides. Polysaccharide A (PSA), the most studied bacterial polysaccharide, is produced by *B. fragilis* and plays an important role in regulating intestinal inflammation. Exogenous administration or bacterial production of PSA can prevent the development of experimental colitis by activating Treg and inhibiting Th17 responses [183–185]. This is mediated by PSA binding to PRRs expressed by DCs, which in turn secrete IL-10 that promotes the development and activation of Tregs. Furthermore, PSA influences the polarisation of Th subsets towards IFN-γ-producing Th cells, an important effector population for anticancer immunity. *B. fragilis* are not the only commensals that regulate inflammation; many other strains, for example, a large number of *Clostridium strains* [186], have been shown to have anti-inflammatory functions. This highlights the fact that the sum of commensals and their metabolites, rather than a defined strain or metabolite, shapes the functionality of the immune system by impacting the polarisation of immune subsets, crucial for clearance of diseases.

4. Conclusions

The link between microbiome disturbances and the development of inflammatory diseases highlights the importance of studying the effects of microbes and their metabolites on immune cell function. Deciphering the effects of microbial metabolites on the immune system in a highly dynamic organ system, such as the GI tract, is inherently difficult. The actions of individual metabolites need to be considered before the complex interplay of microbes, metabolites and cellular components, such as epithelial and immune cells can be investigated. The GI tumour microenvironment is unique in that immunological tolerance is required to maintain a healthy intestinal environment, including maintenance of the "normal" microbiome, yet the presence of regulatory immune cells may impede antitumour immune responses and promote carcinogenesis.

There is increasing evidence from preclinical mouse model systems and human studies that GI tract microbiota, such as *B. fragilis*, *Bifidobacterium*, *Faecalibacterium prausnitzii* and *Akkermansia muciniphila*, can directly influence response to treatment including immunotherapies and survival in some malignancies [187–193]. This effect is potentially mediated by bacteria stimulating activation of innate immune cells and downstream polarisation of Th-cell subsets towards Th1 cells [194]. The species and diversity of bacterium identified as influencing treatment response and survival vary, likely reflecting the complexity of the interactions involved, the diverse malignancies and populations within which those malignancies had arisen, and the number of bacterial species that have immunomodulatory effects mediated through the GI tract.

The influence of infections on initiation and promotion of cancer has been long recognised, but our understanding of the complex network of interactions between the host, the microbiome, the genetics of both the host and microbiome and the metabolome remains superficial. These interactions are not static, which, with the diversity of the GI tract environment, add to the challenge of deciphering what microbial species may be influencing the immune response in a tumour-promoting or tumour-suppressive manner. The complexity of microbial species and indeed the complexity of immune cells and their function mean that practically assaying and identifying individual species of bacteria, or subsets of immune cells, clinically in a prognostic or predictive sense is challenging. The more readily measureable microbial metabolome may provide a more clinically accessible read-out of this interaction. The wide-ranging impact that products of microbial metabolism have on immune cell function and polarity and therefore anticancer immunity has been underappreciated to this point. A greater understanding of how microbial metabolites influence the GI tumour microenvironment has the potential to expand therapeutic options and improve survival of patients with GI cancers.

Conflict of interest

The authors declare no conflict of interest.

Author details

Silke Neumann[1], Estelle M. Peyroux[1], Matt J. Woodall[1], Nick J. Shields[1], Sarah L. Young[1] and Sharon T. Pattison[2]*

1 Department of Pathology, Dunedin School of Medicine, University of Otago, Dunedin, New Zealand

2 Department of Medicine, Dunedin School of Medicine, University of Otago, Dunedin, New Zealand

*Address all correspondence to: sharon.pattison@otago.ac.nz

IntechOpen

© 2019 The Author(s). Licensee IntechOpen. This chapter is distributed under the terms of the Creative Commons Attribution License (http://creativecommons.org/licenses/by/3.0), which permits unrestricted use, distribution, and reproduction in any medium, provided the original work is properly cited.

References

[1] Frank DN et al. Molecular-phylogenetic characterization of microbial community imbalances in human inflammatory bowel diseases. PNAS. 2007;**104**(34):13780-13785

[2] Wen L et al. Innate immunity and intestinal microbiota in the development of Type 1 diabetes. Nature. 2008;**455**(7216):1109-1113

[3] Ley RE et al. Microbial ecology: Human gut microbes associated with obesity. Nature. 2006;**444**(7122):1022-1023

[4] Hsiao EY et al. Microbiota modulate behavioral and physiological abnormalities associated with neurodevelopmental disorders. Cell. 2013;**155**(7):1451-1463

[5] Valles-Colomer M et al. The neuroactive potential of the human gut microbiota in quality of life and depression. Nature Microbiology. 2019;**4**(4):623-632

[6] Kostic AD et al. Genomic analysis identifies association of fusobacterium with colorectal carcinoma. Genome Research. 2012;**22**(2):292-298

[7] Allen-Vercoe E et al. Fusobacterium and Enterobacteriaceae: Important players for CRC? Immunology Letters. 2014;**162**(2 Pt A):54-61

[8] Levy M et al. Metabolites: Messengers between the microbiota and the immune system. Genes & Development. 2016;**30**(14):1589-1597

[9] The Human Microbiome Project C et al. Structure, function and diversity of the healthy human microbiome. Nature. 2012;**486**:207

[10] Turnbaugh PJ et al. A core gut microbiome in obese and lean twins. Nature. 2009;**457**(7228):480-484

[11] Zitvogel L et al. Nutrition, inflammation and cancer. Nature Immunology. 2017;**18**(8):843-850

[12] Proctor LM et al. The integrative human microbiome project. Nature. 2019;**569**(7758):641-648

[13] Zmora N et al. You are what you eat: Diet, health and the gut microbiota. Nature Reviews Gastroenterology & Hepatology. 2019;**16**(1):35-56

[14] Macpherson AJ et al. How nutrition and the maternal microbiota shape the neonatal immune system. Nature Reviews. Immunology. 2017;**17**(8):508-517

[15] Zur Hausen H. The search for infectious causes of human cancers: Where and why. Virology. 2009;**392**(1):1-10

[16] Dąbrowska K et al. Correlations of host genetics and gut microbiome composition. Frontiers in Microbiology. 2016;7:1357

[17] Hillman ET et al. Microbial ecology along the gastrointestinal tract. Microbes and Environments. 2017;**32**(4):300-313

[18] Corless CL et al. Gastrointestinal stromal tumours: Origin and molecular oncology. Nature Reviews. Cancer. 2011;**11**(12):865-878

[19] Cancer Genome Atlas Research N. Comprehensive molecular characterization of gastric adenocarcinoma. Nature. 2014;**513**(7517):202-209

[20] Cancer Genome Atlas Research N et al. Integrated genomic characterization of oesophageal carcinoma. Nature. 2017;**541**(7636):169-175

[21] Cancer Genome Atlas Research Network. Electronic address

aadhe, et al. Integrated genomic characterization of pancreatic ductal adenocarcinoma. Cancer Cell. 2017;**32**(2):185-203 e13

[22] Farshidfar F et al. Integrative genomic analysis of cholangiocarcinoma identifies distinct IDH-mutant molecular profiles. Cell Reports. 2017;**18**(11):2780-2794

[23] Hoshida Y et al. Integrative transcriptome analysis reveals common molecular subclasses of human hepatocellular carcinoma. Cancer Research. 2009;**69**(18):7385-7392

[24] Lawrence B et al. Recurrent loss of heterozygosity correlates with clinical outcome in pancreatic neuroendocrine cancer. NPJ Genomic Medicine. 2018;**3**:18

[25] Liu Y et al. Comparative molecular analysis of gastrointestinal adenocarcinomas. Cancer Cell. 2018;**33**(4):721-735 e8

[26] Scarpa A et al. Whole-genome landscape of pancreatic neuroendocrine tumours. Nature. 2017;**543**(7643):65-71

[27] Yao JC et al. Genomic profiling of NETs: A comprehensive analysis of the RADIANT trials. Endocrine Related Cancer. 2019;**26**(4):391-403

[28] Plummer M et al. Global burden of cancers attributable to infections in 2012: A synthetic analysis. Lancet Global Health. 2016;**4**(9):e609-e616

[29] Cancer Genome Atlas Research Consortium. Comprehensive molecular characterization of gastric adenocarcinoma. Nature. 2014;**513**(7517):202-209

[30] World Health Organization, International Agency for Research on Cancer. Schistosomes, liver flukes and Helicobacter pylori. IARC Working Group on the Evaluation of Carcinogenic Risks to Humans. Lyon, 7-14 June 1994. ARC Mongr Eval Carcinog Risks Hum. 1994;**61**:1-241

[31] Stolte M et al. Helicobacter and gastric MALT lymphoma. Gut. 2002;**50**(Suppl 3):III19-III24

[32] Peek RM Jr et al. *Helicobacter pylori* and gastrointestinal tract adenocarcinomas. Nature Reviews. Cancer. 2002;**2**(1):28-37

[33] Fuccio L et al. Gastric cancer, *Helicobacter pylori* infection and other risk factors. World Journal of Gastrointestinal Oncology. 2010;**2**(9):342-347

[34] Conteduca V et al. *H. pylori* infection and gastric cancer: State of the art (review). International Journal of Oncology. 2013;**42**(1):5-18

[35] Shang F-M et al. Fusobacterium nucleatum and colorectal cancer: A review. World Journal of Gastrointestinal Oncology. 2018;**10**(3):71-81

[36] Dejea CM et al. Patients with familial adenomatous polyposis harbor colonic biofilms containing tumorigenic bacteria. Science. 2018;**359**:592-597

[37] Sripa B et al. Liver fluke induces cholangiocarcinoma. PLoS Medicine. 2007;**4**(7):e201

[38] Chen DS et al. Oncology meets immunology: The cancer-immunity cycle. Immunity. 2013;**39**(1):1-10

[39] Schreiber RD et al. Cancer immunoediting: Integrating Immunity's roles in cancer suppression and promotion. Science. 2011;**331**(6024):1565-1570

[40] Mantovani A et al. Cancer-related inflammation. Nature. 2008;**454**(7203):436-444

[41] Ostrand-Rosenberg S et al. Cross-talk between myeloid-derived suppressor cells (MDSC), macrophages, and dendritic cells enhances tumor-induced immune suppression. Seminars in Cancer Biology. 2012;**22**(4):275-281

[42] Gabrilovich D et al. Myeloid-derived suppressor cells as regulators of the immune system. Nature Reviews Immunology. 2009;**9**:162-174

[43] Hand TW et al. Linking the microbiota, chronic disease, and the immune system. Trends in Endocrinology & Metabolism. 2016;**27**(12):831-843

[44] Piconese S et al. Viral hepatitis, inflammation, and cancer: A lesson for autoimmunity. Journal of Autoimmunity. 2018;**95**:58-68

[45] O'Sullivan J et al. Obesity and gastrointestinal cancer: The interrelationship of adipose and tumour microenvironments. Nature reviews. Gastroenterology & Hepatology. 2018;**15**(11):699-714

[46] Hu B et al. Microbiota-induced activation of epithelial IL-6 signaling links inflammasome-driven inflammation with transmissible cancer. PNAS. 2013;**110**(24):9862-9867

[47] Levy M et al. Dysbiosis and the immune system. Nature Reviews. Immunology. 2017;**17**(4):219-232

[48] Ekbom A et al. Ulcerative colitis and colorectal cancer. New England Journal of Medicine. 1990;**323**(18):1228-1233

[49] Karin M et al. Innate immunity gone awry: Linking microbial infections to chronic inflammation and cancer. Cell. 2006;**124**(4):823-835

[50] Grivennikov SI et al. Adenoma-linked barrier defects and microbial products drive IL-23/IL-17-mediated tumour growth. Nature. 2012;**491**(7423):254-258

[51] Huber S et al. IL-22BP is regulated by the inflammasome and modulates tumorigenesis in the intestine. Nature. 2012;**491**(7423):259-263

[52] Garrett WS et al. Colitis-associated colorectal cancer driven by T-bet deficiency in dendritic cells. Cancer Cell. 2009;**16**(3):208-219

[53] Tosolini M et al. Clinical impact of different classes of infiltrating T cytotoxic and helper cells (Th1, Th2, Treg, Th17) in patients with colorectal cancer. Cancer Research. 2011;**71**(4):1263-1271

[54] Arthur JC et al. Intestinal inflammation targets cancer-inducing activity of the microbiota. Science. 2012;**338**(6103):120-123

[55] Fiehn O. Metabolomics—The link between genotypes and phenotypes. Plant Molecular Biology. 2002;**48**(1-2):155-171

[56] Aguiar-Pulido V et al. Metagenomics, metatranscriptomics, and metabolomics approaches for microbiome analysis. Evolutionary Bioinformatics Online. 2016;**12**(Suppl 1):5-16

[57] Vernocchi P et al. Gut microbiota profiling: Metabolomics based approach to unravel compounds affecting human health. Frontiers in Microbiology. 2016;**7**(1144)

[58] Kumar R et al. Getting started with microbiome analysis: Sample acquisition to bioinformatics. Current Protocols in Human Genetics. 2014;**82**:18.8.1-18.8.29

[59] Aldridge BB et al. Microbial metabolomics: Innovation, application, insight. Current Opinion in Microbiology. 2014;**19**:90-96

[60] Artis D. Epithelial-cell recognition of commensal bacteria and maintenance of immune homeostasis in the gut. Nature Reviews. Immunology. 2008;**8**(6):411-420

[61] Mowat AM. Anatomical basis of tolerance and immunity to intestinal antigens. Nature Reviews. Immunology. 2003;**3**(4):331-341

[62] Izcue A et al. Regulatory T cells suppress systemic and mucosal immune activation to control intestinal inflammation. Immunological Reviews. 2006;**212**:256-271

[63] Bain CC et al. Macrophages in intestinal homeostasis and inflammation. Immunological Reviews. 2014;**260**(1):102-117

[64] Whibley N et al. Regulatory T cell adaptation in the intestine and skin. Nature Immunology. 2019;**20**(4):386-396

[65] Stagg AJ. Intestinal dendritic cells in health and gut inflammation. Frontiers in Immunology. 2018;**9**:2883

[66] Mann ER et al. Intestinal antigen-presenting cells in mucosal immune homeostasis: Crosstalk between dendritic cells, macrophages and B-cells. World Journal of Gastroenterology. 2014;**20**(29):9653-9664

[67] Rios-Covian D et al. Intestinal short chain fatty acids and their link with diet and human health. Frontiers in Microbiology. 2016;7:185

[68] den Besten G et al. The role of short-chain fatty acids in the interplay between diet, gut microbiota, and host energy metabolism. Journal of Lipid Research. 2013;**54**(9):2325-2340

[69] Flint HJ. Gut microbial metabolites in health and disease. Gut Microbes. 2016;7(3):187-188

[70] Louis P et al. Understanding the effects of diet on bacterial metabolism in the large intestine. Journal of Applied Microbiology. 2007;**102**(5):1197-1208

[71] Cummings JH et al. The control and consequences of bacterial fermentation in the human colon. The Journal of Applied Bacteriology. 1991;**70**(6):443-459

[72] Brown AJ et al. The Orphan G protein-coupled receptors GPR41 and GPR43 are activated by propionate and other short chain carboxylic acids. The Journal of Biological Chemistry. 2003;**278**(13):11312-11319

[73] Le Poul E et al. Functional characterization of human receptors for short chain fatty acids and their role in polymorphonuclear cell activation. The Journal of Biological Chemistry. 2003;**278**(28):25481-25489

[74] Zmora N et al. Inflammasomes and intestinal inflammation. Mucosal immunology. 2017;**10**(4):865-883

[75] Elinav E et al. Inflammation-induced cancer: Crosstalk between tumours, immune cells and microorganisms. Nature Reviews. Cancer. 2013;**13**(11):759-771

[76] Elinav E et al. NLRP6 inflammasome regulates colonic microbial ecology and risk for colitis. Cell. 2011;**145**(5):745-757

[77] Hornung V et al. Silica crystals and aluminum salts activate the NALP3 inflammasome through phagosomal destabilization. Nature Immunology. 2008;**9**(8):847-856

[78] Wang Q et al. NLRP6, decreased in gastric cancer, suppresses tumorigenicity of gastric cancer cells. Cancer Managment and Research. 2018;**10**:6431-6444

[79] Normand S et al. Nod-like receptor pyrin domain-containing protein 6 (NLRP6) controls epithelial self-renewal and colorectal carcinogenesis upon injury. PNAS. 2011;**108**(23):9601-9606

[80] Du Q et al. Dietary cholesterol promotes AOM-induced colorectal cancer through activating the NLRP3 inflammasome. Biochemical Pharmacology. 2016;**105**:42-54

[81] Zitvogel L et al. Inflammasomes in carcinogenesis and anticancer immune responses. Nature Immunology. 2012;**13**(4):343-351

[82] van Deventer HW et al. The inflammasome component NLRP3 impairs antitumor vaccine by enhancing the accumulation of tumor-associated myeloid-derived suppressor cells. Cancer Research. 2010;**70**(24):10161-10169

[83] Chow MT et al. NLRP3 suppresses NK cell-mediated responses to carcinogen-induced tumors and metastases. Cancer Research. 2012;**72**(22):5721-5732

[84] Zaki MH et al. The NLRP3 inflammasome protects against loss of epithelial integrity and mortality during experimental colitis. Immunity. 2010;**32**(3):379-391

[85] Dupaul-Chicoine J et al. The Nlrp3 inflammasome suppresses colorectal cancer metastatic growth in the liver by promoting natural killer cell tumoricidal activity. Immunity. 2015;**43**(4):751-763

[86] Karki R et al. Diverging inflammasome signals in tumorigenesis and potential targeting. Nature Reviews Cancer. 2019;**19**(4):197-214

[87] Macia L et al. Metabolite-sensing receptors GPR43 and GPR109A facilitate dietary fibre-induced gut homeostasis through regulation of the inflammasome. Nature Communications. 2015;**6**:6734

[88] Ohira H et al. Butyrate enhancement of interleukin-1β production via activation of oxidative stress pathways in lipopolysaccharide-stimulated THP-1 cells. Journal of Clinical Biochemistry and Nutrition. 2012;**50**(1):59-66

[89] Singh N et al. Activation of Gpr109a, receptor for niacin and the commensal metabolite butyrate. Suppresses Colonic Inflammation and Carcinogenesis. Immunity. 2014;**40**(1):128-139

[90] D'Souza WN et al. Differing roles for short chain fatty acids and GPR43 agonism in the regulation of intestinal barrier function and immune responses. PLoS One. 2017;**12**(7):e0180190

[91] Falkenberg KJ et al. Histone deacetylases and their inhibitors in cancer, neurological diseases and immune disorders. Nature Reviews. Drug Discovery. 2014;**13**(9):673-691

[92] Halsall JA et al. Histone deacetylase inhibitors for cancer therapy: An evolutionarily ancient resistance response may explain their limited success. BioEssays. 2016;**38**(11):1102-1110

[93] Fellows R et al. Microbiota derived short chain fatty acids promote histone crotonylation in the colon through histone deacetylases. Nature Communications. 2018;**9**(1):105

[94] Vander Heiden MG et al. Understanding the Warburg effect: The metabolic requirements of cell proliferation. Science. 2009;**324**(5930):1029-1033

[95] Lupton JR. Microbial degradation products influence colon cancer risk: The butyrate controversy. The Journal of Nutrition. 2004;**134**(2):479-482

[96] Donohoe DR et al. The Warburg effect dictates the mechanism of butyrate-mediated histone acetylation and cell proliferation. Molecular Cell. 2012;**48**(4):612-626

[97] Furusawa Y et al. Commensal microbe-derived butyrate induces the differentiation of colonic regulatory T cells. Nature. 2013;**504**(7480):446-450

[98] Arpaia N et al. Metabolites produced by commensal bacteria promote peripheral regulatory T-cell generation. Nature. 2013;**504**:451

[99] Nastasi C et al. The effect of short-chain fatty acids on human monocyte-derived dendritic cells. Scientific Reports. 2015;**5**:16148

[100] Qiang Y et al. Butyrate and retinoic acid imprint mucosal-like dendritic cell development synergistically from bone marrow cells. Clinical and Experimental Immunology. 2017;**189**(3):290-297

[101] Nastasi C et al. Butyrate and propionate inhibit antigen-specific CD8(+) T cell activation by suppressing IL-12 production by antigen-presenting cells. Scientific Reports. 2017;**7**(1):14516

[102] Kaisar MMM et al. Butyrate conditions human dendritic cells to prime type 1 regulatory T cells via both histone deacetylase inhibition and G protein-coupled receptor 109A signaling. Frontiers in Immunology. 2017;**8**:1429

[103] Ward-Hartstonge KA et al. Regulatory T-cell heterogeneity and the cancer immune response. Clinical & Translational Immunology. 2017;**6**(9):e154

[104] Barnes MJ et al. Regulatory T cells reinforce intestinal homeostasis. Immunity. 2009;**31**(3):401-411

[105] Schmidt A et al. Molecular mechanisms of treg-mediated T cell suppression. Frontiers in Immunology. 2012;**3**:51

[106] Zhang M et al. Butyrate inhibits interleukin-17 and generates Tregs to ameliorate colorectal colitis in rats. BMC Gastroenterology. 2016;**16**(1):84

[107] Howie D et al. Foxp3 drives oxidative phosphorylation and protection from lipotoxicity. JCI insight. 2017;**2**(3):e89160

[108] Smith PM et al. The microbial metabolites, short-chain fatty acids, regulate colonic Treg cell homeostasis. Science. 2013;**341**(6145):569-573

[109] Jaglin M et al. Indole, a signaling molecule produced by the gut microbiota, negatively impacts emotional behaviors in rats. Frontiers in Neuroscience. 2018;**12**:216

[110] Wikoff WR et al. Metabolomics analysis reveals large effects of gut microflora on mammalian blood metabolites. PNAS. 2009;**106**(10):3698-3703

[111] Rothhammer V et al. The aryl hydrocarbon receptor: An environmental sensor integrating immune responses in health and disease. Nature Reviews Immunology. 2019;**19**(3):184-197

[112] Kiss EA et al. Natural aryl hydrocarbon receptor ligands control organogenesis of intestinal lymphoid follicles. Science. 2011;**334**(6062):1561-1565

[113] Shi LZ et al. The aryl hydrocarbon receptor is required for optimal resistance to listeria monocytogenes infection in mice. The Journal of Immunology. 2007;**179**(10):6952-6962

[114] Qiu J et al. The aryl hydrocarbon receptor regulates gut immunity through modulation of innate lymphoid cells. Immunity. 2012;**36**(1):92-104

[115] Lee JS et al. AHR drives the development of gut ILC22 cells and postnatal lymphoid tissues via pathways dependent on and independent of Notch. Nature Immunology. 2011;**13**:144

[116] Zelante T et al. Tryptophan catabolites from microbiota engage aryl hydrocarbon receptor and balance mucosal reactivity via Interleukin-22. Immunity. 2013;**39**(2):372-385

[117] Ebbo M et al. Innate lymphoid cells: Major players in inflammatory diseases. Nature Reviews. Immunology. 2017;**17**(11):665-678

[118] Geremia A et al. IL-23-responsive innate lymphoid cells are increased in inflammatory bowel disease. The Journal of Experimental Medicine. 2011;**208**(6):1127-1133

[119] Veldhoen M et al. The aryl hydrocarbon receptor links TH17-cell-mediated autoimmunity to environmental toxins. Nature. 2008;**453**:106

[120] Andersson P et al. A constitutively active dioxin/aryl hydrocarbon receptor induces stomach tumors. PNAS. 2002;**99**(15):9990-9995

[121] Moennikes O et al. A constitutively active dioxin/aryl hydrocarbon receptor promotes hepatocarcinogenesis in mice. Cancer Research. 2004;**64**(14):4707-4710

[122] Fritz WA et al. The aryl hydrocarbon receptor inhibits prostate carcinogenesis in TRAMP mice. Carcinogenesis. 2007;**28**(2):497-505

[123] Rooks MG et al. Gut microbiota, metabolites and host immunity. Nature Reviews. Immunology. 2016;**16**(6):341-352

[124] Di Martino ML et al. Polyamines: Emerging players in bacteria-host interactions. International Journal of Medical Microbiology. 2013;**303**(8):484-491

[125] Zhang M et al. Spermine inhibition of monocyte activation and inflammation. Molecular Medicine. 1999;**5**(9):595-605

[126] Hasko G et al. Spermine differentially regulates the production of interleukin-12 p40 and interleukin-10 and suppresses the release of the T helper 1 cytokine interferon-gamma. Shock. 2000;**14**(2):144-149

[127] Postler TS et al. Understanding the Holobiont: How microbial metabolites affect human health and shape the immune system. Cell Metabolism. 2017;**26**(1):110-130

[128] Timmons J et al. Polyamines and gut mucosal homeostasis. Journal of Gastrointestinal and Digestive System. 2012;**2**(Suppl 7). pii: 001

[129] Enright EF et al. Microbiome-mediated bile acid modification: Role in intestinal drug absorption and metabolism. Pharmacological Research. 2018;**133**:170-186

[130] Wilson FA et al. Unstirred water layers in intestine: Rate determinant of fatty acid absorption from micellar solutions. Science (New York, N.Y.). 1971;**174**(4013):1031-1033

[131] Copple BL et al. Pharmacology of bile acid receptors: Evolution of bile acids from simple detergents to complex signaling molecules. Pharmacological Research. 2016;**104**:9-21

[132] Gadaleta RM et al. Activation of bile salt nuclear receptor FXR is repressed by pro-inflammatory cytokines activating NF-κB signaling in the intestine. Biochimica et Biophysica Acta (BBA)—Molecular Basis of Disease. 2011;**1812**(8):851-858

[133] Gadaleta RM et al. Farnesoid X receptor activation inhibits inflammation and preserves the intestinal barrier in inflammatory bowel disease. Gut. 2011;**60**(4):463-472

[134] Wang Y-D et al. Farnesoid X receptor antagonizes nuclear fjactor kappaB in hepatic inflammatory response. Hepatology (Baltimore, Md.). 2008;**48**(5):1632-1643

[135] Vavassori P et al. The bile acid receptor FXR is a modulator of intestinal innate immunity. Journal of Immunology. 2009;**183**(10):6251-6261

[136] Haselow K et al. Bile acids PKA-dependently induce a switch of the IL-10/IL-12 ratio and reduce proinflammatory capability of human macrophages. Journal of Leukocyte Biology. 2013;**94**(6):1253-1264

[137] Hao H et al. Farnesoid X receptor regulation of the NLRP3 inflammasome underlies cholestasis-associated sepsis. Cell Metabolism. 2017;**25**(4):856-867.e5

[138] Guo C et al. Bile acids control inflammation and metabolic disorder through inhibition of NLRP3 Inflammasome. Immunity. 2016;**45**(4):802-816

[139] Levy M et al. Microbiota-modulated metabolites shape the intestinal microenvironment by regulating NLRP6 inflammasome signaling. Cell. 2015;**163**(6):1428-1443

[140] Iwase T et al. Isolation and identification of ATP-secreting bacteria from mice and humans. Journal of Clinical Microbiology. 2010;**48**(5):1949-1951

[141] Mempin R et al. Release of extracellular ATP by bacteria during growth. BMC Microbiology. 2013;**13**(1):301

[142] Bergsbaken T et al. Pyroptosis: Host cell death and inflammation. Nature Reviews. Microbiology. 2009;**7**(2):99-109

[143] Forrester T et al. Release of adenosine triphosphate from isolated adult heart cells in response to hypoxia. The Journal of Physiology. 1977;**268**(2):371-390

[144] Di Virgilio F et al. Extracellular purines, purinergic receptors and tumor growth. Oncogene. 2017;**36**(3):293-303

[145] Burnstock G et al. Cellular distribution and functions of P2 receptor subtypes in different systems. International Review of Cytology. 2004;**240**:31-304

[146] Yaron JR et al. K+ regulates Ca2+ to drive inflammasome signaling: Dynamic visualization of ion flux in live cells. Cell Death and Disease. 2015;**6**:e1954

[147] Ghiringhelli F et al. Activation of the NLRP3 inflammasome in dendritic cells induces IL-1beta-dependent adaptive immunity against tumors. Nature Medicine. 2009;**15**(10):1170-1178

[148] Chen Y et al. ATP release guides neutrophil chemotaxis via P2Y2 and A3 receptors. Science (New York, N.Y.). 2006;**314**(5806):1792-1795

[149] Saez PJ et al. ATP promotes the fast migration of dendritic cells through the activity of pannexin 1 channels and P2X7 receptors. Science Signaling. 2017;**10**(506). pii: eaah7107

[150] Muller T et al. The purinergic receptor P2Y2 receptor mediates chemotaxis of dendritic cells and eosinophils in allergic lung inflammation. Allergy. 2010;**65**(12):1545-1553

[151] Junger WG. Immune cell regulation by autocrine purinergic signalling.

Nature Reviews. Immunology. 2011;**11**(3):201-212

[152] Di Virgilio F et al. Extracellular ATP and P2 purinergic signalling in the tumour microenvironment. Nature Reviews Cancer. 2018;**18**(10):601-618

[153] Schnurr M et al. ATP gradients inhibit the migratory capacity of specific human dendritic cell types: Implications for P2Y11 receptor signaling. Blood. 2003;**102**(2):613-620

[154] Trabanelli S et al. Extracellular ATP exerts opposite effects on activated and regulatory CD4+ T cells via purinergic P2 receptor activation. Journal of Immunology (Baltimore, Md.: 1950). 2012;**189**(3):1303-1310

[155] Atarashi K et al. ATP drives lamina propria T(H)17 cell differentiation. Nature. 2008;**455**(7214):808-812

[156] Friedman DJ et al. CD39 deletion exacerbates experimental murine colitis and human polymorphisms increase susceptibility to inflammatory bowel disease. PNAS. 2009;**106**(39):16788-16793

[157] Neves AR et al. Overexpression of ATP-activated P2X7 receptors in the intestinal mucosa is implicated in the pathogenesis of Crohn's disease. Inflammatory Bowel Diseases. 2014;**20**(3):444-457

[158] Lee JS et al. Unfolding role of a danger molecule adenosine signaling in modulation of microbial infection and host cell response. International Journal of Molecular Sciences. 2018;**19**(1). pii: E199

[159] Stagg J et al. CD73-deficient mice have increased antitumor immunity and are resistant to experimental metastasis. Cancer Research. 2011;**71**(8):2892-2900

[160] Stagg J et al. Anti-CD73 antibody therapy inhibits breast tumor growth and metastasis. PNAS. 2010;**107**(4):1547-1552

[161] Young A et al. Co-inhibition of CD73 and A2AR adenosine signaling improves anti-tumor immune responses. Cancer Cell. 2016;**30**(3):391-403

[162] Vijayan D et al. Targeting immunosuppressive adenosine in cancer. Nature Reviews. Cancer. 2017;**17**(12):709-724

[163] Allard B et al. The ectonucleotidases CD39 and CD73: Novel checkpoint inhibitor targets. Immunological Reviews. 2017;**276**(1):121-144

[164] Borges da Silva H et al. The purinergic receptor P2RX7 directs metabolic fitness of long-lived memory CD8(+) T cells. Nature. 2018;**559**(7713):264-268

[165] LeBlanc JG et al. Bacteria as vitamin suppliers to their host: A gut micro-biota perspective. Current Opinion in Biotechnology. 2013;**24**(2):160-168

[166] Song M et al. Nutrients, foods, and colorectal cancer prevention. Gastroenterology. 2015;**148**(6): 1244-60.e16

[167] Eslami M et al. Importance of probiotics in the prevention and treatment of colorectal cancer. Journal of Cellular Physiology. 2019;**234**(10):17127-17143

[168] Kunisawa J et al. A pivotal role of vitamin B9 in the maintenance of regulatory T cells in vitro and in vivo. PLoS One. 2012;7(2):e32094

[169] Kunisawa J et al. Sphingosine 1-phosphate dependence in the regulation of lymphocyte trafficking to the gut epithelium. The Journal of Experimental Medicine. 2007;**204**(10):2335-2348

[170] Schwab SR et al. Lymphocyte sequestration through S1P lyase inhibition and disruption of S1P gradients. Science. 2005;**309**(5741):1735-1739

[171] Treiner E et al. Selection of evolutionarily conserved mucosal-associated invariant T cells by MR1. Nature. 2003;**422**(6928):164-169

[172] Dusseaux M et al. Human MAIT cells are xenobiotic-resistant, tissue-targeted, CD161hi IL-17-secreting T cells. Blood. 2011;**117**(4):1250-1259

[173] Tang XZ et al. IL-7 licenses activation of human liver intrasinusoidal mucosal-associated invariant T cells. Journal of Immunology. 2013;**190**(7):3142-3152

[174] Kjer-Nielsen L et al. An overview on the identification of MAIT cell antigens. Immunology and Cell Biology. 2018;**96**(6):573-587

[175] Le Bourhis L et al. MAIT cells detect and efficiently lyse bacterially-infected epithelial cells. PLoS Pathogens. 2013;**9**(10):e1003681

[176] Gold MC et al. Human mucosal associated invariant T cells detect bacterially infected cells. PLoS Biology. 2010;**8**(6):e1000407

[177] Kurioka A et al. MAIT cells are licensed through granzyme exchange to kill bacterially sensitized targets. Mucosal Immunology. 2014;**8**:429

[178] Kumar V et al. Role of MAIT cells in the immunopathogenesis of inflammatory diseases: New players in old game. International Reviews of Immunology. 2018;**37**(2):90-110

[179] Won EJ et al. Clinical relevance of circulating mucosal-associated invariant T cell levels and their anti-cancer activity in patients with mucosal-associated cancer. Oncotarget. 2016;**7**(46):76274-76290

[180] Ling L et al. Circulating and tumor-infiltrating mucosal associated invariant T (MAIT) cells in colorectal cancer patients. Scientific Reports. 2016;**6**:20358

[181] Sundstrom P et al. Human mucosa-associated invariant T cells accumulate in colon adenocarcinomas but produce reduced amounts of IFN-gamma. Journal of Immunology. 2015;**195**(7):3472-3481

[182] Haeryfar SMM et al. Mucosa-associated invariant T cells in malignancies: A faithful friend or formidable foe? Cancer Immunology, Immunotherapy: CII. 2018;**67**(12):1885-1896

[183] Mazmanian SK et al. A microbial symbiosis factor prevents intestinal inflammatory disease. Nature. 2008;**453**(7195):620-625

[184] Dasgupta S et al. Plasmacytoid dendritic cells mediate anti-inflammatory responses to a gut commensal molecule via both innate and adaptive mechanisms. Cell Host & Microbe. 2014;**15**(4):413-423

[185] Cobb BA et al. Polysaccharide processing and presentation by the MHCII pathway. Cell. 2004;**117**(5):677-687

[186] Atarashi K et al. Induction of colonic regulatory T cells by indigenous clostridium species. Science. 2011;**331**(6015):337-341

[187] Derosa L et al. Negative association of antibiotics on clinical activity of immune checkpoint inhibitors in patients with advanced renal cell and non-small-cell lung cancer. Annals of Oncology. 2018;**29**(6):1437-1444

[188] Gopalakrishnan V et al. Gut microbiome modulates response to anti-PD-1 immunotherapy in melanoma patients. Science. 2018;**359**(6371):97-103

[189] Iida N et al. Commensal bacteria control cancer response to therapy by modulating the tumor microenvironment. Science. 2013;**342**(6161):967-970

[190] Matson V et al. The commensal microbiome is associated with anti-PD-1 efficacy in metastatic melanoma patients. Science. 2018;**359**(6371):104-108

[191] Routy B et al. Gut microbiome influences efficacy of PD-1-based immunotherapy against epithelial tumors. Science (New York, N.Y.). 2018;**359**(6371):91-97

[192] Taur Y et al. The effects of intestinal tract bacterial diversity on mortality following allogeneic hematopoietic stem cell transplantation. Blood. 2014;**124**(7):1174-1182

[193] Viaud S et al. The intestinal microbiota modulates the anticancer immune effects of cyclophosphamide. Science. 2013;**342**(6161):971-976

[194] Routy B et al. The gut microbiota influences anticancer immunosurveillance and general health. Nature Reviews. Clinical Oncology. 2018;**15**(6):382-396

Chapter 4

Dendritic Cells and Their Roles in Anti-Tumour Immunity

Ee Shan Pang, Christophe Macri, Timothy Patton, Mariam Bafit and Meredith O'Keeffe

Abstract

Dendritic cells are rare cells found in blood and throughout all organs of the body as resident or migrating cell populations. Dendritic cells sense danger signals of pathogens and host cell stress through pattern receptors expressed on the cell surface and within organelles of the cell. Ligation of these receptors leads to activation and production of many different chemokines, cytokines and interferons. Key to the function of dendritic cells is their potent capacity to present antigen and activate naïve T cells. These qualities, potent antigen presentation and cytokine production together allow the dendritic cells to be at the forefront of danger responses, linking innate and adaptive immunity. Research over the last 20 years has clarified a role of dendritic cells in anti-tumour responses, and their location within the tumour environment is clear, with both deleterious and beneficial correlations, depending on the subset and tumour type. Harnessing the qualities of dendritic cells to increase anti-tumour immunity is the ultimate goal, although this will require extensive knowledge of different dendritic cell subsets and their regulation through immune checkpoints.

Keywords: dendritic cells, pattern recognition receptors, immune checkpoints, tumour vaccines, plasmacytoid dendritic cell, conventional dendritic cell

1. Introduction to dendritic cells

Dendritic cells (DCs) are professional antigen presenting cells (APCs), the only cells capable of specifically activating naïve T cells and are key orchestrators of an immune response. They are a rare, heterogeneous population of haematopoietic cells that are equipped to capture, process and present antigen (Ag) to the adaptive immune system.

In a non-inflamed or steady state setting, DCs constantly sample the local environment for Ags and have the potential to induce peripheral tolerance via T cell anergy or deletion [1]. DCs recognise danger via pattern recognition receptors (PRR) on their cell surface, the cytoplasm and within cellular organelles [2]. Ligation of PRRs by pathogen associated molecular patterns (PAMPs) or damage associated molecular patterns (DAMPs), activates DC and licences DC to upregulate co-stimulatory marker expression such as CD86 and CD80 on their cell surface and initiate immunogenic T cell priming.

IntechOpen

DCs situated in non-lymphoid tissues, also known as migratory DCs, constantly migrate to draining lymph nodes (LNs), maturing during this process, to present Ag to naïve T cells. Resident DCs in lymphoid organs are immature and maintain tolerance during steady state, but can stimulate naïve T cells when activated *in situ*. The DC maturation process not only involves morphological changes into their characteristic stellate shape with dendritic cytoplasmic processes and increased expression of MHC and co-stimulatory markers, but their Ag acquisition and sampling capabilities are initially upregulated and then rapidly shut down while MHCII expression on the cell's surface is increased due to the simultaneous up- and down-regulation of MHCII synthesis and turnover events respectively [3]. This allows mature DCs to present a snapshot of the Ag profile in its local environment prior to migration and/or activation. Furthermore, activated DCs produce a combination of cytokines that modulate an immune response that is specific to the initial danger signals.

In humans, the majority of DC characterisation studies are of DCs isolated from the blood due to the rarity of the cell type and limited access to human tissue samples, although more investigations on non-lymphoid DCs in the skin, lung and liver have recently emerged [4–7]. DCs in the blood comprise ~1% of total peripheral blood mononuclear cells (PBMCs) and are traditionally identified by the high expression of MHCII (HLA-DR) and the lack of lineage markers CD3, CD14, CD15, CD19, CD20 and CD56, although the latter marker has recently been shown to be expressed on gut and other non-lymphoid DCs [6].

Human blood DCs can be divided into conventional DCs (cDCs) and plasmacytoid DCs (pDCs), which are HLA-DR^{hi}CD11c^{+}123^{-} and HLA-DR^{hi}CD11c^{-}123^{+} respectively. Human blood cDCs are further categorised into cDC1 and cDC2 subsets. Additionally, there are monocyte-derived DCs that originate separately from cDCs and pDC precursors. The recent use of whole population and single cell sequencing techniques has been instrumental in elucidating transcription factors and surface markers that are unique to each DC subset, which has helped identify

	DC subsets		
	cDC1	**cDC2**	**pDC**
Surface phenotype	CD11c^{+}HLA-DR^{+} CD123^{-}CLEC9A^{+} XCR1^{+}Necl2^{+} CD141^{+} CD11b^{-}CD172α^{-}	CD11c^{+}HLA-DR^{+}CD123^{-} CD1c^{+}CD11b^{+}CD172α^{+} CLEC10A^{+} with further subdivision based on CD5^{hi}CD32B^{+}CD163^{-}CD36^{-} or CD5^{lo}CD32B^{-}CD163^{+}CD36^{+}	CD11c^{-}HLA-DR^{+} CD123^{+}CD303^{+} CD304^{+}CD45RA^{+} CD2$^{+/-}$
Transcription factors	*BATF3*, *IRF8*	*IRF4*, *IRF8*	*TCF4*, *SPIB*, *ZEB2*, *IRF4*, *IRF8*, *IRF7*
PRR expression	TLR3, 8	TLR2, cytosolic RNA sensors (RIG-I, MDA-5), STING	TLR7, 9, STING
Ag presentation	Cross-presentation of cellular Ag	Cross-presentation of soluble Ag	CD4^{+} and CD8^{+} T cell priming*
Roles in immunity	Potent producer of Type III IFN (after TLR3 stimulation), CTL priming, Th1 response	Th1, Th17 response	Potent producers of Type I and III IFN and mediating anti-viral immunity

**Previous Ag presentation abilities by pDCs are now suggested to be contributed by contaminating AXL^{+}Siglec6^{+} (AS) DCs.*

Table 1.
Key features of human DC subsets.

relationships between DC subsets across species and tissues as well as corroborate DC functional analyses [6–9], summarised in **Table 1**.

2. Conventional dendritic cells 1 (cDC1)

cDC1s constitute ~0.03% of PBMCs and are found in the blood, tonsil, spleen and non-lymphoid tissues such as the skin. They were classically defined by the high expression of CD141 (blood DC antigen 3 (BDCA3) or thrombomodulin) [10]. However, CD141 is not a completely specific marker for cDC1 as it is also expressed on endothelial cells, monocytes and other DC subsets [8]. Using phenotypic, transcriptional and functional assays, these $CD141^+$ DCs have been further characterised as $CD11c^+HLA\text{-}DR^+CD11b^-CD172a^-$ $CLEC9a^+XCR1^+Necl2^+$ cells that lack monocytic markers CD14 and CD16 [4, 11] identifying them as human cDC1 [12–16].

The dependence of $CD141^+$ DCs on Flt3 ligand (FL), an important DC developmental factor, has been demonstrated *in vitro* and *in vivo* [11, 17–19] and transcription factor *BATF3* is required *in vitro* but not *in vivo* [15]. Another cDC1-defining transcription factor, *IRF8*, is also highly expressed in human cDC1, although patients harbouring mutations in *IRF8* did not exhibit cDC1 deficiencies, suggesting the involvement of other transcription factors as well [6, 20]. Furthermore, genome wide expression profiling and microarray analyses have revealed transcriptional profile clustering between $CD141^+$ DCs in blood and non-lymphoid tissues, as well as between human blood $CD141^+$ DCs and murine $CD8a^+$ and migratory $CD103^+$ DCs [4, 21], firmly establishing $CD141^+$ cDC as cDC1.

PRRs expressed by human cDC1s are predominantly Toll-like receptor (TLR) 3, located in endosomes and which recognises double-stranded RNA and TLR8, also located in endosomes and which recognises bacterial ssRNA and mammalian mitochondrial RNA [10, 22]. In response to TLR3 signals [23] and also HCV *in vivo* [23, 24], the cDC1 produce large amounts of type III interferon (IFN), also known as IFN-lambda (λ).

The cDC1s are superior to other DC subsets in their ability to present ex*ogenous* Ag on MHCI, a process known as cross-presentation [2] and the activation of cytotoxic $CD8^+$ T cells, crucial for anti-tumour responses. In particular, they have a specialised ability to cross-present Ags from dead or necrotic cells to $CD8^+$ T cells, enhanced by Clec9a on cDC1 binding to actin filaments exposed on dead and dying cells [25]. The cDC1 are superior at inducing Th1 differentiation of CD4 helper T cells [11, 16].

3. Conventional dendritic cells 2 (cDC2)

Human cDC2, traditionally known as $CD1c^+$ or $BDCA1^+$ DCs, constitute ~1% of PBMCs and can be identified by the expression of CD11c, CD11b, CD13, CD33, CD172a, HLA-DR and CD45RO [2, 10, 26]. The phenotypic similarities between these DCs and moDCs, as well as the expression of CD1c on B cells and other DC subsets, have made the precise segregation of this subset quite difficult. Although previous studies have used CD64 to exclude monocytes from bonafide $CD1c^+$ DCs in the blood, cDCs express low levels of this marker and cannot be definitively used to separate the cell populations [6, 7]. More recently, the use of single cell RNA sequencing techniques has identified additional surface phenotypic markers, such as *CLEC10A*, *FCGR2B*, *FCER1A*, to distinguish human cDC2 subsets [7, 8]. In particular, *CLEC10A* protein has been proposed as the cDC1 *CLEC9A*-equivalent marker for cDC2s in different species and tissues. However, different isoforms of Clec10A have been found in mice and should be carefully considered when using it across species [27]. Heterogeneity within the human cDC2 subset has been identified using CD5 or CD32B versus CD163 and CD36. The $CD5^{lo}$ or $CD163^{+}CD36^{+}$ 'cDC2' are transcriptionally more related to monocytes than the other cDC2 subset ($CD5^{hi}$ or $CD32B^{+}$) [8, 28]. Like cDC1, $CD1c^{+}$ cDC2s require FL, but also rely on transcription factors *IRF4* and *IRF8*, for development [20, 29].

The cDC2 DCs highly express TLR2 and also express a range of cytosolic viral RNA sensors such as RIG-I [30, 31]. Different proposed cDC2 subsets also seem to have different PRR expression patterns. For example, $CD5^{hi}$ cDC2 express high levels of TLR7 and 8 compared to $CD5^{lo}$ cDC2 and $CD32B^{+}$ cDC2 express higher levels of *TMEM173* (also known as STING) in comparison to $CD163^{+}$ $CD36^{+}$ cDC2 subset [8, 28].

Activated cDC2s can drive Th17 immune response and can also produce high levels of IL-12p70, potentially inducing Th1 differentiation [2, 29]. However, current data suggests Th17 versus Th1 driven responses may be independently driven by $CD5^{+}$ versus $CD5^{lo}$ cDC2 subsets, respectively [8, 28].

Human cDC2s are able to cross-present *soluble* Ag to naïve and memory $CD8^{+}$ T cells at comparable levels with cDC1s [32–35]. However, the mechanism of cross-presentation differs between both subsets [35] and cDC2 do not possess the potent ability to cross-present Ags from dead cells. Human cDC2 are also potent stimulators of $CD4^{+}$ T cells [8, 10, 16].

4. Plasmacytoid dendritic cells (pDC)

The pDCs constitute ~0.01–0.04% of PBMCs and commonly reside in secondary lymphoid organs localising in the follicular cortex, T cell nodules and around high endothelial venules [36, 37]. As their name suggests, pDCs are similar in morphology to that of plasma cells. Under light microscopy, pDCs are observed to be spherical in shape with a rounded nucleus, often predominant endoplasmic reticulum and present as clusters in T-cell rich regions of lymphoid tissue [36–38].

The pDCs, originally identified as 'natural interferon producing cells' (NIPC), are renowned for their ability to drive immense type I and type III IFN production via TLRs 7 and 9 [39–41]. This IFN production is essential to combat viral infection but pDC-derived IFN is also thought to contribute to disease in autoimmune diseases including systemic lupus erythematosus [42]. They are also thought to play a role in Th2 induction and asthma progression in humans [42]. Conversely, pDC have also been shown to play a major role in tolerance *in vivo*, through their production of IDO and TGF-beta [42].

pDCs are recognised as being $CD11c^{-/lo}CD45RA^{+}CD123^{+}CD303^{+}CD304^{+}HLA\text{-}DR^{+}$ and can express CD56 (reviewed in [2]). pDCs may also be identified by their transcription factors including; TCF4 (also known as E2-2), SPIB, ZEB2, IRF8, IRF7 and IRF4 [43–45]. Haploinsufficiency in the *TCF4* gene results in Pitts-Hopkins syndrome, which characteristically generates defective pDCs, illustrating a dependence of this factor for normal human pDC development [46].

The pDCs can be divided into 2 subsets based on CD2 expression [47]. Recent single cell transcriptomic profiling of blood DCs from healthy donors has revealed that $CD2^{+}$ 'pDC' also express AXL and SIGLEC6 (known as AS DCs). These AS DCs can stimulate $CD4^{+}$ and $CD8^{+}$ allogeneic T cell proliferation whereas the segregation of pDCs away from contaminating AS DCs demonstrated potent IFN-α production after TLR9 stimulation and a lack of T cell priming attributes [8]. Whether AS DCs and pDC are 2 distinct cell types or differentiation stages of one another is yet to be defined.

A rare and highly aggressive acute leukaemia known as Blastic Plasmacytoid Dendritic Cell Neoplasm (BPDCN) involves the malignancy of pDC precursors [48], driven, at least in part by the juxtaposition of the pDC-specific RUNX2 enhancer and the MYC promotor due to the chromosomal translocation (6;8) (p21;q24) [49]. The BPDCN can be reliably identified by immunohistochemical staining with TCF4 and CD123 antibodies [50]. BPDCNs most commonly present as skin lesions and may be accompanied by swelling of other organs such as the lymph nodes, bone marrow or spleen. Standard chemotherapy treatments for myeloid neoplasms often result in poor prognosis [51] although a toxin-conjugated anti-CD123 drug, tagraxofusp-erzs, has recently been approved as the first FDA-approved BPDCN-specific treatment [52].

5. Monocyte derived DCs

Monocyte derived DC (moDC) refers to DCs induced from monocytes with GM-CSF *in vitro*. These tissue culture systems originated in the early 1990s based on work showing varying combination of cytokines with GM-CSF could induce the acquisition of antigen presentation capacity in stem cells and $CD34^+$ blood precursors [53–56], and this was optimised with the addition of IL-4 [57]. These systems have been an immensely popular tool for more than two decades for *in vitro* research pertaining to conventional DC biology and immunological function. They have been particularly useful in human research due to the difficulties in obtaining large numbers of *ex vivo* primary human DC for research. However, the feasibility of these models has recently been questioned, detailed analyses of GM-CSF induced DC cultures reveal a heterogeneous population of macrophages and conventional DCs, with the $MHCII^{hi}$ cells the most DC-like [58–61].

It still remains unclear whether the moDC actually represent an *in vivo* equivalent cell subset. They potentially represent an *in vitro* equivalent of an inflammatory monocyte known as TNF/iNOS producing DCs (TipDCs), based on their surface phenotype [62], cytokine profile and a shared precursor [62]. Importantly, high intra-tumoral expression of CD40L, TNF-α and iNOS, key phenotypes of TipDCs, were strongly correlated with substantially higher long term disease free survival rates over 10 years in patients with colorectal cancer [63]. Therefore, moDCs may represent a useful and relevant *in vitro* model of inflammatory DCs.

5.1 MoDC and cancer vaccines

While the *ex vivo* induced moDC do not recapitulate *bona fide* DC subsets, the ease of isolation and culture has made the moDC a popular vaccine candidate in human clinical trials since the late 1990s. However, results from clinical trials using moDC in cancer immunotherapies for various cancer types have been modest at best [64, 65]. In a more recent phase II trial of patients with surgically resectable liver metastatic colon adenocarcinoma, vaccination of patients with autologous tumour lysate pulsed moDC conferred interim protection, demonstrating a 3-fold increase in the median disease free survival compared to the control arm of the study [66]. The continued refinement of moDC preparations and the choice of antigens, may see future improvements of DC cancer vaccines.

The ability to present Ag and activate the adaptive immune response makes DCs an attractive target to re-invigorate anti-cancer immunity. There are different types of DC vaccines, with the most common type involving the *ex vivo* maturation of autologous DCs. In this method, DCs are isolated from patient peripheral blood mononuclear cells (PBMCs) obtained via leukapheresis, incubated with maturation stimuli and tumour Ags, and vaccinated back into the patient. Because this method requires a large number of DCs, and naturally circulating blood DCs are rare, the majority of clinical trials have previously used moDCs for this type of DC vaccine and have been extensively characterised [67, 68].

Thus far, a wide variety of moDC vaccine strategies have been trialled [68]. moDCs have been differentiated and matured using monocyte conditioned medium with various supplements of cytokines (TNF-α, GM-CSF, IL-4, IFN-α), TLR agonists (LPS) and other factors such as prostaglandin E2 [67–69]. There is also variety in the type of Ags loaded into DCs such as peptides from tumour-associated Ags (TAA), TAA-encoding mRNA and whole tumour lysates [67]. More recently, the electroporation of synthetic mRNA encoding DC-maturation factors such as CD40 ligand, constitutively active TLR4 and CD70 together with fusion proteins DC-LAMP and melanoma-associated Ags into autologous moDCs (TriMixDC-MEL) have proven safe and immunogenic in phase 1 clinical trials in metastatic melanoma [70]. However, the variation in the aforementioned vaccine factors as well as the route of DC administration (intranodal, i.v.) and lack of standardised method of moDC generation has shown variable efficacies of moDC vaccines in clinical outcomes.

6. DC vaccines

More recent clinical trials using naturally circulating blood DCs have turned to CliniMACS system by Miltenyi to isolate different DC subsets from patients (**Figure 1**). Two completed Phase I clinical trials have used CD1c$^+$ DCs (cDC2) loaded with TAA peptides in hormone refractory metastatic prostate cancer and metastatic melanoma and observed good safety and immunogenicity [71, 72]. Another completed Phase I trial using pDCs showed the induction of tumour-Ag specific CTL response as well as an IFN signature [33]. On-going clinical trials, as summarised by Bol et al., are not only isolating single DC subsets for vaccination, but are also trying combination vaccines comprised of cDC2 and pDC subsets and using dual-activating maturation agonists such as single stranded RNA that stimulates TLR8 on cDC2 and TLR7 on pDCs (NCT-02993315, NCT-02574377, NCT-02692976) [67]. However, there are still many challenges in using naturally circulating blood DCs in tumour vaccinations. The methodology for isolation of sufficient CD141$^+$ cDC1 DCs, which comprise only 0.03% PBMCs, is still lacking and will be important to harness due to their superior ability to cross-present dead and necrotic Ag. Furthermore, although improved over the years, the duration of DCs spent *ex vivo* can drastically affect DC viability and functionality and the personalised nature of these vaccines can limit the quantity of patient access to these treatments.

Apart from the *ex vivo* maturation of autologous DCs, another strategy of DC vaccines has been receptor targeting (**Figure 1**). This involves the administration of a monoclonal Ab (mAb) specific for endocytic receptors on various DC subsets to deliver tumour Ags to DCs directly *in vivo* [73]. Tumour Ags are conjugated to these DC-targeting mAb either chemically, through genetic fusion, or attachment to nanoparticles and liposomes [74]. Importantly, the administration of adjuvant, such as TLR3 agonist poly I:C, in conjunction with Ag delivery, is necessary to induce immune priming instead of tolerance, as shown in mice [75–77]. Moreover, the targeting of cross-presenting DC subsets has been particularly attractive, due to their ability to activate CTLs. DEC-205, a C-type lectin that is highly expressed on cDC1 can cross-present Ag when targeted and induce tumour Ag NY-ESO-1-specific

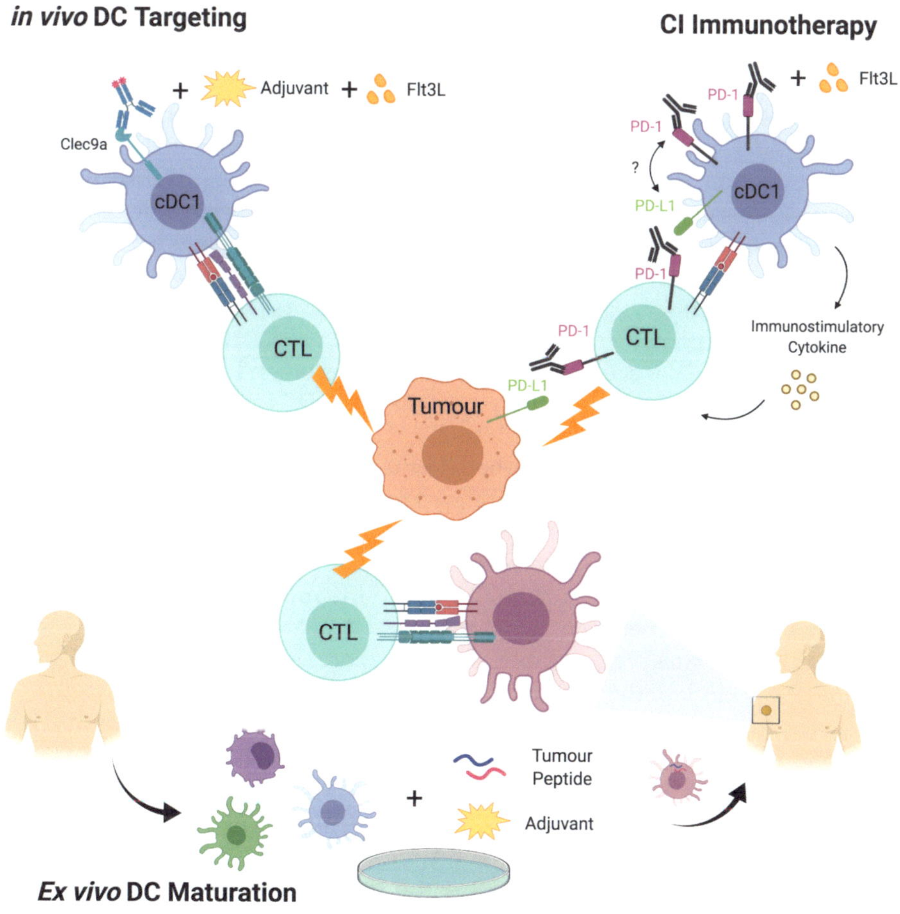

Figure 1.
Overview of potential roles of DC in cancer therapies. To improve current cancer treatments and the activation of tumour-specific CTL, DC may be directly targeted in vivo *(Section 6) or may themselves be the targets of checkpoint immunotherapies (Section 8).* Ex vivo *manipulation of DC (Section 6) may also be beneficial in some cancer patients.* In vivo *targeting strategies may also be combined with Flt3-L treatment to enhance DC numbers, and adjuvants targeting specific PRR to ensure the DC subset of interest are activated. Created with Biorender.com.*

cellular and humoral responses in patients with solid cancers [78, 79]. However, DEC-205 is also expressed on many other cell-types including CD1c$^+$ DCs, pDCs and monocytes which can affect targeting specificities and efficiencies [79–81]. In contrast, another C-type lectin, Clec9a (also known as DNGR-1), is specifically expressed on cDC1 and strategies targeting this molecule have demonstrated highly immunogenic responses without adjuvant in non-human primates, and also superior Ag-specific cross-presentation when targeted *in vitro* and *in vivo* [79, 81, 82]. Based on these pre-clinical studies, the progression of vaccines targeting Clec9a into clinical trials is much anticipated.

7. DC in the tumour microenvironment

The tumour microenvironment (TME) is a complex niche of tumour cells, stromal cells and tumour infiltrating myeloid and lymphoid immune cells. The dynamic nature of this niche varies with different types and stages of cancer, as well as between patients themselves. It has been established that the infiltration of CD8$^+$ cytotoxic T cells have been associated with better treatment outcomes with checkpoint blockade therapies in a number of cancer types including metastatic melanoma [83]. However, the phenotype and role of tumour-infiltrating DCs (TIDCs) are less clear, possibly due to the lack of consistent markers probing DCs within the TME and the lack of distinctions between monocyte and putative DC subsets [84].

Using immunohistochemistry staining, many studies have previously used CD1a and S100 proteins to identify TIDCs. The higher density of these cells within tumours correlated with better clinical outcomes in melanoma and head and neck cancers [84, 85]. However, discrepancies in this correlation were reported in colon, breast, gastric, nasopharyngeal, lung and ovarian cancers [84, 86–88]. One major factor that could explain these reported discrepancies is the markers used to identify DCs. CD1a and S100 are expressed at different levels on Langerhans cells (LCs), interdigitating DCs and moDCs, but not on cDCs or pDCs and the expression of these markers on epithelial-tropic DCs such as LCs could account for the strong correlations observed in only the epithelial cancers [84]. Furthermore, DC activation markers CD83 and DC-LAMP were used to identify mature DCs, though CD83 is not expressed in all DC subsets [7, 84, 89]. In breast adenocarcinoma patients, immature DCs were found to localise within the tumour whereas CD83/DC-LAMP$^+$ mature DCs localised in the peri-tumour edges [90]. Some studies have reported significant correlations between the intratumoral infiltration of mature DCs with better clinical outcomes. For example, a recent report showed that the recruitment of DC-LAMP^{hi} cells into the tumour stroma exhibited strong correlations with significantly higher overall and relapse-free survival in high-grade serous ovarian carcinoma [91]. However, this correlation has also been inconsistent in a number of different cancers [85, 90, 92–94].

More recently, with the establishment of The Cancer Genome Atlas (TCGA) program, scientists are able to compare DC-specific signatures with a publicly available molecular and clinical database of a vast array of cancers. In melanoma and breast cancer patients, DC-specific genes such as *BATF3*, *IRF8*, *CLEC9A* and *FLT3* were associated with higher CTL scores and better overall survival [95–97]. They also exhibited positive correlations with chemokines *CXCL9*, *10* and *11* and chemokine receptor *CCR7* expression [95, 96]. Furthermore, Broz et al. [98] observed strong associations between cDC1-derived genes within the tumour and better overall survival in breast cancer, head-neck squamous cell carcinoma and lung adenocarcinoma. This corroborates mouse tumour models showing that migratory cDC1 subsets are required for cross-presenting tumour Ag in tumour-draining lymph nodes and priming of cytotoxic CD8$^+$ T cells [97, 99].

Whilst the recent data above points towards a benefit of the infiltration of conventional DC into tumour sites, the correlation between tumour infiltrating pDCs and poor survival prognosis is clear. This has been described in breast, head and neck, ovarian and lung cancers [100–103] where it is thought that pDC-induced tolerance and impaired IFN-α production contributes to a suppressive, non-immunogenic TME. Indeed mouse studies point to a role of TGF-β in the tumour environment in preventing an activatory phenotype of pDC and favouring a tolerising, IDO producing phenotype [104].

Further factors within the TME that have been illustrated to correlate with DC infiltration or function include for example, vascular endothelial growth factor (VEGF), a tumour angiogenic factor, inversely correlated with DC density and overall survival in gastric adenocarcinoma tissues [87, 105]. High serum VEGF levels were also associated with low blood cDC1 and cDC2 numbers in colorectal and non-small cell lung cancers and treatment of VEGF decoy receptor, VEGF-Trap, increased the proportion of mature DCs, but not overall numbers or DC priming function in various solid cancer patients [106–108]. Direct evidence of VEGF-induced DC inhibition was also reported in DCs differentiated from $CD34^+$ precursors and moDCs [105, 106, 109]. Other cytokines such as IL-6, IL-10 and TGFβ have also demonstrated DC-inhibitory effects in the TME [104, 110–114].

In metastatic melanoma patients, higher active β-catenin signalling within the tumour was associated with low cDC1 signatures and T cell signatures [115]. Furthermore, the expression of fatty acid synthase was inversely correlated with $CD11c^+$ DC signatures in ovarian, prostate and bladder cancers [116].

8. DC and immune checkpoint inhibitors

Chemotherapy and radiotherapy have remained the core pillars of cancer treatments. However, the combination of these traditional therapies with immunotherapies targeting immune checkpoint receptors has greatly enhanced patient clinical outcomes, especially in patients with immunogenic cancers, summarised in **Table 2**.

Immune checkpoints consist of a family of co-stimulatory and co-inhibitory receptors expressed by T cells that modulate their immune responses. Signalling from these receptors depends on their interaction with specific ligands present at the surface of various immune and non-immune cells. These regulatory pathways are a major cause of immune suppression during cancer due the high levels of co-inhibitory ligands being expressed in the tumour microenvironment, resulting in T cell immunosuppression. Monoclonal antibodies (mAb) blocking programmed cell death 1 (PD-1) and cytotoxic T-lymphocyte-associated protein 4 (CTLA4), two co-inhibitory immune checkpoint receptors have become routine treatment against many malignancies and more therapeutic molecules against members of the immune checkpoint family are being trialled. Here we review the role of DC in the response to immune checkpoint therapies.

8.1 DC and PD-1

PD-1 is expressed by activated T cells and interacts with two ligands, PD-L1 (B7-H1/CD274) and PD-L2 (B7-DC/CD273). PD-1 engagement results in downregulation of T cell proliferation and function [117]. This inhibitory pathway is harnessed by tumour cells to escape attack by T cells through expression of PD-L1 on their cell surface. Anti-PD-1/PD-L1 therapies have shown considerable effects on patients with high PD-L1-expressing tumours, boosting the effector functions of tumour-associated $CD8^+$ T cells inducing tumour regression. To date, two anti-PD-1 mAb (Pembrolizumab, Nivolumab) and three anti-PD-L1 mAb (Atezolizumab, Durvalumab, Avelumab) have been approved for the treatment of cancers including advanced melanoma, non-small-cell lung cancer, head and neck squamous cell carcinoma, Hodgkin lymphoma and renal carcinoma [118].

The ligands for PD-1 are abundant on DC. PD-L1 expression is on pDC and cDC subsets and upregulated in response to inflammatory stimuli and following exposure to platinum-based chemotherapy drugs [84, 119]. Furthermore, PD-L1 is also highly expressed on DC that infiltrate tumours as exemplified by the high PD-L1 expression measured on both pDC and multiple myeloma cells isolated from the bone-marrow of multiple myeloma patients [120]. PD-L2 is detectable at low

Checkpoint inhibitor (CI)	CI cell expression	Ligand	Ligand cell expression	Anti-CI mAb clinical name	Clinical outcome
PD-1	T, B, NK cells, DC	PD-L1/2	PD-L1: DC, monocytes, Treg, cells, tumour; PD-L2: Activated cDC, moDCs	Pembrolizumab, Nivolumab	Approved for metastatic melanoma, renal cell carcinoma, squamous-cell carcinoma of head and neck, Hodgkin's lymphoma, metastatic colorectal, non-small cell lung, Merkel cell and ovarian cancers Improved clinical outcomes in combination with peptide/vector vaccines for advanced solid cancers, metastatic melanoma and HPV-16-related cancers
CTLA4	T cells, activated moDCs	CD80/86 (B7.1/2)	APC	Ipilimumab, Tremelimumab	Approved for metastatic melanoma, renal cell carcinoma and colorectal cancer treatments Mixed results in combination with peptide and moDC vaccines
TIM-3	T, B cells, cDC, myeloid cells	Galectin-9, CEACAM-1, HMGB1, phosphatidylserine	Tumour	— (pre-clinical)	—
LAG-3	Activated T, NK cells, pDCs	MHCII	APC	LAG-3Ig fusion protein	Elevated clinical activity Phase I/II trial in combination with paclitaxel for metastatic breast carcinoma
ICOS	Treg cells, activated T cells	ICOS-L	APC (especially activated pDCs)	MEDI-570	Phase I Trial for T cell lymphoma (National Cancer Institute Clinical Trial NCT02520791)

Table 2.
List of checkpoint inhibitors, their ligands, cell expression and clinical associations.

levels on cDC only after activation and is highly expressed by moDC [121]. Whether PD-L2 is also expressed by DC in different TMEs and the effect of anti-PD-L2 therapies is yet to be defined.

cDC1 play a critical role in the efficacy of anti-PD-1/PD-L1 mAb therapies. Single cell mass spectrometry analyses of PBMC from patients with advanced melanoma, before and after anti-PD-1 therapy revealed that CD141 and CD11c, both expressed by cDC1 are strong predictive biomarkers of clinical response to anti-PD-1 treatments [122]. This is consistent with several mouse studies reporting that cDC1-deficient mice do not respond to immune checkpoint blockade using anti-PD-L1 or a combination of anti-PD-1 anti-CTLA4 mAb [123, 124]. Furthermore, mice that possess cDC1 defective in antigen cross-presentation fail to establish CTL responses and do not respond to anti-PD-1 blockade [125].

The success of anti-PD-1 therapy also depends on a cross-talk between cDC1 and T cells in the TME. In mouse models anti-PD-1 treatment induces IL-12 production by tumour-infiltrating cDC1 [124, 126] which amplifies T cell effector functions. In melanoma patients, the clinical electroporation of an IL-12 plasmid in the tumour lesions enhances the CTL gene signature, thus validating the role of this cytokine in supporting CTL responses [126], **Figure 1**.

In addition to its ligands, expression of the PD-1 receptor on DC has been reported during cancer. In hepatocellular carcinoma patients, detectable levels of PD-1 were reported on peripheral blood cDC1, cDC2 and pDC whereas PD-1 was only present on cDC1 in healthy donors. This was confirmed with microscopy analyses of cancerous liver tissues showing co-expression of PD-1 and the DC marker CD11c [127]. In line with this data, co-expression of PD-1 and PD-L1 was detected on CD11c$^+$ DC isolated from the tumours of non-small cell lung cancer patients [128]. However, in this case, PD-1 was absent from DC isolated from the PBMC of either cancer patients or healthy donors, suggesting that PD-1 is upregulated locally on DC in response to the immunosuppressive tumour environment [128].

Mouse studies support an inhibitory role of PD-1 on DC [127]. This finding however contrasts with a recent study revealing that PD-1 can establish *cis*-interactions with both PD-L1 and PD-L2 at the cell membrane. PD-L1/PD-1 *cis*-interaction disrupts PD-L1 binding to PD-1 on T cells, thus resulting in increased T cell activities. However, whether this mechanism exists in DC in the setting of cancer remains unknown [128]. Similarly, several reports have shown that PD-L1 can interact in *cis* with the immune checkpoint ligand CD80/B7.1 [129–131] and this occurs on several types of APC, including cDC1 and cDC2 [131]. The PD-L1/CD80 *cis*-interaction limits the binding of PD-L1 to PD-1 on T cells and ultimately promotes T cell immune responses [131]. Altogether, these data show that, while *trans*-interactions between PD-L1 and PD-1 at the interface of DC and T cells promote T cell immune suppression, *cis*-interactions between PD-L1 and other molecules on DC show opposite effects and could potentially promote cancer immunity.

Combining anti-PD-1/PD-L1 therapy with DC-based vaccines, or vaccines that target DC *in situ*, or include a DC growth factor, is a logical strategy to increase responses to checkpoint blockade in cancer patients. Several studies in mice have reported that such combination leads to higher protection by boosting the antigen-specific T cell immune response induced by different type of vaccines [18, 123, 132–134]. Several vaccines containing peptides or viral vectors, in combination with anti-PD-1 mAb Pembolizumab or Nivolumab, have shown encouraging results in early clinical trial with patients with advanced solid cancers, melanoma and Human Papillomavirus 16-Related Cancer [135–138].

8.2 DC and CTLA4

The co-inhibitory immune checkpoint CTLA4 (CD152) is constitutively expressed by regulatory T cells (Treg) and by effector T cells upon activation. CTLA4 is highly homologous to the co-stimulatory receptor CD28 and binds the same ligands CD80 and CD86 (B7.2), however with a much higher affinity. As such, CTLA4 outcompetes CD28 for ligand binding and reduces CD28-mediated co-stimulation of T cell functions. CTLA4 blockade promotes anti-tumour immunity by increasing the activation of effector T cells and by depleting Treg in the TME. The CTLA4 blocking mAb Ipilimumab and Tremelimumab have been approved for the treatment of metastatic melanoma, renal cell carcinoma and colorectal cancer [118].

CTLA4 on T cells directly alters DC functions by removing the CTLA4 ligands (CD80/86) from their cell surfaces. When human moDC are co-cultured with CTLA4^{+} T cells, CD80/86 levels on DC decrease rapidly in a CTLA4-dependent manner. This mechanism, named trans-endocytosis, involves the physical capture of CTLA4 ligands by the receptor and their degradation. This process is upregulated by TCR engagement [139, 140]. Mouse *in vivo* studies show that trans-endocytosis is primarily carried out by regulatory T cells and impacts the migratory cDC1 and cDC2 [141]. In addition, CTLA4 interaction with CD80/CD86 on DC induces immunosuppression through reverse signalling. MoDC stimulated with soluble CTLA4 or agonistic anti-CD80/86 Ab produced indoleamine 2,3-dioxygenase (IDO), which is able to inhibit allogenic T cell activation [142]. IDO is expressed by human pDC [143], hence similar immunosuppressive pathways are likely to be induced downstream of CD80/86 in this subset, as reported in mouse pDC [144].

Besides their regulation through CTLA4-CD80/86 interaction, moDC also express the CTLA4 molecule upon activation by TLR stimuli. Treatment of these cells with an agonistic anti-CTLA4 Ab induced increased production of IL-10, reduced expression of IL-8 and IL-12 and decreased T cell stimulation capacity [145]. MoDC are also able to secrete CTLA4 in extracellular microvesicles. Microvesicular CTLA4 has been shown to downregulate CD80 and CD86 on moDC [146].

Combinatorial approaches of anti-CTLA4 mAb with cancer vaccines have been tested in clinics and have yielded mixed results. In melanoma patients, peptide vaccines, in combination with anti-CTLA4 Ipilimumab did not show better clinical outcomes compared to Ipilimumab alone [127, 147, 148]. However, other strategies using DC vaccines have provided promising results. For instance, the co-administration to melanoma patients of autologous moDC that have been pulsed with tumour peptide, together with Tremelimumab, resulted in objective and durable tumour responses [149]. Furthermore, a phase II study using Ipilimumab and moDC electroporated with synthetic mRNA (TriMixDC-MEL) has been tested in advanced melanoma patients and has shown an encouraging rate of highly durable tumour response [150].

8.3 DC and TIM-3

T cell immunoglobulin mucin-3 (TIM-3) is a co-inhibitory immune checkpoint receptor expressed by all T cell populations as well as B cells and a large variety of myeloid cells. Four TIM-3 ligands have been identified, including Galectin-9, CEACAM-1, HMGB1 and phosphatidylserine. Engagement of TIM-3 on tumour-infiltrating T cells induces exhaustion and suppresses tumour immunity. Preclinical studies have reported high therapeutic activities of blocking anti-TIM-3 antibodies against various types of malignancies and clinical trials with TIM-3 inhibitors are currently underway [128].

High TIM-3 expression has been reported on cDC1 and cDC2 from peripheral blood [151–153] and on tumour-associated cDC1 and cDC2 from mammary tumour biopsies [152]. Mouse models indicated that blocking TIM-3 on cDC1 leads to an increase in the T cell chemoattractant CXCL9. Moreover, cDC1 expressing TIM-3 correlated with CXCL9 expression in human breast cancer biopsies and was positively associated with $CD8^+$ T cell infiltration. These data suggest that TIM-3 blocking in these cancers could potentially enhance $CD8^+$ T cell recruitment to the TME [152].

8.4 DC and LAG-3

Lymphocyte activation gene-3 (LAG-3) is a co-inhibitory immune checkpoint receptor expressed on activated T cells and NK cells that recognise MHCII molecules on APCs as a ligand. LAG3 negatively regulates T cell activation and is frequently co-expressed with PD-1 on exhausted T cells in the TME. Several LAG-3-targeting cancer immunotherapies are currently in different phases of clinical development [154].

The interaction between MHCII and LAG-3 not only has effects in T cells, but also induces reverse signalling in DCs that is stimulatory. This was shown using the soluble LAG-3-Ig fusion protein that activates moDC, as indicated by the upregulation of co-stimulatory molecules, the production of several pro-inflammatory cytokines and chemokines and increased allogenic T cell activation. However, Ab-mediated MHCII ligation does not activate moDC, thus showing that the MHCII: LAG-3 interaction is required in this process [155–157]. Soluble LAG-3-Ig fusion protein in combination with the chemotherapy drug Paclitaxel has demonstrated elevated clinical activity in metastatic breast carcinoma during a phase I/II trial. This treatment also strongly stimulated the patients' APC, as evidenced by the increase in the number and activation of monocytes, pDC and cDCs [158].

Notably, LAG-3 itself has been found expressed by DC, specifically by a subpopulation of circulating pDC in healthy donors. $LAG\text{-}3^+$ pDC are also found in the tumour lesions and in the tumour-draining lymph nodes of melanoma patients and are thought to contribute to the immunosuppressive environment. Engagement of LAG-3 on pDC provides an activating signal, independent of TLR signalling, inducing low IFN-α and high IL-6 expression [159]. Hence, LAG-3-specific mAb in cancer immunotherapies may enhance the anti-tumour immune response by inhibiting LAG-3 signalling in both T cells and DC.

8.5 DC and ICOS

Inducible T cell costimulatory (ICOS) belongs to the co-stimulatory immune checkpoint receptor family and similarly to CD28, enhances the proliferation and effector functions of T cells. ICOS is expressed on activated T cells and constitutively on a subpopulation of Treg [160] while ICOS-L is present at the surface of APC. High ICOS expression on T cells has been particularly observed during anti-CTLA4 therapies and the co-administration of agonistic ICOS-specific mAb further improves the efficacy to CTLA4 blockade [161].

pDC are able to induce immunosuppression though ICOS stimulation. ICOS-L is strongly upregulated by human blood pDC, but not $CD11c^+$ cDC, in response to TLR stimuli or IL-3 [162]. Co-cultures of pDC with allogenic T cells induced IL-10 expression through a mechanism mediated by ICOS-L-ICOS interaction [162] and similar observations were reported with pDC isolated from ovarian carcinoma [163]. Furthermore, pDC are able to induce Treg proliferation though ICOS stimulation [160] and this mechanism likely explains the dramatic accumulation of $ICOS^+$ Treg in ovarian, breast, liver and gastric tumour tissues, in close proximity with ICOS-L^+ pDC [101, 164–166].

9. Summary

DCs are rare, heterogeneous cells with clear roles in anti-tumour immunity. As summarised in **Figure 1**, understanding how best to activate DC to gain optimal anti-tumour adaptive immune responses will likely involve careful optimisation of adjuvants, checkpoint immunotherapies and DC targeting strategies. Emerging studies will likely examine checkpoint receptors and their ligands on DC, lymphocytes and other cells in tumour environments, in order to design targeted therapies for optimal antigen presentation, DC activation and anti-tumour response.

Author details

Ee Shan Pang[1], Christophe Macri[2], Timothy Patton[1], Mariam Bafit[1] and Meredith O'Keeffe[1]*

1 Infection and Immunity Program, Monash Biomedicine Discovery Institute and Department of Biochemistry and Molecular Biology, Monash University, Clayton, Victoria, Australia

2 Department of Biochemistry and Molecular Biology, Bio21 Institute, The University of Melbourne, Parkville, VIC, Australia

*Address all correspondence to: meredith.okeeffe@monash.edu

IntechOpen

© 2020 The Author(s). Licensee IntechOpen. This chapter is distributed under the terms of the Creative Commons Attribution License (http://creativecommons.org/licenses/by/3.0), which permits unrestricted use, distribution, and reproduction in any medium, provided the original work is properly cited. CC BY

References

[1] Banchereau J, Steinman RM. Dendritic cells and the control of immunity. Nature. 1998;**392**:245-252. DOI: 10.1038/32588

[2] Macri C, Pang ES, Patton T, O'Keeffe M. Dendritic cell subsets. Seminars in Cell & Developmental Biology. 2018;**84**:11-21. DOI: 10.1016/j.semcdb.2017.12.009

[3] Villadangos JA, Schnorrer P, Wilson NS. Control of MHC class II antigen presentation in dendritic cells: A balance between creative and destructive forces. Immunological Reviews. 2005;**207**:191-205. DOI: 10.1111/j.0105-2896.2005.00317.x

[4] Haniffa M, Shin A, Bigley V, McGovern N, Teo P, See P, et al. Human tissues contain CD141hi cross-presenting dendritic cells with functional homology to mouse CD103+ nonlymphoid dendritic cells. Immunity. 2012;**37**:60-73. DOI: 10.1016/j.immuni.2012.04.012

[5] Baharom F, Thomas S, Rankin G, Lepzien R, Pourazar J, Behndig AF, et al. Dendritic cells and monocytes with distinct inflammatory responses reside in lung mucosa of healthy humans. The Journal of Immunology. 2016;**196**:4498. DOI: 10.4049/jimmunol.1600071

[6] Guilliams M, Dutertre C-A, Scott CL, McGovern N, Sichien D, Chakarov S, et al. Unsupervised high-dimensional analysis aligns dendritic cells across tissues and species. Immunity. 2016;**45**:669-684. DOI: 10.1016/j.immuni.2016.08.015

[7] Heidkamp GF, Sander J, Lehmann CHK, Heger L, Eissing N, Baranska A, et al. Human lymphoid organ dendritic cell identity is predominantly dictated by ontogeny, not tissue microenvironment. Science Immunology. 2016;**1**:eaai7677. DOI: 10.1126/sciimmunol.aai7677

[8] Villani A-C, Satija R, Reynolds G, Sarkizova S, Shekhar K, Fletcher J, et al. Single-cell RNA-seq reveals new types of human blood dendritic cells, monocytes, and progenitors. Science. 2017;**356**:eaah4573. DOI: 10.1126/science.aah4573

[9] See P, Dutertre C-A, Chen J, Günther P, McGovern N, Irac SE, et al. Mapping the human DC lineage through the integration of high-dimensional techniques. Science. 2017;**356**:eaag3009. DOI: 10.1126/science.aag3009

[10] O'Keeffe M, Mok WH, Radford KJ. Human dendritic cell subsets and function in health and disease. Cellular and Molecular Life Sciences. 2015;**72**:4309-4325. DOI: 10.1007/s00018-015-2005-0

[11] Poulin LF, Salio M, Griessinger E, Anjos-Afonso F, Craciun L, Chen J-L, et al. Characterization of human DNGR-1+ BDCA3+ leukocytes as putative equivalents of mouse CD8α+ dendritic cells. The Journal of Experimental Medicine. 2010;**207**:1261. DOI: 10.1084/jem.20092618

[12] Caminschi I, Proietto AI, Ahmet F, Kitsoulis S, Shin Teh J, Lo JCY, et al. The dendritic cell subtype-restricted C-type lectin Clec9A is a target for vaccine enhancement. Blood. 2008;**112**:3264. DOI: 10.1182/blood-2008-05-155176

[13] Huysamen C, Willment JA, Dennehy KM, Brown GD. CLEC9A is a novel activation C-type Lectin-like receptor expressed on BDCA3+ dendritic cells and a subset of monocytes. Journal of Biological Chemistry. 2008;**283**:16693-16701. DOI: 10.1074/jbc.M709923200

[14] Sancho D, Mourão-Sá D, Joffre OP, Schulz O, Rogers NC, Pennington DJ, et al. Tumor therapy in mice via antigen targeting to a novel, DC-restricted C-type lectin. The Journal of Clinical Investigation. 2008;**118**:2098-2110. DOI: 10.1172/JCI34584

[15] Poulin LF, Reyal Y, Uronen-Hansson H, Schraml BU, Sancho D, Murphy KM, et al. DNGR-1 is a specific and universal marker of mouse and human Batf3-dependent dendritic cells in lymphoid and nonlymphoid tissues. Blood. 2012;**119**:6052. DOI: 10.1182/blood-2012-01-406967

[16] Jongbloed SL, Kassianos AJ, McDonald KJ, Clark GJ, Ju X, Angel CE, et al. Human CD141+ (BDCA-3)+ dendritic cells (DCs) represent a unique myeloid DC subset that cross-presents necrotic cell antigens. The Journal of Experimental Medicine. 2010;**207**:1247. DOI: 10.1084/jem.20092140

[17] Proietto AI, Mittag D, Roberts AW, Sprigg N, Wu L. The equivalents of human blood and spleen dendritic cell subtypes can be generated in vitro from human CD34+ stem cells in the presence of fms-like tyrosine kinase 3 ligand and thrombopoietin. Cellular and molecular immunology. 2012;**9**:446. DOI: 10.1038/cmi.2012.48

[18] Ding Y, Wilkinson A, Idris A, Fancke B, O'Keeffe M, Khalil D, et al. FLT3-ligand treatment of humanized mice results in the generation of large numbers of CD141+ and CD1c+ dendritic cells In vivo. The Journal of Immunology. 2014;**192**:1982. DOI: 10.4049/jimmunol.1302391

[19] Galibert L, Diemer GS, Liu Z, Johnson RS, Smith JL, Walzer T, et al. Nectin-like protein 2 defines a subset of T-cell zone dendritic cells and is a ligand for class-I-restricted T-cell-associated molecule. Journal of Biological Chemistry. 2005;**280**:21955-21964. DOI: 10.1074/jbc.M502095200

[20] Hambleton S, Salem S, Bustamante J, Bigley V, Boisson-Dupuis S, Azevedo J, et al. IRF8 mutations and human dendritic-cell immunodeficiency. New England Journal of Medicine. 2011;**365**:127-138. DOI: 10.1056/NEJMoa1100066

[21] Robbins SH, Walzer T, Dembélé D, Thibault C, Defays A, Bessou G, et al. Novel insights into the relationships between dendritic cell subsets in human and mouse revealed by genome-wide expression profiling. Genome Biology. 2008;**9**:R17. DOI: 10.1186/gb-2008-9-1-r17

[22] Krüger A, Oldenburg M, Chebrolu C, Beisser D, Kolter J, Sigmund AM, et al. Human TLR8 senses UR/URR motifs in bacterial and mitochondrial RNA. EMBO Reports. 2015;**16**:1656-1663. DOI: 10.15252/embr.201540861

[23] Lauterbach H, Bathke B, Gilles S, Traidl-Hoffmann C, Luber CA, Fejer G, et al. Mouse CD8α+ DCs and human BDCA3+ DCs are major producers of IFN-λ in response to poly IC. The Journal of Experimental Medicine. 2010;**207**:2703. DOI: 10.1084/jem.20092720

[24] Yoshio S, Kanto T, Kuroda S, Matsubara T, Higashitani K, Kakita N, et al. Human blood dendritic cell antigen 3 (BDCA3)+ dendritic cells are a potent producer of interferon-λ in response to hepatitis C virus. Hepatology. 2013;**57**:1705-1715. DOI: 10.1002/hep.26182

[25] Zhang JG, Czabotar PE, Policheni AN, et al. The dendritic cell receptor Clec9A binds damaged cells via exposed actin filaments. Immunity. 2012;**36**(4):646-657. DOI: 10.1016/j.immuni.2012.03.009

[26] Collin M, Ginhoux F. Human dendritic cells. Seminars in Cell & Developmental Biology. 2019;**86**:1-2. DOI: 10.1016/j.semcdb.2018.04.015

[27] Heger L, Balk S, Lühr JJ, et al. CLEC10A is a specific marker for human CD1c+ dendritic cells and enhances their toll-like receptor 7/8-induced cytokine secretion. Frontiers in Immunology. 2018;**9**:744. DOI: 10.3389/fimmu.2018.00744 [Published: 27 April 2018]

[28] Yin X, Yu H, Jin X, Li J, Guo H, Shi Q, et al. Human blood CD1c+ dendritic cells encompass CD5high and CD5low subsets that differ significantly in phenotype, gene expression, and functions. The Journal of Immunology. 2017;**198**:1553. DOI: 10.4049/jimmunol.1600193

[29] Schlitzer A, McGovern N, Teo P, Zelante T, Atarashi K, Low D, et al. IRF4 transcription factor-dependent CD11b+ dendritic cells in human and mouse control mucosal IL-17 cytokine responses. Immunity. 2013;**38**:970-983. DOI: 10.1016/j.immuni.2013.04.011

[30] Luber CA, Cox J, Lauterbach H, Fancke B, Selbach M, Tschopp J, et al. Quantitative proteomics reveals subset-specific viral recognition in dendritic cells. Immunity. 2010;**32**:279-289. DOI: 10.1016/j.immuni.2010.01.013

[31] Worah K, Mathan TSM, Vu Manh TP, Keerthikumar S, Schreibelt G, Tel J, et al. Proteomics of human dendritic cell subsets reveals subset-specific surface markers and differential Inflammasome function. Cell Reports. 2016;**16**:2953-2966. DOI: 10.1016/j.celrep.2016.08.023

[32] Mittag D, Proietto AI, Loudovaris T, Mannering SI, Vremec D, Shortman K, et al. Human dendritic cell subsets from spleen and blood are similar in phenotype and function but modified by donor health status. The Journal of Immunology. 2011;**186**:6207. DOI: 10.4049/jimmunol.1002632

[33] Tel J, Aarntzen EHJG, Baba T, Schreibelt G, Schulte BM, Benitez-Ribas D, et al. Natural human plasmacytoid dendritic cells induce antigen-specific T-cell responses in melanoma patients. Cancer Research. 2013;**73**:1063. DOI: 10.1158/0008-5472.CAN-12-2583

[34] Chun I, Yu CB, Wang Y, Marches F, Helft J, Leboeuf M, et al. Human CD1c+ dendritic cells drive the differentiation of CD103+ CD8+ mucosal effector T cells via the cytokine TGF-β. Immunity. 2013;**38**:818-830. DOI: 10.1016/j.immuni.2013.03.004

[35] Chiang M-C, Tullett KM, Lee YS, Idris A, Ding Y, McDonald KJ, et al. Differential uptake and cross-presentation of soluble and necrotic cell antigen by human DC subsets. European Journal of Immunology. 2016;**46**:329-339. DOI: 10.1002/eji.201546023

[36] Colonna M, Trinchieri G, Liu Y-J. Plasmacytoid dendritic cells in immunity. Nature Immunology. 2004;**5**:1219

[37] Facchetti F, Vermi W, Mason D, Colonna M. The plasmacytoid monocyte/interferon producing cells. Virchows Archiv. 2003;**443**:703-717

[38] Grouard G, Rissoan M-C, Filgueira L, Durand I, Banchereau J, Liu Y-J. The enigmatic plasmacytoid T cells develop into dendritic cells with interleukin (IL)-3 and CD40-ligand. The Journal of Experimental Medicine. 1997;**185**:1101-1112

[39] Coccia EM, Severa M, Giacomini E, Monneron D, Remoli ME, Julkunen I, et al. Viral infection and Toll-like receptor agonists induce a differential expression of type I and λ interferons in human plasmacytoid and monocyte-derived dendritic cells. European Journal of Immunology. 2004;**34**:796-805. DOI: 10.1002/eji.200324610

[40] Gilliet M, Cao W, Liu Y-J. Plasmacytoid dendritic cells: Sensing

nucleic acids in viral infection and autoimmune diseases. Nature Reviews Immunology. 2008;**8**:594. DOI: 10.1038/nri2358

[41] Swiecki M, Colonna M. The multifaceted biology of plasmacytoid dendritic cells. Nature Reviews. 2015;**15**:471-485. DOI: 10.1038/nri3865

[42] Alculumbre S, Raieli S, Hoffmann C, Chelbi R, Danlos F-X, Soumelis V. Plasmacytoid pre-dendritic cells (pDC): From molecular pathways to function and disease association. Seminars in Cell & Developmental Biology. 2019;**86**:24-35. DOI: 10.1016/j.semcdb.2018.02.014

[43] Murphy TL, Grajales-Reyes GE, Wu X, Tussiwand R, Briseño CG, Iwata A, et al. Transcriptional control of dendritic cell development. Annual Review of Immunology. 2016;**34**:93-119. DOI: 10.1146/annurev-immunol-032713-120204

[44] Musumeci A, Lutz K, Winheim E, Krug AB. What makes a pDC: Recent advances in understanding plasmacytoid DC development and heterogeneity. Frontiers in Immunology. 2019;**10**:1222. DOI: 10.3389/fimmu.2019.01222 [Published: 29 May 2019]

[45] Wu X, Briseño CG, Grajales-Reyes GE, Haldar M, Iwata A, Kretzer NM, et al. Transcription factor Zeb2 regulates commitment to plasmacytoid dendritic cell and monocyte fate. Proceedings of the National Academy of Sciences. 2016;**113**:14775-14780. DOI: 10.1073/pnas.1611408114

[46] Cisse B, Caton ML, Lehner M, Maeda T, Scheu S, Locksley R, et al. Transcription factor E2-2 is an essential and specific regulator of plasmacytoid dendritic cell development. Cell;**135**:37-48. DOI: 10.1016/j.cell.2008.09.016

[47] Matsui T, Connolly JE, Michnevitz M, Chaussabel D, Yu C-I, Glaser C, et al. CD2 distinguishes two subsets of human plasmacytoid dendritic cells with distinct phenotype and functions. The Journal of Immunology. 2009;**182**:6815-6823

[48] Owczarczyk-Saczonek A, Sokołowska-Wojdyło M, Olszewska B, Malek M, Znajewska-Pander A, Kowalczyk A, et al. Clinicopathologic retrospective analysis of blastic plasmacytoid dendritic cell neoplasms. Postepy Dermatologii i Alergologii. 2018;**35**:128-138. DOI: 10.5114/ada.2017.72269

[49] Kubota S, Tokunaga K, Umezu T, Yokomizo-Nakano T, Sun Y, Oshima M, et al. Lineage-specific RUNX2 super-enhancer activates MYC and promotes the development of blastic plasmacytoid dendritic cell neoplasm. Nature Communications. 2019;**10**:1653. DOI: 10.1038/s41467-019-09710-z

[50] Sukswai N, Aung PP, Yin CC, Li S, Wang W, Wang SA, et al. Dual expression of TCF4 and CD123 is highly sensitive and specific for blastic plasmacytoid dendritic cell neoplasm. The American Journal of Surgical Pathology. 2019;**43**:1429-1437. DOI: 10.1097/pas.0000000000001316

[51] Sullivan JM, Rizzieri DA. Treatment of blastic plasmacytoid dendritic cell neoplasm. Hematology-American Society of Hematology Education Program. 2016;**2016**(1):16-23. DOI: 10.1182/asheducation-2016.1.16

[52] Jen EY, Gao X, Li L, Zhuang L, Simpson NE, Aryal B, et al. FDA approval summary: Tagraxofusp-erzs for treatment of blastic plasmacytoid dendritic cell neoplasm. Clinical Cancer Research. 2020;**26**:532-536. DOI: 10.1158/1078-0432.ccr-19-2329

[53] Cavanagh L, Saal R, Grimmet K, Thomas R. Proliferation in monocyte-derived dendritic cell cultures is caused by progenitor cells capable

of myeloid differentiation. Blood. 1998;**92**:1598-1607

[54] Reid CD, Stackpoole A, Meager A, Tikerpae J. Interactions of tumor necrosis factor with granulocyte-macrophage colony-stimulating factor and other cytokines in the regulation of dendritic cell growth in vitro from early bipotent CD34+ progenitors in human bone marrow. Journal of Immunology. 1992;**149**:2681-2688

[55] Santiago-Schwartz F, Belilos E, Diamond B, Carsons S. TNF in combination with GM-CSF enhances the differentiation of neonatal cord bloods cells into dendritic cells and macrophages. Journal of Leukocyte Biology. 1992;**52**:274-281

[56] Gabrilovich D, Nadaf S, Corak J, Berzofsky J, Carbone D. Dendritic cells in antitumor immune responses II. Dendritic cells grown from bone marrow precursors, but not mature DC from tumor-bearing mice, are effective antigen carriers in the therapy of established tumors. Cellular Immunology. 1996;**170**:111-119

[57] Sallusto F, Lanzavecchia A. Efficient presentation of soluble antigen by cultured human dendritic cells is maintained by granulocyte/macrophage colony-stimulating factor plus interleukin 4 and downregulated by tumor necrosis factor alpha. The Journal of Experimental Medicine. 1994;**179**:1109-1118. DOI: 10.1084/jem.179.4.1109

[58] Helft J, Bottcher J, Chakravarty P, Zelenay S, Huotari J, Schraml BU, et al. GM-CSF mouse bone marrow cultures comprise a heterogeneous population of CD11c(+)MHCII(+) macrophages and dendritic cells. Immunity. 2015;**42**:1197-1211. DOI: 10.1016/j.immuni.2015.05.018

[59] Guilliams M, Malissen B. A death notice for in-vitro-generated GM-CSF dendritic cells? Immunity. 2015;**42**:988-990. DOI: 10.1016/j.immuni.2015.05.020

[60] Lutz MB, Inaba K, Schuler G, Romani N. Still alive and kicking: In-vitro-generated GM-CSF dendritic cells! Immunity. 2016;**44**:1-2. DOI: 10.1016/j.immuni.2015.12.013

[61] Helft J, Bottcher JP, Chakravarty P, Zelenay S, Huotari J, Schraml BU, et al. Alive but confused: Heterogeneity of CD11c(+) MHC class II(+) cells in GM-CSF mouse bone marrow cultures. Immunity. 2016;**44**:3-4. DOI: 10.1016/j.immuni.2015.12.014

[62] Xu Y, Zhan Y, Lew AM, Naik SH, Kershaw MH. Differential development of murine dendritic cells by GM-CSF versus Flt3 ligand has implications for inflammation and trafficking. The Journal of Immunology. 2007;**179**:7577-7581. DOI: 10.4049/jimmunol.179.11.7577

[63] Marigo I, Zilio S, Desantis G, Mlecnik B, Agnellini AHR, Ugel S, et al. T cell cancer therapy requires CD40-CD40L activation of tumor necrosis factor and inducible nitric-oxide-synthase-producing dendritic cells. Cancer Cell. 2016;**30**:377-390. DOI: 10.1016/j.ccell.2016.08.004

[64] Kumar C, Kohli S, Bapsy PP, Vaid AK, Jain M, Attili VSS, et al. Immune modulation by dendritic-cell-based cancer vaccines. Journal of Biosciences. 2017;**42**:161-173. DOI: 10.1007/s12038-017-9665-x

[65] Murphy GP, Tjoa BA, Simmons SJ, Jarisch J, Bowes VA, Ragde H, et al. Infusion of dendritic cells pulsed with HLA-A2-specific prostate-specific membrane antigen peptides: A phase II prostate cancer vaccine trial involving patients with hormone-refractory metastatic disease. Prostate. 1999;**38**:73-78

[66] Rodriguez J, Castanon E, Perez-Gracia JL, Rodriguez I, Viudez A,

Alfaro C, et al. A randomized phase II clinical trial of dendritic cell vaccination following complete resection of colon cancer liver metastasis. Journal for Immunotherapy of Cancer. 2018;**6**:96. DOI: 10.1186/s40425-018-0405-z

[67] Bol KF, Schreibelt G, Rabold K, Wculek SK, Schwarze JK, Dzionek A, et al. The clinical application of cancer immunotherapy based on naturally circulating dendritic cells. Journal for Immunotherapy of Cancer. 2019;7:109-109. DOI: 10.1186/s40425-019-0580-6

[68] Mody N, Dubey S, Sharma R, Agrawal U, Vyas SP. Dendritic cell-based vaccine research against cancer. Expert Review of Clinical Immunology. 2015;**11**:213-232. DOI: 10.1586/1744666X.2015.987663

[69] Reddy A, Sapp M, Feldman M, Subklewe M, Bhardwaj N. A monocyte conditioned medium is more effective than defined cytokines in mediating the terminal maturation of human dendritic cells. Blood. 1997;**90**:3640

[70] Wilgenhof S, Van Nuffel AMT, Benteyn D, Corthals J, Aerts C, Heirman C, et al. A phase IB study on intravenous synthetic mRNA electroporated dendritic cell immunotherapy in pretreated advanced melanoma patients. Annals of Oncology. 2013;**24**:2686-2693. DOI: 10.1093/annonc/mdt245

[71] Schreibelt G, Bol KF, Westdorp H, Wimmers F, Aarntzen EHJG, Boer T D-d, et al. Effective clinical responses in metastatic melanoma patients after vaccination with primary myeloid dendritic cells. Clinical Cancer Research. 2016;**22**:2155. DOI: 10.1158/1078-0432.CCR-15-2205

[72] Prue RL, Vari F, Radford KJ, Tong H, Hardy MY, D'Rozario R, et al. A phase I clinical trial of CD1c (BDCA-1)+ dendritic cells pulsed with HLA-A*0201 peptides for immunotherapy of metastatic hormone refractory prostate cancer. Journal of Immunotherapy. 2015;**38**:71-76. DOI: 10.1097/cji.0000000000000063

[73] Macri C, Dumont C, Johnston AP, Mintern JD. Targeting dendritic cells: A promising strategy to improve vaccine effectiveness. Clinical & Translational Immunology. 2016;**5**:e66-e66. DOI: 10.1038/cti.2016.6

[74] Caminschi I, Maraskovsky E, Heath W. Targeting dendritic cells in vivo for cancer therapy. Frontiers in Immunology. 2012;**3**:13

[75] Bonifaz LC, Bonnyay DP, Charalambous A, Darguste DI, Fujii S-I, Soares H, et al. In vivo targeting of antigens to maturing dendritic cells via the DEC-205 receptor improves T cell vaccination. The Journal of Experimental Medicine. 2004;**199**:815-824. DOI: 10.1084/jem.20032220

[76] Hawiger D, Inaba K, Dorsett Y, Guo M, Mahnke K, Rivera M, et al. Dendritic cells induce peripheral T cell unresponsiveness under steady state conditions in vivo. The Journal of Experimental Medicine. 2001;**194**:769-779. DOI: 10.1084/jem.194.6.769

[77] Mahnke K, Ring S, Johnson TS, Schallenberg S, Schönfeld K, Storn V, et al. Induction of immunosuppressive functions of dendritic cells in vivo by CD4+CD25+ regulatory T cells: Role of B7-H3 expression and antigen presentation. European Journal of Immunology. 2007;**37**:2117-2126. DOI: 10.1002/eji.200636841

[78] Dhodapkar MV, Sznol M, Zhao B, Wang D, Carvajal RD, Keohan ML, et al. Induction of antigen-specific immunity with a vaccine targeting NY-ESO-1 to the dendritic cell receptor DEC-205. Science Translational Medicine. 2014;**6**:232ra251. DOI: 10.1126/scitranslmed.3008068

[79] Tullett KM, Leal Rojas IM, Minoda Y, Tan PS, Zhang J-G, Smith C, et al. Targeting CLEC9A delivers antigen to human CD141(+) DC for CD4(+) and CD8(+)T cell recognition. JCI Insight. 2016;**1**:e87102-e87102. DOI: 10.1172/jci.insight.87102

[80] Kato M, McDonald KJ, Khan S, Ross IL, Vuckovic S, Chen K, et al. Expression of human DEC-205 (CD205) multilectin receptor on leukocytes. International Immunology. 2006;**18**:857-869. DOI: 10.1093/intimm/dxl022

[81] Schreibelt G, Klinkenberg LJJ, Cruz LJ, Tacken PJ, Tel J, Kreutz M, et al. The C-type lectin receptor CLEC9A mediates antigen uptake and (cross-) presentation by human blood BDCA3+ myeloid dendritic cells. Blood. 2012;**119**:2284. DOI: 10.1182/blood-2011-08-373944

[82] Li J, Ahmet F, Sullivan LC, Brooks AG, Kent SJ, De Rose R, et al. Caminschi, antibodies targeting Clec9A promote strong humoral immunity without adjuvant in mice and non-human primates. European Journal of Immunology. 2015;**45**:854-864. DOI: 10.1002/eji.201445127

[83] Spranger S, Gajewski TF. Impact of oncogenic pathways on evasion of antitumour immune responses. Nature Reviews Cancer. 2018;**18**:139. DOI: 10.1038/nrc.2017.117

[84] Karthaus N, Torensma R, Tel J. Deciphering the message broadcast by tumor-infiltrating dendritic cells. The American Journal of Pathology. 2012;**181**:733-742. DOI: 10.1016/j.ajpath.2012.05.012

[85] Ladányi A, Kiss J, Somlai B, Gilde K, Fejős Z, Mohos A, et al. Density of DC-LAMP+ mature dendritic cells in combination with activated T lymphocytes infiltrating primary cutaneous melanoma is a strong independent prognostic factor. Cancer Immunology, Immunotherapy. 2007;**56**:1459-1469. DOI: 10.1007/s00262-007-0286-3

[86] Coventry B, Heinzel S. CD1a in human cancers: A new role for an old molecule. Trends in Immunology. 2004;**25**:242-248. DOI: 10.1016/j.it.2004.03.002

[87] Saito H, Tsujitani S, Ikeguchi M, Maeta M, Kaibara N. Relationship between the expression of vascular endothelial growth factor and the density of dendritic cells in gastric adenocarcinoma tissue. British Journal of Cancer. 1998;**78**:1573-1577. DOI: 10.1038/bjc.1998.725

[88] Hilly O, Rath-Wolfson L, Koren R, Mizrachi A, Hamzany Y, Bachar G, et al. CD1a-positive dendritic cell density predicts disease-free survival in papillary thyroid carcinoma. Pathology—Research and Practice. 2015;**211**:652-656. DOI: 10.1016/j.prp.2015.05.009

[89] Coventry BJ, Lee PL, Gibbs D, Hart DNJ. Dendritic cell density and activation status in human breast cancer—CD1a, CMRF-44, CMRF-56 and CD-83 expression. British Journal of Cancer. 2002;**86**:546-551. DOI: 10.1038/sj.bjc.6600132

[90] Bell D, Chomarat P, Broyles D, Netto G, Harb GM, Lebecque S, et al. In breast carcinoma tissue, immature dendritic cells reside within the tumor, whereas mature dendritic cells are located in peritumoral areas. The Journal of Experimental Medicine. 1999;**190**:1417

[91] Truxova I, Kasikova L, Hensler M, Skapa P, Laco J, Pecen L, et al. Mature dendritic cells correlate with favorable immune infiltrate and improved prognosis in ovarian carcinoma patients. Journal for Immunotherapy of

Cancer. 2018;**6**:139-139. DOI: 10.1186/s40425-018-0446-3

[92] Lewko B, Zółtowska A, Stepinski J, Roszkiewicz A, Moszkowska G. Dendritic and cancer cells in the breat tumours—An immunohistochemical study: Short communication. Medical Science Monitor. 2000;**6**:892-895

[93] Lespagnard L, Gancberg D, Rouas G, Leclercq G, de Saint-Aubain Somerhausen N, Di Leo A, et al. Tumor-infiltrating dendritic cells in adenocarcinomas of the breast: A study of 143 neoplasms with a correlation to usual prognostic factors and to clinical outcome. International Journal of Cancer. 1999;**84**:309-314. DOI: 10.1002/(SICI)1097-0215(19990621)84:3<309::AID-IJC19>3.0.CO;2-3

[94] Hillenbrand EE, Neville AM, Coventry BJ. Immunohistochemical localization of CD1a-positive putative dendritic cells in human breast tumours. British Journal of Cancer. 1999;**79**:940-944. DOI: 10.1038/sj.bjc.6690150

[95] Roberts EW, Broz ML, Binnewies M, Headley MB, Nelson AE, Wolf DM, et al. Critical role for CD103+/CD141+ dendritic cells bearing CCR7 for tumor antigen trafficking and priming of T cell immunity in melanoma. Cancer Cell. 2016;**30**:324-336. DOI: 10.1016/j.ccell.2016.06.003

[96] Spranger S, Dai D, Horton B, Gajewski TF. Tumor-residing Batf3 dendritic cells are required for effector T cell trafficking and adoptive T cell therapy. Cancer Cell. 2017;**31**:711, e714-723. DOI: 10.1016/j.ccell.2017.04.003

[97] Böttcher JP, Bonavita E, Chakravarty P, Blees H, Cabeza-Cabrerizo M, Sammicheli S, et al. NK cells stimulate recruitment of cDC1 into the tumor microenvironment promoting cancer immune control. Cell. 2018;**172**:1022, e1014-1037. DOI: 10.1016/j.cell.2018.01.004

[98] Broz ML, Binnewies M, Boldajipour B, Nelson AE, Pollack JL, Erle DJ, et al. Dissecting the tumor myeloid compartment reveals rare activating antigen-presenting cells critical for T cell immunity. Cancer Cell. 2014;**26**:638-652. DOI: 10.1016/j.ccell.2014.09.007

[99] Daniel S, Chen IM. Oncology meets immunology: The cancer-immunity cycle. Immunity. 2013;**39**:1-10. DOI: 10.1016/j.immuni.2013.07.012

[100] Treilleux I, Blay J-Y, Bendriss-Vermare N, Ray-Coquard I, Bachelot T, Guastalla J-P, et al. Dendritic cell infiltration and prognosis of early stage breast cancer. Clinical Cancer Research. 2004;**10**:7466. DOI: 10.1158/1078-0432.CCR-04-0684

[101] Conrad C, Gregorio J, Wang Y-H, Ito T, Meller S, Hanabuchi S, et al. Plasmacytoid dendritic cells promote immunosuppression in ovarian cancer via ICOS Costimulation of Foxp3+ T-regulatory cells. Cancer Research. 2012;**72**:5240. DOI: 10.1158/0008-5472.CAN-12-2271

[102] Sisirak V, Faget J, Gobert M, Goutagny N, Vey N, Treilleux I, et al. Impaired IFN-α production by plasmacytoid dendritic cells favors regulatory T-cell expansion that may contribute to breast cancer progression. Cancer Research. 2012;**72**:5188. DOI: 10.1158/0008-5472.CAN-11-3468

[103] Mitchell D, Chintala S, Dey M. Plasmacytoid dendritic cell in immunity and cancer. Journal of Neuroimmunology. 2018;**322**:63-73. DOI: 10.1016/j.jneuroim.2018.06.012

[104] Terra M, Oberkampf M, Fayolle C, Rosenbaum P, Guillerey C, Dadaglio G, et al. Tumor-derived TGFβ alters the ability of plasmacytoid dendritic cells to respond to innate immune signaling. Cancer Research.

2018;**78**:3014-3026. DOI: 10.1158/0008-5472.can-17-2719

[105] Takahashi A, Kono K, Ichihara F, Sugai H, Fujii H, Matsumoto Y. Vascular endothelial growth factor inhibits maturation of dendritic cells induced by lipopolysaccharide, but not by proinflammatory cytokines. Cancer Immunology, Immunotherapy. 2004;**53**:543-550. DOI: 10.1007/s00262-003-0466-8

[106] Della Porta M, Danova M, Rigolin GM, Brugnatelli S, Rovati B, Tronconi C, et al. Dendritic cells and vascular endothelial growth factor in colorectal cancer: Correlations with clinicobiological findings. Oncology. 2005;**68**:276-284. DOI: 10.1159/000086784

[107] H. B FXH, Dong QG, Sha HF, Bao GL, Liao ML. Ascular endothelial growth factor inhibits dendritic cells from patients with non-small cell lung carcinoma. Zhonghua Jie He He Hu Xi Za Zhi. 2003;**26**:539-543

[108] Fricke I, Mirza N, Dupont J, Lockhart C, Jackson A, Lee J-H, et al. Vascular endothelial growth factor-trap overcomes defects in dendritic cell differentiation but does not improve antigen-specific immune responses. Clinical Cancer Research. 2007;**13**:4840. DOI: 10.1158/1078-0432.CCR-07-0409

[109] Gabrilovich DI, Chen HL, Girgis KR, Cunningham HT, Meny GM, Nadaf S, et al. Production of vascular endothelial growth factor by human tumors inhibits the functional maturation of dendritic cells. Nature Medicine. 1996;**2**:1096-1103. DOI: 10.1038/nm1096-1096

[110] Thepmalee C, Panya A, Junking M, Chieochansin T, Yenchitsomanus P-t. Inhibition of IL-10 and TGF-β receptors on dendritic cells enhances activation of effector T-cells to kill cholangiocarcinoma cells. Human Vaccines & Immunotherapeutics. 2018;**14**:1423-1431. DOI: 10.1080/21645515.2018.1431598

[111] Bharadwaj U, Li M, Zhang R, Chen C, Yao Q. Elevated Interleukin-6 and G-CSF in human pancreatic cancer cell conditioned medium suppress dendritic cell differentiation and activation. Cancer Research. 2007;**67**:5479. DOI: 10.1158/0008-5472.CAN-06-3963

[112] Fu C, Jiang A. Dendritic cells and CD8 T cell immunity in tumor microenvironment. Frontiers in Immunology. 2018;**9**:3059

[113] Zong J, Keskinov AA, Shurin GV, Shurin MR. Tumor-derived factors modulating dendritic cell function. Cancer Immunology, Immunotherapy. 2016;**65**:821-833. DOI: 10.1007/s00262-016-1820-y

[114] Kitamura H, Ohno Y, Toyoshima Y, Ohtake J, Homma S, Kawamura H, et al. Interleukin-6/STAT3 signaling as a promising target to improve the efficacy of cancer immunotherapy. Cancer Science. 2017;**108**:1947-1952. DOI: 10.1111/cas.13332

[115] Spranger S, Bao R, Gajewski TF. Melanoma-intrinsic β-catenin signalling prevents anti-tumour immunity. Nature. 2015;**523**:231. DOI: 10.1038/nature14404

[116] Jiang L, Fang X, Wang H, Li D, Wang X. Ovarian cancer-intrinsic fatty acid synthase prevents anti-tumor immunity by disrupting tumor-infiltrating dendritic cells. Frontiers in Immunology. 2018;**9**:2927

[117] Freeman GJ, Long AJ, Iwai Y, Bourque K, Chernova T, Nishimura H, et al. Engagement of the PD-1 immunoinhibitory receptor by a novel B7 family member leads to negative regulation of lymphocyte activation.

The Journal of Experimental Medicine. 2000;**192**:1027-1034. DOI: 10.1084/jem.192.7.1027

[118] Seidel JA, Otsuka A, Kabashima K. Anti-PD-1 and anti-CTLA-4 therapies in cancer: Mechanisms of action, efficacy, and limitations. Frontiers in Oncology. 2018;**8**:86. DOI: 10.3389/fonc.2018.00086

[119] Pulko V, Liu X, Krco CJ, Harris KJ, Frigola X, Kwon ED, et al. TLR3-stimulated dendritic cells up-regulate B7-H1 expression and influence the magnitude of CD8 T cell responses to tumor vaccination. Journal of Immunology. 2009;**183**:3634-3641. DOI: 10.4049/jimmunol.0900974

[120] Ray A, Das DS, Song Y, Richardson P, Munshi NC, Chauhan D, et al. Targeting PD1-PDL1 immune checkpoint in plasmacytoid dendritic cell interactions with T cells, natural killer cells and multiple myeloma cells. Leukemia. 2015;**29**:1441-1444. DOI: 10.1038/leu.2015.11

[121] Brown JA, Dorfman DM, Ma FR, Sullivan EL, Munoz O, Wood CR, et al. Blockade of programmed death-1 ligands on dendritic cells enhances T cell activation and cytokine production. Journal of Immunology. 2003;**170**:1257-1266. DOI: 10.4049/jimmunol.170.3.1257

[122] Krieg C, Nowicka M, Guglietta S, Schindler S, Hartmann FJ, Weber LM, et al. High-dimensional single-cell analysis predicts response to anti-PD-1 immunotherapy. Nature Medicine. 2018;**24**:144-153. DOI: 10.1038/nm.4466

[123] Salmon H, Idoyaga J, Rahman A, Leboeuf M, Remark R, Jordan S, et al. Expansion and activation of CD103(+) dendritic cell progenitors at the tumor site enhances tumor responses to therapeutic PD-L1 and BRAF inhibition. Immunity. 2016;**44**:924-938. DOI: 10.1016/j.immuni.2016.03.012

[124] Beavis PA, Henderson MA, Giuffrida L, Davenport AJ, Petley EV, House IG, et al. Dual PD-1 and CTLA-4 checkpoint blockade promotes antitumor immune responses through CD4(+) Foxp3(−) cell-mediated modulation of CD103(+) dendritic cells. Cancer Immunology Research. 2018;**6**:1069-1081. DOI: 10.1158/2326-6066.CIR-18-0291

[125] Alloatti A, Rookhuizen DC, Joannas L, Carpier JM, Iborra S, Magalhaes JG, et al. Critical role for Sec22b-dependent antigen cross-presentation in antitumor immunity. The Journal of Experimental Medicine. 2017;**214**:2231-2241. DOI: 10.1084/jem.20170229

[126] Garris CS, Arlauckas SP, Kohler RH, Trefny MP, Garren S, Piot C, et al. Successful anti-PD-1 cancer immunotherapy requires T cell-dendritic cell crosstalk involving the cytokines IFN-gamma and IL-12. Immunity. 2018;**49**:1148-1161e1147. DOI: 10.1016/j.immuni.2018.09.024

[127] Bjoern J, Iversen TZ, Nitschke NJ, Andersen MH, Svane IM. Safety, immune and clinical responses in metastatic melanoma patients vaccinated with a long peptide derived from indoleamine 2,3-dioxygenase in combination with ipilimumab. Cytotherapy. 2016;**18**:1043-1055. DOI: 10.1016/j.jcyt.2016.05.010

[128] He Y, Cao J, Zhao C, Li X, Zhou C, Hirsch FR. TIM-3, a promising target for cancer immunotherapy. Oncotargets and Therapy. 2018;**11**:7005-7009. DOI: 10.2147/OTT.S170385

[129] Butte MJ, Keir ME, Phamduy TB, Sharpe AH, Freeman GJ. Programmed death-1 ligand 1 interacts specifically with the B7-1 costimulatory molecule to inhibit T cell responses. Immunity. 2007;**27**:111-122. DOI: 10.1016/j.immuni.2007.05.016

[130] Chaudhri A, Xiao Y, Klee AN, Wang X, Zhu B, Freeman GJ. PD-L1

binds to B7-1 only In Cis on the same cell surface. Cancer Immunology Research. 2018;**6**:921-929. DOI: 10.1158/2326-6066.CIR-17-0316

[131] Sugiura D, Maruhashi T, Okazaki IM, Shimizu K, Maeda TK, Takemoto T, et al. Restriction of PD-1 function by cis-PD-L1/CD80 interactions is required for optimal T cell responses. Science. 2019;**364**: 558-566. DOI: 10.1126/science.aav7062

[132] Sierro SR, Donda A, Perret R, Guillaume P, Yagita H, Levy F, et al. Combination of lentivector immunization and low-dose chemotherapy or PD-1/PD-L1 blocking primes self-reactive T cells and induces anti-tumor immunity. European Journal of Immunology. 2011;**41**:2217-2228. DOI: 10.1002/eji.201041235

[133] Li B, VanRoey M, Wang C, Chen TH, Korman A, Jooss K. Anti-programmed death-1 synergizes with granulocyte macrophage colony-stimulating factor—Secreting tumor cell immunotherapy providing therapeutic benefit to mice with established tumors. Clinical Cancer Research. 2009;**15**:1623-1634. DOI: 10.1158/1078-0432.CCR-08-1825

[134] Rice AE, Latchman YE, Balint JP, Lee JH, Gabitzsch ES, Jones FR. An HPV-E6/E7 immunotherapy plus PD-1 checkpoint inhibition results in tumor regression and reduction in PD-L1 expression. Cancer Gene Therapy. 2015;**22**:454-462. DOI: 10.1038/cgt.2015.40

[135] Chung V, Kos FJ, Hardwick N, Yuan Y, Chao J, Li D, et al. Evaluation of safety and efficacy of p53MVA vaccine combined with pembrolizumab in patients with advanced solid cancers. Clinical & Translational Oncology. 2019;**21**:363-372. DOI: 10.1007/s12094-018-1932-2

[136] Massarelli E, William W, Johnson F, Kies M, Ferrarotto R, Guo M, et al. Combining immune checkpoint blockade and tumor-specific vaccine for patients with incurable human papillomavirus 16-related cancer: A phase 2 clinical trial. JAMA Oncology. 2019;**5**:67-73. DOI: 10.1001/jamaoncol.2018.4051

[137] Weber JS, Kudchadkar RR, Yu B, Gallenstein D, Horak CE, Inzunza HD, et al. Safety, efficacy, and biomarkers of nivolumab with vaccine in ipilimumab-refractory or -naive melanoma. Journal of Clinical Oncology. 2013;**31**:4311-4318. DOI: 10.1200/JCO.2013.51.4802

[138] Gibney GT, Kudchadkar RR, DeConti RC, Thebeau MS, Czupryn MP, Tetteh L, et al. Safety, correlative markers, and clinical results of adjuvant nivolumab in combination with vaccine in resected high-risk metastatic melanoma. Clinical Cancer Research. 2015;**21**:712-720. DOI: 10.1158/1078-0432.CCR-14-2468

[139] Qureshi OS, Zheng Y, Nakamura K, Attridge K, Manzotti C, Schmidt EM, et al. Trans-endocytosis of CD80 and CD86: A molecular basis for the cell-extrinsic function of CTLA-4. Science. 2011;**332**:600-603. DOI: 10.1126/science.1202947

[140] Hou TZ, Qureshi OS, Wang CJ, Baker J, Young SP, Walker LS, et al. A transendocytosis model of CTLA-4 function predicts its suppressive behavior on regulatory T cells. Journal of Immunology. 2015;**194**:2148-2159. DOI: 10.4049/jimmunol.1401876

[141] Ovcinnikovs V, Ross EM, Petersone L, et al. CTLA-4-mediated transendocytosis of costimulatory molecules primarily targets migratory dendritic cells. Science Immunology. 2019;**4**(35):eaaw0902. DOI: 10.1126/sciimmunol.aaw0902

[142] Munn DH, Sharma MD, Mellor AL. Ligation of B7-1/B7-2 by human CD4+ T cells triggers

indoleamine 2,3-dioxygenase activity in dendritic cells. Journal of Immunology. 2004;**172**:4100-4110. DOI: 10.4049/jimmunol.172.7.4100

[143] Chen W, Liang X, Peterson AJ, Munn DH, Blazar BR. The indoleamine 2,3-dioxygenase pathway is essential for human plasmacytoid dendritic cell-induced adaptive T regulatory cell generation. Journal of Immunology. 2008;**181**:5396-5404. DOI: 10.4049/jimmunol.181.8.5396

[144] Mellor AL, Chandler P, Baban B, Hansen AM, Marshall B, Pihkala J, et al. Specific subsets of murine dendritic cells acquire potent T cell regulatory functions following CTLA4-mediated induction of indoleamine 2,3 dioxygenase. International Immunology. 2004;**16**:1391-1401. DOI: 10.1093/intimm/dxh140

[145] Laurent S, Carrega P, Saverino D, Piccioli P, Camoriano M, Morabito A, et al. CTLA-4 is expressed by human monocyte-derived dendritic cells and regulates their functions. Human Immunology. 2010;**71**:934-941. DOI: 10.1016/j.humimm.2010.07.007

[146] Halpert MM, Konduri V, Liang D, Chen Y, Wing JB, Paust S, et al. Dendritic cell-secreted cytotoxic T-lymphocyte-associated Protein-4 regulates the T-cell response by Downmodulating bystander surface B7. Stem Cells and Development. 2016;**25**:774-787. DOI: 10.1089/scd.2016.0009

[147] Hodi FS, O'Day SJ, McDermott DF, Weber RW, Sosman JA, Haanen JB, et al. Improved survival with ipilimumab in patients with metastatic melanoma. The New England Journal of Medicine. 2010;**363**:711-723. DOI: 10.1056/NEJMoa1003466

[148] Sarnaik AA, Yu B, Yu D, Morelli D, Hall M, Bogle D, et al. Extended dose ipilimumab with a peptide vaccine: Immune correlates associated with clinical benefit in patients with resected high-risk stage IIIc/IV melanoma. Clinical Cancer Research. 2011;**17**:896-906. DOI: 10.1158/1078-0432.CCR-10-2463

[149] Ribas A, Comin-Anduix B, Chmielowski B, Jalil J, de la Rocha P, McCannel TA, et al. Dendritic cell vaccination combined with CTLA4 blockade in patients with metastatic melanoma. Clinical Cancer Research. 2009;**15**:6267-6276. DOI: 10.1158/1078-0432.CCR-09-1254

[150] Wilgenhof S, Corthals J, Heirman C, van Baren N, Lucas S, Kvistborg P, et al. Phase II study of autologous monocyte-derived mRNA electroporated dendritic cells (TriMixDC-MEL) plus Ipilimumab in patients with pretreated advanced melanoma. Journal of Clinical Oncology. 2016;**34**:1330-1338. DOI: 10.1200/JCO.2015.63.4121

[151] Anderson AC, Anderson DE, Bregoli L, Hastings WD, Kassam N, Lei C, et al. Promotion of tissue inflammation by the immune receptor Tim-3 expressed on innate immune cells. Science. 2007;**318**:1141-1143. DOI: 10.1126/science.1148536

[152] de Mingo Pulido A, Gardner A, Hiebler S, Soliman H, Rugo HS, Krummel MF, et al. TIM-3 regulates CD103(+) dendritic cell function and response to chemotherapy in breast cancer. Cancer Cell. 2018;**33**:60-74e66. DOI: 10.1016/j.ccell.2017.11.019

[153] Fromm PD, Kupresanin F, Brooks AE, Dunbar PR, Haniffa M, Hart DN, et al. A multi-laboratory comparison of blood dendritic cell populations. Clinical & Translational Immunology. 2016;**5**:e68. DOI: 10.1038/cti.2016.5

[154] Long L, Zhang X, Chen F, Pan Q, Phiphatwatchara P, Zeng Y, et al. The promising immune checkpoint

LAG-3: From tumor microenvironment to cancer immunotherapy. Genes & Cancer. 2018;**9**:176-189. DOI: 10.18632/genesandcancer.180

[155] Andreae S, Piras F, Burdin N, Triebel F. Maturation and activation of dendritic cells induced by lymphocyte activation gene-3 (CD223). Journal of Immunology. 2002;**168**:3874-3880. DOI: 10.4049/jimmunol.168.8.3874

[156] Avice MN, Sarfati M, Triebel F, Delespesse G, Demeure CE. Lymphocyte activation gene-3, a MHC class II ligand expressed on activated T cells, stimulates TNF-alpha and IL-12 production by monocytes and dendritic cells. Journal of Immunology. 1999;**162**:2748-2753

[157] Buisson S, Triebel F. MHC class II engagement by its ligand LAG-3 (CD223) leads to a distinct pattern of chemokine and chemokine receptor expression by human dendritic cells. Vaccine. 2003;**21**:862-868

[158] Brignone C, Gutierrez M, Mefti F, Brain E, Jarcau R, Cvitkovic F, et al. First-line chemoimmunotherapy in metastatic breast carcinoma: Combination of paclitaxel and IMP321 (LAG-3Ig) enhances immune responses and antitumor activity. Journal of Translational Medicine. 2010;**8**:71. DOI: 10.1186/1479-5876-8-71

[159] Camisaschi C, De Filippo A, Beretta V, Vergani B, Villa A, Vergani E, et al. Alternative activation of human plasmacytoid DCs in vitro and in melanoma lesions: Involvement of LAG-3. The Journal of Investigative Dermatology. 2014;**134**:1893-1902. DOI: 10.1038/jid.2014.29

[160] Ito T, Hanabuchi S, Wang YH, Park WR, Arima K, Bover L, et al. Two functional subsets of FOXP3+ regulatory T cells in human thymus and periphery. Immunity. 2008;**28**:870-880. DOI: 10.1016/j.immuni.2008.03.018

[161] Marinelli O, Nabissi M, Morelli MB, Torquati L, Amantini C, Santoni G. ICOS-L as a potential therapeutic target for cancer immunotherapy. Current Protein & Peptide Science. 2018;**19**:1107-1113. DOI: 10.2174/1389203719666180608093913

[162] Ogata M, Ito T, Shimamoto K, Nakanishi T, Satsutani N, Miyamoto R, et al. Plasmacytoid dendritic cells have a cytokine-producing capacity to enhance ICOS ligand-mediated IL-10 production during T-cell priming. International Immunology. 2013;**25**:171-182. DOI: 10.1093/intimm/dxs103

[163] Wei S, Kryczek I, Zou L, Daniel B, Cheng P, Mottram P, et al. Plasmacytoid dendritic cells induce CD8+ regulatory T cells in human ovarian carcinoma. Cancer Research. 2005;**65**:5020-5026. DOI: 10.1158/0008-5472.CAN-04-4043

[164] Faget J, Bendriss-Vermare N, Gobert M, Durand I, Olive D, Biota C, et al. ICOS-ligand expression on plasmacytoid dendritic cells supports breast cancer progression by promoting the accumulation of immunosuppressive CD4+ T cells. Cancer Research. 2012;**72**:6130-6141. DOI: 10.1158/0008-5472.CAN-12-2409

[165] Huang XM, Liu XS, Lin XK, Yu H, Sun JY, Liu XK, et al. Role of plasmacytoid dendritic cells and inducible costimulator-positive regulatory T cells in the immunosuppression microenvironment of gastric cancer. Cancer Science. 2014;**105**:150-158. DOI: 10.1111/cas.12327

[166] Pedroza-Gonzalez A, Zhou G, Vargas-Mendez E, Boor PP, Mancham S, Verhoef C, et al. Tumor-infiltrating plasmacytoid dendritic cells promote immunosuppression by Tr1 cells in human liver tumors. Oncoimmunology. 2015;**4**:e1008355. DOI: 10.1080/2162402X.2015.1008355

Chapter 5

What Are the New Challenges of the Current Cancer Biomarkers?

Jie Chen, Liqiong Yang, Yuxi Duan, Tinging Pu, Sha Zheng, Fangfang Liu, Kun Huang, Greg Mirt and Fan Xu

Abstract

Biomarkers are emerging research filed in the past decade. Even though numerous biomarkers were reported, the efficiency of cancer therapy remains low. So the question emerges as to how much can we trust the current biomarkers on cancer therapy? In this upcoming chapter, we would like to illustrate the outcomes of classical cancer therapies on advanced pancreatic cancer disclosed successful, neutral and failed in clinical trials. The analysis will be carried on the perspective interdisciplinary on the biomarkers including anatomy, physiology, pharmacology, biochemistry, history path and development of pharmacy. Particular in-depth insight may open a window for new researches and lighting the therapies.

Keywords: advanced pancreatic cancer, biomarker, clinical trials

1. Introduction

Advance pancreatic cancer (APC) is a highly lethal tumor. Most patients with APC remain asymptomatic until the disease reaches an advanced stage [1]. The incidence rate was 5.5 for men and 4.0 for women per 100,000 people. The mortality rate was 5.1 for men and 3.8 for women per 100,000 people around the world, according to data, from 2018 [2]. For the incidence rate, Asia is at 48.4%, Europe at 23.4%, and the Americas is at 21.0%. As for the mortality rate, Asia is at 57.3%, Europe at 20.3%, and the Americas is at 14.3% [3].

Our previous study disclosed that there were more than 19 chemotherapy regimens combinations in clinical practice available [4]. The advantages and disadvantages of each therapy regimens are clear. Briefly, to lengthen the overall survival and to reduce the treatment-related toxicity we must consider the outclass selection. There are more than 14 treatment-related toxicities in gastrointestinal, constitutional, skin, hepatotoxicity, infection, vascular, neuropathy, mental, pain, renal, electrolytes and pulmonary of human body in current dominant chemotherapy regimens. To broaden the balance requires expertise and professional medical training based on evidence.

2. Long period run in research and development in pharmacy

The development of drugs is based on the determination of new therapeutic targets, the pharmacological receptors. This concept was first proposed by Paul

IntechOpen

Ehrlich in 1908 [5]. Normal cells replicate their DNA with great accuracy, but cancer has a large number of mutations that show up in cancer cells that make them pharmacological targets [6]. From the initial concept of molecular targets, drug targets were discovered and validated, which successful translated the most drugs into practice [7].

Excellent and reliable targets identification and validation can increase the credibility of the relationship between intentions and diseases, this may strength the effectively of drugs. Drugs are usually developed only when specific drug target for the action of these drugs are analyzed and examined. Sufficient potential targets have been discovered rapidly for the drug discovery process.

Numerous data including identified gene and drug discovery cycles have been generated exponentially. This may forge the difficultness in decision making and becomes more and more difficult for drug R&D. Thanks to rapid bioinformatic discoveries, more and more biopharmaceutical targets can be identified and analyzed [8].

Validation from cross-species a bioeffect is performed after the drug target is determined and verified. Rodents and non-human primates provide appropriate animal models for screening and evaluation of a new drug. Most of current cancer in vivo experiments use rodent experimental animals such as mice and rats. Because they are small, rapid reproduction, clear genetic background and mature genetic modification technology can be done. However, due to the distant relationship between rodents and humans, many of the results obtained from rodent models cannot be reproduced in humans. Moreover, non-human primates are highly similar to humans in terms of genetic evolution, immunity, physiology and metabolism. They are theoretically more suitable for cancer researches [9].

Clinical trials are the best channel to tie up pharmaceutical targets to reliable drugs. The goal is to determine whether a candidate drug is safe and effective. There are four phases in clinical trials. More specific biomarker studies are based on data from prospective studies [10]. In the study of cancer biomarkers, retrospective studies and prospective studies help to identify potential biomarkers, which may be validated in the future studies, however, the reliability of evidence remains controversial.

3. Can we trust the current biomarkers of cancer?

Unfortunately, the overall survival of APC patients has not revised assuredly. There are too many choices in clinical practice and evidence-based medicine is a permanent challenge. Which of the modern biomarkers is reliable? Are we ever going to detect precise pharmaceutical targets on APC [11]?

4. Validation method

In order to clarify this question, we collected the raw data source (http://clinicaltrials.gov) and searched all the drug treatments on APC. We refined all the data which had results and were published. Briefly, a total of 2726 recordings were found since May 2019. Hundred and fifteen recordings which finished clinical trials, further we ruled out irrelevant 32 recordings and 56 unclear results. Finally, 27 recordings kept comprising the following three tables. Raw data are free, please follow the link 10.6084/m9.figshare.8275190.

5. What can data tell us?

Total, there are 18 biomarkers used among these results. For details please see **Table 1**. The results from 27 clinical trials could be divided into three categories (a) rank of the effectiveness (b) rank of intervention and (c) quality of life improved.

5.1 Estimation of clinical trials with success outcome on advanced pancreatic cancer

Total, we found 10 publications where the author declares the successful outcome on the treatment of APC from 2011 to 2019, **Table 2**. These clinical trials recruited 1080 patients with APC (611 male and 469 female). The average overall survival month is 11.62 and progress-free survival month is 10.79. Briefly, Lutz et al. tests the GVAX pancreatic cancer vaccine via GPI biomarkers The OS and PFS approach got the highest point, 24.8 and 17.3, respectively Similarly, Phan et al. tested the pazopanib hydrochloride via VEGF biomarkers. This approach had a higher OS and PFS points. Survival months are 25 and 14.4. Furthermore, Hong et al. disclosed the capecitabine may put the OS and PFS to 17.3 and 10.4 survival months; the remain studies presented similar results, the OS and PFS were lower than 10 months.

Biomarkers	Abbreviation
Vascular endothelial growth factor*	VEGF
Thymidine phosphorylase	TP
Epidermal growth factor receptor*	EGFR
Tumor necrosis factor α	TNF-α
Topoisomerase I inhibitor	TIH
Sonic hedgehog	SHH
Severe hypoxia intracellular reductases	SHIR
Secreted protein acid rich in cysteine	SPARC
Platelet-derived growth factor	PDGF
MEK1/2-dependent effector proteins	ERK1/2
Kirsten rat sarcoma viral oncogene homolog*	KRAS
Interleukin 6/interleukin 8	IL-6/IL-8
Heat shock protein 27	Hsp27
Glycosyl-phosphatidylinositol	GPI
Double-strand breaks in DNA	—
Checkpoint kinase 1	CHK1
Microtubule-associated protein light chain 3- II	LC3- II
Circulating free DNA	cfDNA
Dihydropyrimidine dehydrogenase	DPD

NCCN Recommend: National Comprehensive Cancer Network.

Table 1.
Potential biomarkers used in advanced pancreatic cancer.

Year	Author	N	M	F	Drug	OS	PFS	Biomarkers
2011	Hill [12]	21	8	13	Capecitabine; docetaxel; gemcitabine	7.4	5.8	TP
2011	Lutz [13]	60	37	23	GVAX pancreatic cancer Vaccine	24.8	17.3	GPI
2011	Raymond [14]	86	42	44	Sunitinib	9	30	VEGF
		85	40	45	Sunitinib	21	51	
2013	Hosein [15]	19	9	10	Abraxane	7.3	1.7	SPARC
2014	Soares [16]	43	21	22	Capecitabine; docetaxel	5.3	3.7	TP
2014	Ban [17]	33	30	3	Belotaxel; belloxa	10.9	3.6	Double-strand breaks in DNA
2014	Borad [18]	69	40	29	TH-302 with gemcitabine; Gemcitabine	6.9	3.6	Severe hypoxia Intracellular reductases
		71	44	27	TH-303 with gemcitabine; gemcitabine	8.7	5.6	
		74	42	32	TH-304 with gemcitabine; gemcitabine	9.2	6	
2015	Phan [19]	32	22	10	Pazopanib hydrochloride	25	14.4	VEGF
		20	12	8	Pazopanib hydrochloride	18.5	12.2	
2019	Wang-Gillam [20]	151	87	64	MM-398	4.9	2.7	Topoisomerase I inhibitor
		149	81	68	5 Fluorouracil; leucovorin	4.2	1.6	
		117	69	48	MM-398; 5 fluorouracil; leucovorin	6.2	3.1	

Table 2.
Clinical trials with a successful outcome on pancreatic cancer.

Year	Author	N	M	F	Drug	OS	PFS	Biomarkers
2008	Spano [21]	69	35	34	Gemcitabine	5.6	3.7	VEGF
		34	16	18	Gemcitabine; AG-013736	6.9	4.2	
2015	Hobday [22]	58	29	29	Bevacizumab; temsirolimus	34	13.2	VEGF
2016	Stein [23]	37	21	16	MPC modified FOLFIRINOX	10.2	6.1	DPD
		31	20	11	LAPC modified FOLFIRINOX	26.6	17.8	

Table 3.
Clinical trial with neutral outcomes on pancreatic cancer.

5.2 Estimation of clinical trials with the neutral outcome on advanced pancreatic cancer

Here are three studies clarified neural results in OS and PFS result, ranged from 2008 to 2016, totally recruited 229 APC patients (121 male and 108 female). For details please see **Table 3**. Averagely the OS is 16.6 months and PFS is 9 months in neutral studies. For example, Jean in 2008 reported gemcitabine plus AG-013736 achieved better OS and PFS (6.9 and 4.2) than gemcitabine single used.

5.3 Estimation of clinical trials with the failed outcome on advanced pancreatic cancer

Regarding the failed outcomes, there are 14 studies ranged from 2011 to 2018, recruited 2448 APC patients (1385 male and 1063 female) for clinical trials. For details please see **Table 1**. Averagely the OS is 8.25 months and PFS is 4.39 months. It is evident that Faivre et al. in 2016 tested sunitinib malate to treat APC and achieved 38.6 months of OS and 12.6 months of PFS. However, Brian reported that hydroxychloroquine cures APC, unfortunately, there were 1.8 months both in OS and PFS negativity. Even though many combination tests, the benefit for APC patient is low.

6. Different perspectives on biomarkers

6.1 Vascular endothelial growth factor, VEGF

VEGF is a highly specific vascular endothelial cell mitogen and an angiogenic factor associated with platelet-derived growth factor (PDGF) structure. It is also known as vascular permeability factor (VPF), due to its permeabilization of blood vessels [24]. It is a subfamily of growth factors and belongs to a family of platelet-derived growth factors of cystine knot growth factor. VEGF is divided into the following groups: VEGF-A, VEGF-B, VEGF-C, VEGF-D, VEGF-E and placental growth factor. VEGF binds to three transmembrane receptors (VEGFR1, VEGFR2 and VEGFR3). This receptor initiates downstream signaling through intracellular tyrosine kinase activity [25]. In fact, VEGF family members are playing an important role in the physiological angiogenesis of adults. Like wound healing, ovulation and pregnancy [26].

Activation of the VEGF/VEGF receptor (VEGFR) axis may trigger multiple signaling networks. Consequently, this may lead to endothelial cell survival, mitosis, migration and differentiation, vascular permeability and mobilization of endothelial progenitor cells (EPCs) from the bone marrow into the peripheral circulation [27]. On ligand binding, VEGFR-2 dimerization results in kinase activation and autophosphorylation of tyrosine residues. Activation of PKC may stimulate the Raf/MEK/ERK pathway, which accelerates the cell proliferation. Ca^{2+} mobilization and PKC activation are playing the key role in signaling events for VEGF-A-induced vascular permeability through activation of endothelial nitric oxide synthase activity [28].

The sword has double sides. VEGF participates in the pathogenesis of cancer, proliferative retinopathy and rheumatoid arthritis [29]. Its antibodies have shown therapeutic potential to inhibit tumor growth in vivo by inhibiting tumor-induced angiogenesis [30]. VEGF overexpression is associated with a variety of tumor progression and poor prognosis, including colorectal cancer [31], pancreatic cancer [32], gastric cancer [33], breast cancer [34], lung cancer [35], prostate cancer [36] and melanoma [37]. This unique protein aids tumors grow and can be used for cancer treatment if used properly.

Early in 1971, Folkman first proposed the idea of angiogenesis. He believed that tumor growth and proliferation are closely related to angiogenesis and could be used as a targeted tumor therapy procedure [38]. Subsequently, countless scientists gathered in the field of VEGF to study the molecular mechanism of VEGF in tumor angiogenesis. They have also used it as a drug target to block the formation of blood vessels, thereby inhibiting tumor growth [39]. Studies have shown that the mechanism of anti-VEGF inhibitors may involve a variety of signaling pathways, such as FGF, D114, PGF/VEGFR1 and VEGF-C/VEGFR2. At least some of these pathways can increase the efficacy of VEGF inhibitors [40]. The anti-tumor drugs were developed with VEGF as the main target area. Like anti-VEGF humanized monoclonal antibody, VEGF-targeted antibody, protein kinase inhibitor and tumor vaccine [41, 42]. However, in the clinical application of anti-antigenic drugs, reliable biomarkers have not been found to screen the target population before patient improvement.

Our data disclosed that there were two studies reporting successful outcomes [14, 19], two studies reported neutral outcomes [21, 22] and four studies reported negative outcomes [43–46]. The results from the above eight trials remain controversial.

Regarding successful outcomes, Raymond et al. found that neuroendocrine tumors may be particularly sensitive to the combined inhibition of VEGFR and PDGFR. As for the neutral outcomes [14], Spano et al. used the gemcitabine + axitinib to treat the APC [21]. However, results differ from the results of Phase III trials in which erlotinib + gemcitabine confers the greatest survival advantage for patients with ECOG status 2 and metastatic disease, it possibly due to the mechanism of action between different EGFR and VEGFR inhibitors. Moreover, Hobday et al. found that the median PFS in the gefitinib trial was only 3.7 months which was even lower than the placebo group in the phase III trial [22].

With respect to the failed outcomes, Kindler et al. found that the effect of axitinib and gemcitabine on APC was limited to improve the survival period in patients with locally APC [43]. In fact, the results may be related to the gene locus of the VEGF receptor 1 tyrosine kinase domain. Furthermore, Ropugier et al. found that PFS was not significantly improved between the treatment arms. It indicates that blocking the VEGF/VEGFR axis does not lead to the survival of a patient with APC [45]. Nooan et al. study shows that pelareorep combination chemotherapy is not a sufficient solution to overcome the severe immunosuppression prevalent in PCA patients [46].

6.2 Epidermal growth factor receptor, EGFR

EGFR is one of the transmembrane receptors of epidermal growth factor family members of extracellular protein ligands. Its main function is to regulate various cellular functions including proliferation, movement and differentiation. Its mechanism can be described as the binding of the ligand to EGFR leading to dimerization followed by autophosphorylation of EGFR and activation of downstream signaling pathways. Activation of EGFR triggers multiple signal cascades within the cell, ultimately leading to gene transcription and biological responses [47]. Recently, studies have shown that dimerization occurs even in the absence of ligands, particularly when EGFR is overexpressed, possibly limited to a subset of dimers. Moreover, overexpressed EGFR can dimerize and become tyrosine phosphorylated without ligand [48].

EGFR signal transduction pathway can directly participate in tumor pathogenesis and progression [49]. EGFR overexpression plays a major role in carcinogenesis in cancer development [50]. Overexpression of EGFR accounts for 90% in pancreatic cancer cells [51]. Specifically, the aberrant activity of EGFR may impact the development and growth of tumor cells [52].

Mutation of EGFR may induce the resistance of tyrosine kinase inhibitors (TKIs) [53]. Notably, in tumor angiogenesis, vascular endothelial growth factor receptor-2 (VEGFR-2) plays a key role, and inhibition of VEGFR-2 signaling pathway has become an attractive cancer treatment method [54]. The binding of VEGF to VEGFR-2 stimulates the signaling pathway (PI3K/Akt, p38MAPK) that mediates several cellular functions. Besides, glycoproteins, EGFR and VEGFR-2 are in close correlation. Inhibition of EGFR can also reduce VEGF expression, while VEGFR-2 targeting can enhance the anticancer activity of EGFR inhibitors. Therefore, the dual inhibition treatment of EGFR and VEGFR-2 has a good effect and represents a promising cancer treatment. Recently, several EGFR/VEGFR-2 dual inhibitors have been discovered, such as vandetanib showing effective inhibitory activity on EGFR and VEGFR-2 [55].

A receptor tyrosine kinase is associated with cell proliferation and survival. Epidermal Growth Factor Receptor, EGFR, is overactive in many epithelial-derived tumors. It has been reported that EGFR is not related to its kinase activity, but rather maintains basal intracellular glucose levels to prevent autophagic death of cells. Despite the presence of chemotherapeutic drugs and tyrosine kinase inhibitors, this function of EGFR allows tumor cells to have higher viability [56]. EGFR inhibitors for cancer therapy are rapidly evolving in the broad context of cancer therapy, and in those patients achieving significant tumor response to EGFR inhibitors. Most patients will eventually exhibit disease progression, suggesting acquired resistance. This reminds us that increasing our ability to recognize tumors that depend on EGFR signaling growth is critical for the best choice of treating patients [57].

Unfortunately, two clinical trials showed that the results failed via EGFR. Studies by Ko et al. showed that subjects treated by cetuximab, bevacizumab and gemcitabine had 5.41 months in OS and 4.17 months in PFS. Propper et al. in 2014 tested Erlotinib to treat APC, and only achieved 4.0 months of OS and 1.5 months of PFS, **Table 4** [44, 58]. Ko reported the incidence of severe (grades 3–5) toxicity, comparable to the use of gemcitabine as a single agent in this patient population which may reflect a relatively short duration of treatment due to lack of efficacy. Moreover, it is difficult to explain the quality of life analysis based on the number of patients completing the series of questionnaires and the overall time the patients stayed in the study [44]. Propper concluded that there is limited evidence to support the use of predictive biomarkers for patients with pancreatic cancer who could benefit from targeted therapies [58].

6.3 Kirsten rat sarcoma viral oncogene homolog, KRAS

KRAS protein plays a key role in human cancer but has not yet succumbed to therapeutic attacks [59]. The search is now focused on targeting alternative pathways that are activated in mtKRAS cells, to circumvent or prevent drug resistance [60].

There are currently no therapeutic interventions for KRAS. Pharmacological agents that are speculated to inhibit KRAS include farnesyltransferase inhibitors that block the binding of KRAS to the cell membrane. These drugs have failed in clinical studies. Antisense oligonucleotides and engineered microRNAs (miRNAs) have been used as an alternative to targeted mutations in KRAS without disrupting

Year	Author	N	M	F	Drug	OS	PFS	Biomarkers
2011	Kindler [43]	314	191	123	Gemcitabine; AG-013736	8.5	4.4	VEGF
		316	188	128	Gemcitabine; placebo	8.3	4.4	
2012	Ko [44]	29	18	11	Cetuximab; bevacizumab gemcitabine	5.41	4.17	EGFR VEGF
		29	14	15	Cetuximab; bevacizumab	3.55	1.91	
2013	Rougier [45]	275	157	118	Placebo; gemcitabine	7.8	3.7	VEGF
		271	160	111	Aflibercept; gemcitabine	6.5	3.7	
2013	Wu [61]	30	16	14	Etanercept; gemcitabine	5.43	0.3	TNF-α
		8	3	5	Gemcitabine	8.1	1.8	
2014	Propper [58]	104	59	45	Erlotinib	4.0	1.5	EGFR
		103	59	44	Placebo	3.1	1.5	
2014	Infante [62]	80	39	41	Gemcitabine; GSK1120212	8.4	16.1	cfDNA
		80	46	34	Placebo; gemcitabine	6.7	15.1	
2014	Wolpin [63]	10	5	5	Hydroxychloroquine 400 mg	1.8	1.8	LC3-II
		10	6	4	Hydroxychloroquine 600 mg	3.0	1.6	
2015	Catenacci [64]	53	27	26	Gemcitabine hydrochloride; Placebo	6.1	2.5	SHH
		53	31	22	Gemcitabine hydrochloride; vismodegib	6.9	4.0	
2016	Noonan [46]	36	22	14	wild-type reovirus; carboplatin; paclitaxel	7.31	4.94	VEGF; IL-6; IL-8
		37	19	18	Carboplatin; paclitaxel	8.77	5.2	
2017	Chung [65]	62	22	40	Fluorouracil; oxaliplatin	6.7	2.0	KRAS protein
		58	35	23	Akt inhibitor MK2206; selumetinib	3.9	1.9	
2017	Faivre [66]	86	42	44	Sunitinib malate	38.6	12.6	VEGF; PDGF
		85	40	45	Placebo	29.1	5.8	
2017	Ko [67]	66	38	28	OGX-427	6.9	3.8	Hsp27
		66	37	29	Placebo	5.3	2.7	
2017	Laquente [68]	65	42	23	LY2603618; gemcitabine	7.8	3.5	CHK1
		34	20	14	Gemcitabine	8.3	5.6	
2018	Van Cutsem [69]	44	22	22	Gemcitabine; placebo	7.6	2.8	ERK 1/2
		44	27	17	Gemcitabine; pimasertib	7.3	3.7	

Table 4.
Clinical trial failed outcome on pancreatic cancer.

the expression of non-mutant KRAS and have achieved some success in preclinical trials [70].

In recent years, many studies have suggested that the oncogene KRAS plays a major role in controlling cancer metabolism by coordinating multiple metabolic changes [71]. Furthermore, combined inhibition of therapeutic effects and feedback pathways is promising in KRAS mutant cancers. Moreover, it is unclear what specific pathways should be used to optimize treatment response [72].

Unfortunately, Chung et al. tested pharmaceutical target via KRAS protein, whereas the result was unsuccessful. The results showed that the OS and PFS of patients treated by Akt Inhibitor MK2206 and selumetinib were 3.9 and 1.9 months, respectively, see **Table 4** [65]. The results indicated that the strategy of utilizing two or more kinase inhibitors is subject to the challenge of toxicity overlap. These toxicities will significantly block the delivery of effective inhibitory amounts of both drugs in vivo. However, a major disadvantage factor is the delay in toxicity-related treatment and the frequency of dose reduction in the experimental group through damaging sustained signal suppression [65].

7. Conclusion

APC reserves unpredictable mechanisms to maintain a highly resistant phenotype. The genetic and epigenetic alterations of the APC lead to the resistance of the chemotherapy.

Nowadays, many biomarkers have been on board to improve the clinical treatment outcome of advanced pancreatic cancer. Although these successful biomarkers have provided notable therapeutic effects on advanced pancreatic cancer, the outcomes remain unsatisfactory to the patients and health providers. With the development of the biology of advanced pancreatic cancer, we now expect better biomarkers and conduct therapy by unveiling the tumor microenvironment and the mechanism of the mutations (**Figure 1**).

We can assume that with the development of truly effective treatments and clinically useful markers for early detection of the disease, better combination of markers to advanced pancreatic cancer. In the meanwhile, researchers are trying to detect magnificently predictive biomarkers to decide the treatment strategy and permit practitioners to adequately evaluate and propose individualized treatment protocols which would give a greater survival rate.

Clearly, there is a need to better understand the underlying signaling networks that drive pancreatic cancer progression and potential escape mechanisms. In addition, it is necessary to improve the role of preclinical models of pancreatic cancer

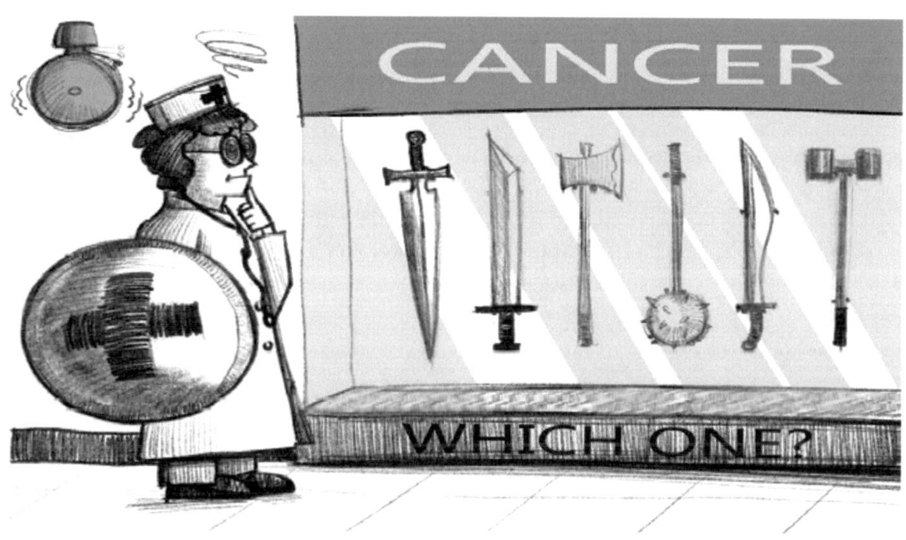

Figure 1.
Difficulties in decision making both for R&D and doctors.

and the optimal transformation of preclinical success into experimental design. The genetic and proteomic technologies show great potential to detect the novel biomarkers in cancer research. We place great expectations on these technologies to personalize treatment for advanced pancreatic cancer patients.

Acknowledgements

This work was supported by the Chengdu Medical College Natural Science Foundation (CYZ18-08, CYZ18-20, CYZ18-33), the Sichuan Provincial Education Department (17ZA0134), the Sichuan Medical Association (S18023), and Sichuan undergraduate innovation and startup program funding support (S201913705080, S201913705130, S201913705059).

Authors' contribution

XF developed the general idea and drafted the manuscript with CJ; YLQ and DYX searched the reference, HK sort the clinical trials data, PTT and ZS participated in drafting process and double check the data; LFF drew the figure; GM proofread the manuscript and ensure the general quality.

Competing interests

The authors declare that they have no competing interests.

Ethics statement

Not applicable.

Consent for publication

Not applicable.

Availability of data and material

All data will be made available upon reasonable request.

Author details

Jie Chen[1,2†], Liqiong Yang[3†], Yuxi Duan[3†], Tinging Pu[3], Sha Zheng[3], Fangfang Liu[4], Kun Huang[5], Greg Mirt[6] and Fan Xu[7*]

1 School of Chinese Medicine, Li Ka Shing Faculty of Medicine, The University of Hong Kong, Hong Kong, China

2 Department of Orthopedics, Shanghai Institute of Traumatology and Orthopedics, Ruijin Hospital, Shanghai Jiaotong University School of Medicine, Shanghai, China

3 School of Pharmacy, Chengdu Medical College, Sichuan, China

4 Art College, Southwest Minzu University, Chengdu, Sichuan, China

5 Department of Software, Chengdu TME Co., Ltd, China

6 Neuro Occupational Activity Centre Novo Mesto, Slovenia

7 Department of Public Health, Chengdu Medical College, Sichuan, China

*Address all correspondence to: xufan@cmc.edu.cn

† These authors contributed equally.

IntechOpen

© 2019 The Author(s). Licensee IntechOpen. This chapter is distributed under the terms of the Creative Commons Attribution License (http://creativecommons.org/licenses/by/3.0), which permits unrestricted use, distribution, and reproduction in any medium, provided the original work is properly cited. CC BY

References

[1] Kamisawa T, Wood LD, Itoi T, et al. Pancreatic cancer. Lancet. 2016;**388**: 73-85

[2] Bray F, Ferlay J, Soerjomataram I, et al. Global cancer statistics 2018: GLOBOCAN estimates of incidence and mortality worldwide for 36 cancers in 185 countries. CA: A Cancer Journal for Clinicians. 2018;**68**:394-424

[3] Ferlay J, Colombet M, Soerjomataram I, et al. Estimating the global cancer incidence and mortality in 2018: GLOBOCAN sources and methods. International Journal of Cancer. 2019;**144**:1941-1953

[4] Chen J, Chen L, Yu J, et al. Metaanalysis of current chemotherapy regimens in advanced pancreatic cancer to prolong survival and reduce treatmentassociated toxicities. Molecular Medicine Reports. 2019;**19**: 477-489

[5] Drews J. Paul Ehrlich: magister mundi. Nature Reviews. Drug Discovery. 2004;**3**:797-801

[6] Prindle MJ, Fox EJ, Loeb LA. The mutator phenotype in cancer: Molecular mechanisms and targeting strategies. Current Drug Targets. 2010;**11**: 1296-1303

[7] Andrade EL, Bento AF, Cavalli J, et al. Non-clinical studies required for new drug development - part I: Early in silico and in vitro studies, new target discovery and validation, proof of principles and robustness of animal studies. Brazilian Journal of Medical and Biological Research. 2016;**49**:e5644

[8] Katara P. Role of bioinformatics and pharmacogenomics in drug discovery and development process. Network Modeling and Analysis in Health Informatics and Bioinformatics. 2013;**2**: 225-230

[9] Xia HJ, Chen CS. Progress of non-human primate animal models of cancers. Dongwuxue Yanjiu. 2011;**32**: 70-80

[10] Ballman KV. Introduction to clinical trials, clinical trial designs, and statistical terminology used for predictive biomarker research and validation. In: Badve S, Kumar GL, editors. Predictive Biomarkers in Oncology: Applications in Precision Medicine. Cham: Springer International Publishing; 2019. pp. 19-36

[11] Bharali D, Banerjee BD, Bharadwaj M, et al. Expression analysis of MicroRNA-21 and MicroRNA-122 in hepatocellular carcinoma. Journal of Clinical and Experimental Hepatology. 2019;**9**:294-301

[12] Hill ME, Li X, Kim S, et al. A phase I study of the biomodulation of capecitabine by docetaxel and gemcitabine (mGTX) in previously untreated patients with metastatic adenocarcinoma of the pancreas. Cancer Chemotherapy and Pharmacology. 2011; **67**:511-517

[13] Lutz E, Yeo CJ, Lillemoe KD, et al. A lethally irradiated allogeneic granulocyte-macrophage colony stimulating factor-secreting tumor vaccine for pancreatic adenocarcinoma. A phase II trial of safety, efficacy, and immune activation. Annals of Surgery. 2011;**253**:328-335

[14] Raymond E, Dahan L, Raoul JL, et al. Sunitinib malate for the treatment of pancreatic neuroendocrine tumors. The New England Journal of Medicine. 2011;**364**:501-513

[15] Hosein PJ, de Lima Lopes G Jr, Pastorini VH, et al. A phase II trial of nab-paclitaxel as second-line therapy in patients with advanced pancreatic

cancer. American Journal of Clinical Oncology. 2013;**36**:151-156

[16] Soares HP, Bayraktar S, Blaya M, et al. A phase II study of capecitabine plus docetaxel in gemcitabine-pretreated metastatic pancreatic cancer patients: CapTere. Cancer Chemotherapy and Pharmacology. 2014;**73**:839-845

[17] Ban H, Kim KS, Oh IJ, et al. Efficacy and safety of docetaxel plus oxaliplatin as a first-line chemotherapy in patients with advanced or metastatic non-small cell lung cancer. Thoracic Cancer. 2014; **5**:525-529

[18] Borad MJ, Reddy SG, Bahary N, et al. Randomized phase II trial of gemcitabine plus TH-302 versus gemcitabine in patients with advanced pancreatic cancer. Journal of Clinical Oncology. 2015;**33**: 1475-1481

[19] Phan AT, Halperin DM, Chan JA, et al. Pazopanib and depot octreotide in advanced, well-differentiated neuroendocrine tumours: A multicentre, single-group, phase 2 study. The Lancet Oncology. 2015;**16**:695-703

[20] Wang-Gillam A, Hubner RA, Siveke JT, et al. NAPOLI-1 phase 3 study of liposomal irinotecan in metastatic pancreatic cancer: Final overall survival analysis and characteristics of long-term survivors. European Journal of Cancer. 2019;**108**:78-87

[21] Spano JP, Chodkiewicz C, Maurel J, et al. Efficacy of gemcitabine plus axitinib compared with gemcitabine alone in patients with advanced pancreatic cancer: An open-label randomised phase II study. Lancet. 2008;**371**:2101-2108

[22] Hobday TJ, Qin R, Reidy-Lagunes D, et al. Multicenter phase II trial of temsirolimus and bevacizumab in pancreatic neuroendocrine tumors. Journal of Clinical Oncology. 2015;**33**: 1551-1556

[23] Stein SM, James ES, Deng Y, et al. Final analysis of a phase II study of modified FOLFIRINOX in locally advanced and metastatic pancreatic cancer. British Journal of Cancer. 2016; **114**:737-743

[24] Neufeld G, Tessler S, Gitay-Goren H, et al. Vascular endothelial growth factor and its receptors. Progress in Growth Factor Research. 1994;**5**:89-97

[25] Stewart W, Vascular Endothelial M. Growth factor (VEGF) biochemistry and development of inhibitory drugs. Current Drug Therapy. 2012;**7**:80-89

[26] Hicklin DJ, Ellis LM. Role of the vascular endothelial growth factor pathway in tumor growth and angiogenesis. Journal of Clinical Oncology. 2005;**23**:1011-1027

[27] Koch S, Claesson-Welsh L. Signal transduction by vascular endothelial growth factor receptors. Cold Spring Harbor Perspectives in Medicine. 2012; **2**:a006502-a006502

[28] Cross MJ, Dixelius J, Matsumoto T, et al. VEGF-receptor signal transduction. Trends in Biochemical Sciences. 2003;**28**:488-494

[29] Aiello LP, Avery RL, Arrigg PG, et al. Vascular endothelial growth factor in ocular fluid of patients with diabetic retinopathy and other retinal disorders. The New England Journal of Medicine. 1994;**331**:1480-1487

[30] Kim KJ, Li B, Winer J, et al. Inhibition of vascular endothelial growth factor-induced angiogenesis suppresses tumour growth in vivo. Nature. 1993;**362**:841-844

[31] Lee JC, Chow NH, Wang ST, et al. Prognostic value of vascular endothelial growth factor expression in colorectal

cancer patients. European Journal of Cancer. 2000;**36**:748-753

[32] Fujimoto K, Hosotani R, Wada M, et al. Expression of two angiogenic factors, vascular endothelial growth factor and platelet-derived endothelial cell growth factor in human pancreatic cancer, and its relationship to angiogenesis. European Journal of Cancer. 1998;**34**:1439-1447

[33] Takahashi Y, Cleary KR, Mai M, et al. Significance of vessel count and vascular endothelial growth factor and its receptor (KDR) in intestinal-type gastric cancer. Clinical Cancer Research. 1996;**2**:1679-1684

[34] Berns EM, Klijn JG, Look MP, et al. Combined vascular endothelial growth factor and TP53 status predicts poor response to tamoxifen therapy in estrogen receptor-positive advanced breast cancer. Clinical Cancer Research. 2003;**9**:1253-1258

[35] Fontanini G, Lucchi M, Vignati S, et al. Angiogenesis as a prognostic indicator of survival in non-small-cell lung carcinoma: A prospective study. Journal of the National Cancer Institute. 1997;**89**:881-886

[36] George DJ, Halabi S, Shepard TF, et al. Prognostic significance of plasma vascular endothelial growth factor levels in patients with hormone-refractory prostate cancer treated on cancer and leukemia group B 9480. Clinical Cancer Research. 2001;**7**: 1932-1936

[37] Gorski DH, Leal AD, Goydos JS. Differential expression of vascular endothelial growth factor-a isoforms at different stages of melanoma progression. Journal of the American College of Surgeons. 2003;**197**:408-418

[38] Folkman J. Tumor angiogenesis: Therapeutic implications. The New England Journal of Medicine. 1971;**285**: 1182-1186

[39] Chou HF, Lin MF, Chen CY, et al. Three-dimensional brain images in preterm children with periventricular leukomalacia. Pediatrics and Neonatology. 2012;**53**:45-48

[40] Ferrara N. Pathways mediating VEGF-independent tumor angiogenesis. Cytokine & Growth Factor Reviews. 2010;**21**:21-26

[41] Semenza GL. Defining the role of hypoxia-inducible factor 1 in cancer biology and therapeutics. Oncogene. 2010;**29**:625-634

[42] Hoeben A, Landuyt B, Highley MS, et al. Vascular Endothelial growth factor and angiogenesis. Pharmacological Reviews. 2004;**56**:549

[43] Kindler HL, Ioka T, Richel DJ, et al. Axitinib plus gemcitabine versus placebo plus gemcitabine in patients with advanced pancreatic adenocarcinoma: A double-blind randomised phase 3 study. The Lancet Oncology. 2011;**12**:256-262

[44] Ko AH, Youssoufian H, Gurtler J, et al. A phase II randomized study of cetuximab and bevacizumab alone or in combination with gemcitabine as first-line therapy for metastatic pancreatic adenocarcinoma. Investigational New Drugs. 2012;**30**:1597-1606

[45] Rougier P, Riess H, Manges R, et al. Randomised, placebo-controlled, double-blind, parallel-group phase III study evaluating aflibercept in patients receiving first-line treatment with gemcitabine for metastatic pancreatic cancer. European Journal of Cancer. 2013;**49**:2633-2642

[46] Noonan AM, Farren MR, Geyer SM, et al. Randomized phase 2 trial of the oncolytic virus Pelareorep (Reolysin) in upfront treatment of metastatic pancreatic adenocarcinoma. Molecular Therapy. 2016;**24**:1150-1158

[47] Guo G, Gong K, Wohlfeld B, et al. Ligand-independent EGFR signaling. Cancer Research. 2015;**75**:3436-3441

[48] Chung I, Akita R, Vandlen R, et al. Spatial control of EGF receptor activation by reversible dimerization on living cells. Nature. 2010;**464**:783-787

[49] Habban Akhter M, Sateesh Madhav N, Ahmad J. Epidermal growth factor receptor based active targeting: A paradigm shift towards advance tumor therapy. Artificial Cells, Nanomedicine, and Biotechnology. 2018;**46**:1188-1198

[50] Chakraborty S, Li L, Puliyappadamba VT, et al. Constitutive and ligand-induced EGFR signalling triggers distinct and mutually exclusive downstream signalling networks. Nature Communications. 2014;**5**:5811

[51] Tuan Anh HL, Tran PT, Thao DT, et al. Degalactotigonin, a steroidal glycoside from *Solanum nigrum*, induces apoptosis and cell cycle arrest via inhibiting the EGFR signaling pathways in pancreatic cancer cells. BioMed Research International. 2018;**2018**: 3120972

[52] Seshacharyulu P, Ponnusamy MP, Haridas D, et al. Targeting the EGFR signaling pathway in cancer therapy. Expert Opinion on Therapeutic Targets. 2012;**16**:15-31

[53] Wu K, Guo C, Li R. Clinical characterization of icotinib-induced chemoresistance in erlotinib-treated lung adenocarcinoma patient with EGFR mutations: A case report. Medicine (Baltimore). 2019;**98**:e15489

[54] Sun W, Hu S, Fang S, et al. Design, synthesis and biological evaluation of pyrimidine-based derivatives as VEGFR-2 tyrosine kinase inhibitors. Bioorganic Chemistry. 2018;**78**:393-405

[55] Mghwary AE, Gedawy EM, Kamal AM, et al. Novel thienopyrimidine derivatives as dual EGFR and VEGFR-2 inhibitors: Design, synthesis, anticancer activity and effect on cell cycle profile. Journal of Enzyme Inhibition and Medicinal Chemistry. 2019;**34**:838-852

[56] Weihua Z, Tsan R, Huang WC, et al. Survival of cancer cells is maintained by EGFR independent of its kinase activity. Cancer Cell. 2008;**13**:385-393

[57] Wheeler DL, Dunn EF, Harari PM. Understanding resistance to EGFR inhibitors-impact on future treatment strategies. Nature Reviews. Clinical Oncology. 2010;**7**:493-507

[58] Propper D, Davidenko I, Bridgewater J, et al. Phase II, randomized, biomarker identification trial (MARK) for erlotinib in patients with advanced pancreatic carcinoma. Annals of Oncology. 2014;**25**:1384-1390

[59] McCormick F. KRAS as a therapeutic target. Clinical Cancer Research. 2015;**21**:1797-1801

[60] Charitou T, Srihari S, Lynn MA, et al. Transcriptional and metabolic rewiring of colorectal cancer cells expressing the oncogenic KRAS(G13D) mutation. British Journal of Cancer. 2019;**121**:37-50

[61] Wu C, Fernandez SA, Criswell T, et al. Disrupting cytokine signaling in pancreatic cancer: A phase I/II study of etanercept in combination with gemcitabine in patients with advanced disease. Pancreas. 2013;**42**:813-818

[62] Infante JR, Somer BG, Park JO, et al. A randomised, double-blind, placebo-controlled trial of trametinib, an oral MEK inhibitor, in combination with gemcitabine for patients with untreated metastatic adenocarcinoma of the pancreas. European Journal of Cancer. 2014;**50**:2072-2081

[63] Wolpin BM, Rubinson DA, Wang X, et al. Phase II and pharmacodynamic

study of autophagy inhibition using hydroxychloroquine in patients with metastatic pancreatic adenocarcinoma. The Oncologist. 2014;**19**:637-638

[64] Catenacci DV, Junttila MR, Karrison T, et al. Randomized phase Ib/II study of gemcitabine plus placebo or vismodegib, a hedgehog pathway inhibitor, in patients with metastatic pancreatic cancer. Journal of Clinical Oncology. 2015;**33**: 4284-4292

[65] Chung V, McDonough S, Philip PA, et al. Effect of selumetinib and MK-2206 vs oxaliplatin and fluorouracil in patients with metastatic pancreatic cancer after prior therapy: SWOG S1115 study randomized clinical trial. JAMA Oncology. 2017;**3**:516-522

[66] Faivre S, Niccoli P, Castellano D, et al. Sunitinib in pancreatic neuroendocrine tumors: Updated progression-free survival and final overall survival from a phase III randomized study. Annals of Oncology. 2017;**28**:339-343

[67] Ko AH, Murphy PB, Peyton JD, et al. A randomized, double-blinded, phase II trial of gemcitabine and nab-paclitaxel plus apatorsen or placebo in patients with metastatic pancreatic cancer: The RAINIER trial. The Oncologist. 2017;**22**:1427-e1129

[68] Laquente B, Lopez-Martin J, Richards D, et al. A phase II study to evaluate LY2603618 in combination with gemcitabine in pancreatic cancer patients. BMC Cancer. 2017;**17**:137

[69] Van Cutsem E, Hidalgo M, Canon JL, et al. Phase I/II trial of pimasertib plus gemcitabine in patients with metastatic pancreatic cancer. International Journal of Cancer. 2018; **143**:2053-2064

[70] Gober MK, Flight RM, Lambert J, et al. Deregulation of a network of mRNA and miRNA genes reveals that CK2 and MEK inhibitors may synergize to induce apoptosis KRAS-active NSCLC. Cancer Informatics. 2019;**18**: 1176935119843507

[71] Kawada K, Toda K, Sakai Y. Targeting metabolic reprogramming in KRAS-driven cancers. International Journal of Clinical Oncology. 2017;**22**: 651-659

[72] Anderson GR, Winter PS, Lin KH, et al. A landscape of therapeutic cooperativity in KRAS mutant cancers reveals principles for controlling tumor evolution. Cell Reports. 2017;**20**: 999-1015

Section 2

Clinical Challenges

Chapter 6

An Overview of Pediatric CNS Malignancies

Neha Sharma and Deepti Sharma

Abstract

Central nervous system tumours are the most common solid tumours and second most common malignancy in pediatric age group. They are the leading cause of cancer related morbidity and mortality. It accounts for 3.5% of all deaths in the 1–14 years age group. Childhood central nervous system (CNS) tumors differ significantly from adult brain tumors in reference to their sites of origin, clinical presentation, tendency to disseminate early, histological features and their biological behaviour. Supratentorial tumors are more common in infants and children up to 3 years of age and again after age 10, whereas between ages 4 and 10 infratentorial tumors are more common. The initial workup of patients with brain tumors must include a complete history, physical examination, imaging and biopsy confirmation of primary. The management of pediatric brain tumours is important due to their high incidence, challenging aspects of surgery and high mortality. Many CNS malignancies, which were once universally fatal are now curable with multimodality approaches that integrate surgery, chemotherapy and radiotherapy. In this chapter, we will discuss these issues in detail and summarize the ongoing efforts to reduce the morbidity and mortality in pediatric CNS tumours.

Keywords: CNS, pediatric, adjuvant, radiation therapy

1. Overview

Tumors of the central nervous system are the most common solid tumors in the pediatric age group and the second most common childhood malignancy. They are the leading cause of morbidity and mortality associated with cancer. Although it affects all ages, the incidence peaks among children between the ages of 3 and 7. In adults and older children, most tumours are supratentorial in location while in young children they are more commonly infratentorial in location [1].

2. Incidence

The incidence of childhood CNS tumor varies from 1.12 to 5.14 cases per 100,000 individuals [2]. Based upon data from the Central Brain Tumor Registry of the United States (CBTRUS), the estimated incidence of primary non-malignant and malignant CNS tumors for children and adolescents up to 19 years of age was 7.18 cases per 100,000 person-year in 2016 [3]. More than 100 different

Location	Tumor type	Relative frequency (%) in 0–17 years old
Supratentorial	Pilocytic astrocytoma	23.5
	Fibrillary astrocytoma	5
	Gangliogangl ioma	2.5
	Dysembryoplastic neuroepithelial tumor	0.6
	Desmoplastic infantile ganglioglioma	0.6
	Choroid plexus papilloma	0.9
	Ependymoma	3.8
	Anaplastic ependymoma	3.8
	Anaplastic astrocytoma	7.2
	Glioblastoma	7.2
	Supratentorial PNET	1.9
	Choroid plexus carcinoma	0.6
Posterior fossa	Medulloblastoma	16.3
	ATRT	1.3
	Pilocytic astrocytoma	23.5
	Ependymoma	3.8
	Brainstem glioma	10–20
Pineal tumours	Germ cell tumour	2.5
	Pineal parenchymal tumour	1.9
Suprasellar	Craniopharyngioma	5.6
	Optic hypothalamic glioma	3–6

Table 1.
Common brain tumor types with location and frequency [5].

histological subtypes of CNS tumours are recognized but their incidence varies with age. Incidence in Africa is around 11 per 10,00,000 and in Japan and Europe it ranges from 20 to 30 per 1,000,000. The male to female ratio is 1.25:1, as slightly higher frequency of medulloblastoma and CNS germinoma is seen in boys [4]. The most common histological subtypes along with location are mentioned below (**Table 1**).

3. Etiology and pathogenesis

Development of brain tumours occurs as a consequence of cellular genetic alterations that allow them to evade normal regulatory mechanisms and destruction by the immune system. These changes may be caused by an inherited or acquired (chemical, physical or biological neuro-carcinogens) cause. Overall, only a very small percentage of brain tumors can be ascribed to the effect of inherited inclination (**Table 2**). The different environmental factors involved and alleged typically involve ionizing radiation, non-ionizing radiation, N-nitroso compounds, viral infections (JC virus, cytomegalovirus, HIV, SV-40, varicella-zoster, chicken pox) and head injury [6].

Syndrome	Gene locus	Gene	Type of CNS tumour
NF type 1	17q11	NF1	Neurofibroma, meningioma, optic nerve glioma
NF2	22q12	NF2	Meningioma, schwannoma
TS	9q34, 16p13	TSc1/TSC2	SEGA
VHL	3p35	VHL	Haemangioblastoma
Li-Fraumani	17q13	p53	Glioma
Gorlin's syndrome	9q31		PNET

Table 2.
CNS tumour along with gene involved.

4. Pathology and classification

Astrocytic tumors

- subependymal giant cell astrocytoma
- pilocytic astrocytoma
- Pilomyxoid astrocytoma
- diffuse astrocytoma
- pleomorphic xanthoastrocytoma
- anaplastic astrocytoma
- glioblastoma
- giant cell glioblastoma
- gliosarcoma

Oligodendroglial tumors

- oligodendroglioma
- anaplastic oligodendroglioma

Oligoastrocytic tumors

- oligoastrocytoma
- anaplastic oligoastrocytoma

Ependymal tumors

- subependymoma

- myxopapillary ependymoma
- ependymoma
- anaplastic epedymoma

Choroid plexus tumors

- choroid plexus papilloma
- atypical choroid plexus papilloma
- choroid plexus carcinoma

Other neuroepithelial tumors

- astroblastoma
- angiocentric glioma
- chordoid glioma of the third ventricle

Neuronal and mixed neuronal-glial tumors

- gangliocytoma
- ganglioglioma
- Anplastic ganglioglioma
- desmoplastic infantile astrocytoma and ganglioglioma
- dysembryplastic neuroepithelial tumor
- central neurocytoma
- extraventricular neurocytoma
- cerebellar liponeurocytoma
- paraganglioma of the spinal cord
- papillary glioneuronal tumor
- Rosette-forming glioneuronal tumor of the fourth ventricle

Pineal tumors

- pineocytoma
- pineal parenchymal tumor of intermediate differentiation

- pineoblastoma
- papillary tumor of the pineal region

Embryonal tumors

- medulloblastoma
- CNS primitive neuroectodermal tumors
- atypical teratoid/rhabdoid tumor

Tumors of cranial and paraspinal nerves

- Schwannoma
- neurofibroma
- perineuroma
- malignant peripheral nerve sheath tumors

Meningeal tumors

- tumors of meningothelial cells
- mesenchymal tumors
- primary melanocytic lesions
- other neoplasms related to the meninges
- hemangioblastoma

Lymphoma and hematopoietic neoplasms

- malignant lymphoma
- plasmacytoma
- granulocytic sarcoma

Germ cell tumors

- germinoma
- embryonal carcinoma
- yolk-sac tumors
- choriocarcinoma

- teratoma
- mixed germ cell tumor

Tumors of the sellar region

- craniopharyngioma
- granular cell tumor of the neurohypophysis
- pituicytoma
- spindle cell oncocytoma of the adenohypophysis

Metastatic tumors
Modified from the WHO Classification of Tumors of the CNS, 2007 [7].

5. Clinical manifestations

The most common presenting symptoms of pediatric brain tumours are due to increased intracranial pressure. Headache and vomiting are two well-known symptoms associated with elevated intracranial pressure. Other signs, which reflect the increase in intracranial pressure, include drowsiness, confusion, nausea, sixth nerve palsy, papilledema, generalized seizures, and cognitive impairment. Focal signs and symptoms reflect the effect of the tumor on specific structures [8].

6. Radiological diagnosis

The features that play an important role in establishing the diagnosis are the age of the patient, location of the tumor and the imaging characteristics. Supratentorial tumors are more common in neonates and infants up to 2 years old, whereas infratentorial tumors are more common in children older than 2 years. Although some tumors may be found both supra- and infratentorially. Tumors that are considered mostly supratentorial and intraaxial include astrocytomas, such as diffuse astrocytoma, anaplastic astrocytoma, pleomorphic xanthoastrocytoma (PXA), subependymal giant cell astrocytoma (SEGA), and glioblastoma multi-forme (GBM); oligodendrocytoma; primitive neuroectodermal tumor (PNET); dysembryo-plastic neuroepithelial tumor (DNET); ganglioglioma; and desmoplastic infantile ganglioglioma. Some supratentorial extraaxial masses include arachnoid cysts, pineal region masses, and choroid plexus tumors.

Imaging is an important aspect in the management of patients with brain tumors. Imaging workup is largely based upon CT and MRI of the lesion. The technical development of CT and MRI methods has greatly enhanced brain tumor detection and sophisticated neuroimaging offers extra data by determining the metabolism and physiology of these lesions, which helps to diagnose and monitor brain neoplasms [9].

7. Computed tomography (CT)

CT scan plays an important role in establishing diagnosis of brain tumours. It can detect both blood and calcification. But some tumors, particularly tumors of the brainstem, cerebellum, and suprasellar region as well as infiltrative tumors of the white matter, can be missed on CT neuroimaging [10].

7.1 MRI

It is the standard of care in children for imaging of suspected brain tumours.

The most useful imaging studies are T1-weighted sagittal images, gadolinium (Gd)-enhanced and unenhanced T1 axial images, T2-weighted axial images, and fluid-attenuated inversion recovery (FLAIR) sequences.

T1 images usually are better at demonstrating anatomy and areas of contrast enhancement. T2 and FLAIR images are more sensitive for detecting edema and infiltrative tumor.

7.2 Perfusion MRI

It plays an important role In differentiating low-grade tumors from high-grade tumors. It evaluates several hemodynamic parameters including cerebral blood volume (CBV), cerebral blood flow (CBF), and mean transit time (MTT); however, CBV has been shown to be the most useful parameter for the evaluation of intracranial masses [11].

7.3 Functional MRI

It detects functional areas of the brain by identifying areas of brain activation which have increased blood flow and changes in cerebral metabolism. It is used to determine the extent of resection as it can prevent any functional compromise. It is essential for planning function-preserving surgery in patients with brain tumours [12].

7.4 Magnetic resonance spectroscopy

It is useful in the evaluation of brain tumors in pediatric patients by helping determine the diagnosis, grade, and extent of the tumor. MRS can also differentiate radiation necrosis from tumor recurrence because normal metabolite levels after treatment favor edema and postsurgical changes [13].

7.5 Positron emission tomography (PET)

PET has clearly defined roles in primary brain tumor imaging. The FDG uptake of high-grade gliomas is more as compared with low-grade or well-differentiated neoplasms, and FDG-PET can be useful in making a distinction between low- and high-grade gliomas [14].

A few limitations of FDG-PET as a cerebral imaging agent are that normal brain tissue has high physiologic glucose metabolic rate producing a high FDG uptake which may mask smaller lesions. Another issue is in the detection of tumors with only modest increases in glucose metabolism, such as low-grade tumors which may be difficult to interpret [15]. 18F-fluoroethyl-L-thyrosin (18F-FET) is a promising radiotracer in determining the grade of brain tumors.

7.6 Cerebral fluid analysis

Chemistry and cytology of the cerebral fluid are used to determine the spread of the tumor. Findings may be important in subsequent treatment approaches.

8. Histologic confirmation of diagnosis

Histopathologic diagnosis of brain tumours is necessary for decision making regarding appropriate management. Stereotactic biopsy has emerged as a comparatively safe method of histological diagnosis and has significantly reduced the risks associated with brain biopsy [16]. Tissue sampling can be obtained either with stereotactic, open, or endoscopic procedures and, overall, provides.

Greater than 90% diagnostic yield, while it may be significantly lower (60–70%) in small (<1 cm^3) and/or heterogeneous lesions [17].

8.1 Open biopsy

It is performed as an open technique by intraoperative neuronavigation. Typically, it is asserted for surface brain lesion, where hemostasis is critically vital or a surgical resection depending on frozen section histopathology is arranged. Although morbidity and mortality of open biopsy is more as compared to stereotactic biopsy but neoplastic tissue yield is better and it influences the likelihood of an accurate diagnosis.

8.2 Stereotactic biopsy

It can be frame based and frameless. The frame-based method is focused on the fixation of the stereotactic frame on the patient's head, whereupon the localizer is attached to the frame with many N-shaped posts. Under stereotactic circumstances, neuroimaging (CT, MRI, positron emission tomography [PET], etc.) is carried out and radiological information is transmitted to the specialized computer platform. The localizer posts are used as space coordinate references. For optimizing the target location and defining the ideal trajectory for biopsy, multiple pictures are combined.

The frameless biopsies are generally technically easier and require less preparatory efforts in comparison to frame-based ones [18].

8.3 Endoscopic biopsy

It is recommended for intra- and periventricular tumors and can be done with or without frameless stereotactic guidance. The advantages of this technique are

1. direct visualization of the lesion

2. vascular structures can be seen during tissue sampling

3. more pathological specimens can be taken.

4. cerebrospinal fluid (CSF) samples can be taken for tumor marker analysis

In case obstructive hydrocephalus, third ventriculostomy can be simultaneously done [10].

Exception may be produced in chosen patients such as patients with known active systemic cancer and numerous lesions radiographically associated with brain metastases, patients with classic clinical and MRI results of brain stem glioma or optic nerve meningioma, HIV-positive patients with CT or MRI results consistent with primary CNS lymphoma and positive Epstein-Barr virus polymerase chain reaction in the CSF, or patients with secretory germ-cell tumors [19].

9. Differential diagnosis

9.1 Infectious

Abscess-fever, acutely ill, ±systemic infection, ct findings show cyst cavity with smooth thin walls and restricted diffusion within cavity.

Cerebritis-fever, acutely ill, ±systemic infection, mri findings show diffuse T2 change, no mass meningitis-diffuse enhancement of meninges on T1-weighted imaging.

9.2 Vascular

Infarct—MRI findings show Gray and white matter involvement, wedge like vascular distribution associated with restricted diffusion and low signal.

Subdural hematoma: anemia, retinal hemorrhage.

Bleeding—homogenous, clears quickly, residual hemosiderin ring.

Treatment-related necrosis—central hypodensity, edema, >6 months after radiation therapy or chemotherapy, metabolic scan shows low activity.

9.3 Neoplasm

Primary-solitary, no prior cancer.

Metastatic-multiple, prior cancer, ++edema, located at gray/white junction hydrocephalus: headache, vomiting, subarachnoid hemorrhage, Guillain-Barré syndrome tuberculoma: exposure to tuberculosis.

Pseudotumor cerebri: after otitis media, hormonal abnormalities.

10. General management

A focused history and symptom-based neurological examination is required which may be sufficient to raise brain tumor suspicion. Mental status assessment, cranial nerves, motor skills, sensory examination, coordination, and gait are key components of the neurological examination.

Preoperative laboratory testing which includes a complete blood cell count, renal and hepaic profile. A baseline ophthalmologic evaluation, including visual field testing and fundoscopic evaluation, is important in preoperative evaluations because most patients do not complain of visual field deficits at presentation. Glucocorticoids are used to control neurologic signs and symptoms caused by cerebral edema.

Although there is little evidence to support the use of corticosteroids with regard to overall outcome, corticosteroids can relieve headache, nausea, and vomiting and remain a generally accepted treatment.

In assessing a child suspected of having a brain tumor, a thorough neurological examination is of critical importance. Most kids diagnosed with a brain tumor have abnormal results on the presentation of neurological examination [20].

11. Neurosurgical procedure

Surgery remains the main treatment modality for most pediatric brain tumors. Depending on tumor type, the goals of surgical intervention are:

- Tissue diagnosis
- Re-establishment of normal CSF pathways

- Diversion of CSF (shunting)
- Tumor debulking
- Complete tumor resection [5]

In the literature, overall surgical morbidity rates vary from 10 to 54%. The rates highly depend on the location of the tumour, grade and propensity to disseminate [21].

12. Radiotherapy

Radiotherapy plays an important role in the management of pediatric brain tumours. It can be used either as adjuvant treatment in case of resectable tumours or as a definitive management option in case of unresectable tumours [22].

The most common long term side effect of radiotherapy in pediatric age group is neurocognitive dysfunction and upto 20–60% patients suffer from neurocognitive deficit as a long term sequelae of radiotherapy [23]. Sophisticated radiotherapy techniques are warranted for to avoid future negative impacts of radiation on pediatric brain development.

Use of better immobilization and more suitable imaging techniques like high-resolution brain imaging with computed tomography (CT) and magnetic resonance imaging (MRI) to accurately define the tumour limits and precisely assess the normal brain structures has greatly improved the degree of efficacy achieved by radiotherapy without increasing the side effects [24].

Technological advancements like use of conformal radiotherapy allows high radiation dose distributions within targeted tissues while simultaneously attempting to reduce dose to surrounding normal tissues. Conformal radiotherapy can be accomplished through a variety of techniques, including intensity-modulated radiotherapy (IMRT), stereotactic radiotherapy and proton beam therapy.

IMRT has shown promise in the treatment of a number of disease sites and is now being investigated in the use of pediatric tumors to reduce long-term toxicity. Stereotactic technique has the ability to reduce the treatment volume as it delivers highly conformal radiation to brain tumours and minimum dose to surrounding brain tissue. It can be delivered as stereotactic radiosurgery in which the entire dose is delivered as a single fraction or as fractionated stereotactic radiotherapy (FSRT) in which the treatment is delivered over weeks with multiple daily fractions. Only small margins of several millimeters are used for brain tumors, greatly reducing the volume of normal brain parenchyma receiving high doses of radiation.

13. Chemotherapy

High-dose chemotherapy with or without support by autologous stem cell transplantation, especially in children below the age of 3 years [25].

Palliative chemotherapy:

- May induce transient remission
- Increases the quality of life
- The benefits of chemotherapy or other treatments must be balanced by consideration of the toxicities

14. Special tumor types astrocytic tumor

Astrocytomas are the most common pediatric brain tumors, accounting for 7–8% of all childhood cancers [26]. Approximately 40% of all pediatric brain tumours are low grade astrocytoma, whereas most common primary CNS malignancy in adults being high grade astrocytoma [7]. Pediatric brain tumors are typically infratentorial, localized predominantly in the posterior fossa and brainstem [27].

Pediatric astrocytic tumours are further sub-classified by WHO grades (**Table 3**).

14.1 Genomic alterations low grade glioma

1. Most common genomic modification in cases of pilocytic astrocytoma involves activation of *BRAF* and the ERK/MAPK pathway [29]

2. Alternative *BRAF* gene fusions, *RAF1* rearrangements, *RAS* mutations, and *BRAF* V600E point mutations are less commonly observed in such cases [30].

3. Presence of the *BRAF-KIAA1549* fusion gene shows better progression-free survival (PFS) and overall survival (OS) [31].

4. Other pediatric low-grade gliomas (e.g., pilomyxoid astrocytoma) are also associated with *BRAF* activation through the *BRAF-KIAA1549* fusion [32].

5. In 53% pediatric grade II diffuse astrocytomas, the most common alterations reported are rearrangements in the MYB family of transcription factors [33].

Children having mutation in one of two tuberous sclerosis genes (*TSC1*/hamartin or *TSC2*/tuberin) are at a risk of developing Subependymal giant cell astrocytomas, cortical tubers, and subependymal nodules, as either of these mutations results in activation of the mammalian target of rapamycin (mTOR) complex 1 [34].

14.2 High grade glioma

The following pediatric high-grade glioma subgroups were identified on the basis of their DNA methylation patterns, and they show distinctive molecular and clinical characteristics:

1. Histone K27 mutation: **H3.3 (*H3F3A*) and H3.1 (*HIST1H3B* and, rarely, *HIST1H3C*) mutation at K27.** These cases occur predominantly in mid

Astrocytic tumour	Grade
Subependymal giant cell astrocytoma Pilocytic astrocytoma	I
Pilomyxoid astrocytoma Diffuse astrocytoma Pleomorphic xanthoastrocytoma	II
Anaplastic astocytoma	III
Glioblastoma giant glioblastoma gliosarcoma	IV

Table 3.
WHO grades of pediatric astrocytic tumours [28].

childhood (median age, approximately 10 years). They are almost exclusively midline, usually present in the thalamus, brain stem, and spinal cord, and carry a very poor prognosis.

H3.3K27M cases are usually present between ages 5 and 10 years, accounting for approximately 60% of cases in the midline and pons. The prognosis for H3.3K27M patients is extremely poor, with a median survival of <1 year [35].

H3.1K27M cases present at a younger age than H3.3K27M cases and are approximately 5 times less frequent. These cases have a slightly more favorable prognosis than do H3.3K27M cases (median survival, 15 vs. 11 months).

2. **H3.3 (*H3F3A*) mutation at G34**: The H3.3G34 subtype is associated with mutations in *TP53* and *ATRX* which show widespread hypomethylation across the whole genome. It is common in older children and young adults (median age, 14–18 years) and arises exclusively in the cerebral cortex [36].

About 5% pediatric high-grade gliomas have *IDH1*-mutation. They are almost exclusively common in older adolescents (median age in a pediatric population, 16 years).

Pleomorphic xanthoastrocytoma (PXA)-like: Approximately 10% of pediatric high-grade gliomas have DNA methylation patterns that are PXA-like [37].

15. Treatment

15.1 Low-grade astrocytomas

Low-grade astrocytomas (grade I [pilocytic] and grade II) spread by direct extension; dissemination to other CNS sites is uncommon. Complete excision is the treatment of choice and the outcome is favorable especially if the tumor is circumscribed [38].

Markers of poor prognosis for childhood low-grade astrocytomas are:

1. Young age.

2. Diffuse histology, especially IDH-mutant.

3. Inability to obtain a complete resection.

4. Diencephalic syndrome.

5. Intracranial hypertension at initial presentation [39].

6. Metastases.

15.2 High-grade astrocytomas

Gross total resection is recommended for anaplastic astrocytomas. Local invasion of adjacent brain tissue is relatively common. Prognosis is poor for younger patients.

Depending on the degree of resectability, other treatment options are:

- Radiotherapy usually causes short-term and partial remission.

- Multiagent chemotherapy improve survivability with variable long-term remission
- Effective drugs alone or in combination: cisplatin, carboplatin, cyclophosphamide, ifosfamide, etoposide, topotecan, procarbazine, temozolomide, lomustine (CCNU), carmustine (BCNU) [40].

15.3 Optic-hypothalamic glioma

Optic pathway-hypothalamic gliomas are rare astrocytic tumors that are more among young children. They comprise approximately 2% of all central nervous system tumors and account for 3–5% of pediatric intracranial tumors.

OPG was classified by Dodge et al. into the following three stages: (A) limited to the optic nerve; (B) involving optic chiasma (with or without extension to the optic nerve) and (C) involvement of hypothalamus and other structures [41].

The tumours do not produce symptoms at an early stage. The symptoms can be due to impingement on optic nerve or chiasma which leads to visual disturbances, involvement of hypothalamus causing endocrinopathies and hypothalamic dysfunction such as the diencephalic syndrome. It can also cause csf outflow block leading to hydrocephalus [42].

Surgery has a limited role in the treatment of these tumours as they lie close to critical structures. It is usually limited to establishing a histopathological diagnosis or debulking in case of large tumours. Although Gross total resection of low-grade glioma is strongly associated with improvement of both OS and PFS but Aggressive resection, often leads to blindness, hypothalamic damage and cognitive dysfunctions [43].

15.3.1. Chemotherapy

Carboplatin and Vincristine is the most frequently recommended first-line chemotherapy, and it is considered to be the standard treatment of OPG [44].

15.3.2. Radiation

Radiotherapy is considered as a treatment option for OPG but at a cost of long term complications of neurocognitive dysfunction and visual disturbances [45]. Radiation may therefore be useful for an adjuvant treatment in the case of chemotherapy refractory tumors. Prognosis depends upon the age of the patient and location of the tumour. Young age and tumour located in optic pathway and hypothalamus are considered as poor prognostic factors.

16. Brain stem tumors

Pediatric brainstem gliomas occur as two major types:

Focal brainstem gliomas, usually WHO grade I–II tumors.

Diffuse intrinsic pontine gliomas, range from WHO grade III–IV [46]. They usually arise in the medulla, pons, or midbrain.

Focal brainstem gliomas (FBSG): constitutes approximately 20% of pediatric brainstem gliomas and usually occur outside the pons. Most are either pilocytic astrocytomas (grade I) or fibrillary astrocytomas (grade II) [47].

FBSG is usually insidious in nature and the symptoms are related to site of tumour location. Most common symptoms include neck stiffness, cranial nerve deficit and contralateral hemiparesis.

Hydrocephalus is uncommon except in posterior exophytic tumours [48].

On MRI, FBSG can be seen with defined borders, lack of surrounding edema, iso- or hypointensity on T1, hyperintensity on T2, and homogeneous contrast enhancement [49].

Surgical resection has emerged as treatment of choice due to development of modern imaging and neurosurgical techniques. FBSG confined to cervicomedullary region and/ or exophytic are amenable to complete resection [50] even with incomplete resection, the long-term prognosis for this patient population is excellent.

Chemotherapy can be used as adjuvant after complete or incomplete tumour resection or in cases of tumour progression. Most commonly used chemotherapy regimen is vincristine and carboplatin, which achieves at least stable disease in 68–75% of patients, and a positive response in about 40% [51]. Other regimens comprise of 6-thioguanine, procarbazine, lomustine, and vincristine (TPCV), vinblastine [52], bevacizumab with or without irinotecan [53], everolimus [54], and a metronomic, oral, anti-angiogenic regimen consisting of celecoxib, thalidomide, fenofibrate, cyclosphosphamide, and etoposide [55].

Radiation therapy (RT), while often effective in inducing prolonged remission in FBSG, has severe associated toxicities, especially for young children.

Diffuse intrinsic pontine gliomas (DIPG) account for approximately 80% of pediatric brainstem tumors and with male to female ratio as 1:1. It is more common in younger age group. These tumors are almost always highly malignant and fatal [56].

The patients have DIPG have a more lethal and shorter duration course than FBSG as it is more aggressive disease. Patients usually present within 3 months of tumour development. The most common symptoms are cranial nerve palsies, most often of cranial nerves VI and VII but sometimes including III, IV, IX, and/or X, as well as long tract signs like hemiparesis.

On CT scan, DIPG appears isodense or hypodense, without calcifications. On MRI, DIPG is most often hypointense on T1 and hyperintense on T2. Contrast enhancement is variable in both modalities but is usually not diffusely uniform, as it often is in FBSG. Diffusion is most often increased [57].

Apart from medical management starting with dexamethsone, aimed to relieve neurological symptoms, not many treatment options are available. RT is the only therapy proven to prolong survival of patients, that too it is palliative in nearly every case.

Currently, RT is given at a dose of 54–59 Gy at 1.8 Gy daily fractions for 30–33 days locally, to the area of the tumor plus a 1–2 cm surrounding margin.

Chemotherapy has not shown any benefit in concurrent, adjuvant or palliative form.

The prognosis for DIPG patients remains devastatingly poor. Recent studies have shown median progression free survival of 7 months and an overall survival of 9–11 months. In one large series, 77% of patients responded to treatment, and it was for a transient period as the therapy is rarely curative [58]. Poor prognostic marker at diagnosis or post treatment is the presence of leptomeningeal disease and no studies confirm these patients will benefit from craniospinal irradiation [59].

17. Medulloblastoma

Medulloblastoma is the second most common central nervous system tumour of childhood, most commonly occurring between 4 and 7 years of age. It usually arises from the roof of the fourth ventricle or from the midline structures of the brain [60].

Etiology: for most patients the etiology is unknown but is associated with certain genetic disorders (i.e., Gorlin syndrome, Turcot syndrome, Li-Fraumeni syndrome, Rubinstein-Taybi syndrome, and ataxia telangiectasia) [61].

It has the propensity to disseminate along the cerebrospinal fluid (CSF) pathway, and metastatic disease at diagnosis is found in approximately 30% of patients. Spread outside the central nervous system (CNS) is very rare at diagnosis.

WHO classification 2007 categorises medulloblastoma as grade IV neoplasms under the group of embryonal neuroepithelial tumours. There are several histopathological subtypes of medulloblastoma. In addition to classic variant, other subtypes include desmoplastic/nodular medulloblastoma, medulloblastoma with extensive nodularity (MBEN), anaplastic medulloblastoma, and large cell medulloblastoma [25].

Molecular subgrouping of medulloblastoma divides it into four distinct subgroups which are identified on the basis of transcriptional profiling studies as wingless (Wnt), sonic hedgehog (Shh), Group 3, and Group 4 (**Table 4**). Each subgroup is defined by a unique set of demographic and clinical features, genetics, and gene expression [63].

Signs and symptoms: usually due to increased intracranial tension, hydrocephalus and cerebellar dysfunction, and comprise vomiting, macrocephalus, loss of developmental achievements in infants, and headache, vomiting, ataxia, and cranial nerve palsy in older patients.

Management: biopsy has no role in the diagnosis if it is radiographically supported. Medulloblastomas have distinct imaging characteristics on both computed tomography (CT) and magnetic resonance imaging (MRI). Since 75% of medulloblastomas arise from the cerebellar vermis, they tend to protrude into the fourth ventricle in pediatric age group. On CT scan, in case of young patients, effacement of the fourth ventricle is seen along with its dilatation which is secondary to obstructive hydrocephalus. In case of older patients, they are most commonly seen as a hyperdense mass arising from the vermis with cyst formation or necrosis.

On MRI, medulloblastomas are hypointense to grey matter on T1-weighted imaging with heterogeneous gadolinium enhancement on T2-weighted imaging

	WNT	SHH	GROUP 3	GROUP 4
Percentage	10%	30%	25%	35%
Age	Children and adults	Mainly infants and adults	Mainly infants and children	Mainly children and adults
Somatic nucleotide variant	*CTNNB1, DDX3, SMARCA4, CREBBP, TP53**	*PTCH1, SUFU, SMO, TERT, IDH1, TP53, KMT2D*	*SMARCA4, CTDNEP1, KMT2D, KBTBD4*	*KDM6A, KMT2C*
Somatic copy number alterations		*MYCN, GLI2*	*MYC, PVT1, OTX2, GFI1/1b*	*SNCAIP, MYCN, CDK6, GFI1/1b*
Cytogenetics	Monosomy 6	Gain of 3q, 9p, loss of 9q, 10q, 14q, 17p	i17q, loss of 8, 10q, 11, 16p, 17p, gain of 1q, 7, 17q, 18q	i17q, loss of 8p, 11p, X, gain of 7q, 18q
Prognosis	Very good	Intermediate	Poor	Intermediate
Incidence of metastasis	5–10%	10–15%	40–45%	35–40%
Pattern of relapse	Local and distal	Local	Distal	Distal

**It shows characterstics of each molecular subgroups of medulloblastoma.*

Table 4.
Molecular subgroups of medulloblastoma [62].

	Average risk	High risk
Residual postoperative tumour volume	<1.5 cm^2	≥1.5
CSF cytology/evidence of disease dissemination on MRI in brain and spine	Absent	Present

Table 5.
Risk stratification of medulloblastoma.

they appear iso- to hyperintense to grey matter and can seem heterogeneous due to cyst formation, calcification and necrosis. MR spectroscopy shows elevated choline peaks and decreased creatine and N-acetyl acetate peaks, with occasional elevation in lactic acid and lipid peaks [64].

Maximal safe resection is recommended in all medulloblastoma patients. Apart from surgical resection, the current standards of radiation therapy and medical management vary by extent of disease and age of the patient. Radiation therapy can be used to decrease the risk of recurrence but neurocognitive effects of radiation therapy have to be considered by weighing the risk benefit ratio.

Patients who are 3 years of age or older are stratified as either "average-risk" or "high-risk" depending upon postoperative residual tumor volume and the presence or absence of disseminated disease (**Table 5**).

Patients who are younger than 3 years of age, are treated without upfront radiation therapy due to the unacceptably high risk of severe neurocognitive impairment [65].

In the postoperative setting, average-risk patients >3 years old were previously treated with 36 Gy craniospinal irradiation (CSI) but now a boost to the posterior fossa is given for a total dose of 54 Gy due to the high rate of relapse within the posterior fossa. CSI dose of 23.4–24 Gy can be given with the addition of chemotherapy as supported by Studies conducted by the International Society of Pediatric Oncology (SIOP) and the Children's Oncology Group [66].

Current recommendations for post-radiation chemotherapy in average-risk patients include approximately 1 year of therapy consisting of 8 cycles at 6-week intervals of cisplatin, lomustine (CCNU), and vincristine. The St. Jude Medulloblastoma-96 trial has demonstrated a similar event-free survival of 83% when an alkylator-based, dose-intensive chemotherapy regimen consisting of four 4-week cycles of cyclophosphamide, cisplatin, and vincristine with autologous stem cell rescue was employed following each cycle [67].

For high risk medulloblastoma cases in children 3 years or older, the treatment is surgical resection followed by post-operative "standard dose" RT (36 Gy CSI with a boost to both the posterior fossa and focal sites of metastatic disease to 55.8 Gy) as well as adjuvant chemotherapy.

The most common adverse effect of craniospinal irradiation in children <3 years age is neurocognitive deficit. Therefore radiotherapy is either delayed or omitted in this subset of patients. There is evidence that regimens consisting of surgery and chemotherapy without RT can be successful in specific subsets of medulloblastoma patients. Outcomes in patients with relapsed disease are generally poor, with reported 5-year survival rates of approximately 25% [68]. Unfavorable prognostic factors include large tumor, csf dissemination, age <4 years, subtotal tumour resection (<90%), chromosome deletion 17p, c-*MYC* amplification.

18. Atypical teratoid rhabdoid tumors (ATRT)

Atypical teratoid rhabdoid tumours (ATRTs) are the most common malignant central nervous system tumours in children ≤1 year of age and represent approximately 1–2% of all pediatric brain tumours [69]. ATRT is a primarily monogenic disease characterized by the bi-allelic loss of the *SMARCB1* gene, which encodes the hSNF5 subunit of the SWI/SNF chromatin remodeling complex [70]. The most common site of ATRT is posterior fossa, mainly cerebellar hemispheres (⅔ cases) [71]. It can also occupy fourth ventricle causing its displacement and compression by invading the adjacent cisternal space.

In patients <3 years of age, the most common treatment is high dose chemotherapy with autologous stem cell rescue, so that CSI can be avoided in young patients as poor outcomes are seen due radiotherapy induced neurocognitive impairment [72].

Despite using chemotherapy and radiotherapy as treatment options, ATRT has poor survival outcomes due to early dissemination and progression of the tumours [73].

19. Pineal tumors

Incidence of pineal tumours in children ranges from 2.7 to 11% [74]. Germ cell tumors (GCTs) account for nearly 50–75% of all pineal tumors [75], Pineal parenchymal tumors account for nearly 15–27% of pineal tumors and include pineocytoma, parenchymal tumor of intermediate differentiation, pineoblastoma and papillary tumor of the pineal region. Other described pineal tumors include glioma, ependymoma and atypical teratoid or rhabdoid tumors [76].

Preferred treatment strategy of different pineal region tumours [77] (**Table 6**).

Pineoblastoma <3 years	Radiotherapy is avoided Induction chemotherapy followed by consolidation myeloablative chemotherapy with stem cell rescue
Pineoblastoma 3–6 years	Induction chemotherapy followed by consolidation myeloablative chemotherapy with stem cell rescue
Pineoblastoma >6 years	Full-dose craniospinal irradiation (36 Gy) plus boost (total of 54 Gy) to the primary site along with concomitant daily carboplatin and weekly vincristine followed by 6 cycles of maintenance chemotherapy
Germinoma	Four cycles of chemotherapy with carboplatin and etoposide followed by whole ventricular irradiation to 23.4 Gy plus a boost to the primary site to a total dose of 30 Gy
Non-germinomatous germ cell tumour	Six cycles of chemotherapy with carboplatin, ifosfamide and etoposide followed by 30 Gy whole ventricular irradiation plus a boost to the primary site to a total dose of 50 Gy in patients with a radiographic and serologic complete response

Table 6.
Treatment strategies of different pineal tumours.

20. Ependymoma

Ependymoma accounts for 6–12% of all brain tumors in childhood. It represents the third most common brain tumor in this age group, following astrocytomas and medulloblastomas [78]. Ependymoma are classified according to the WHO pathological grading system (**Table 7**).

They are usually located in or adjacent to ventricles within the parenchyma. In pediatric age group majority of intracranial ependymoma are located at infratentorial region in posterior fossa, usually arising at the floor of fourth ventricle.

Prognostic factors include tumor location, size, surrounding anatomical structures, tumor appearance, genotype, comorbidities, clinical symptoms, and patient age [79].

Tumour type	Grade
Subependymoma (benign) myxopapillary ependymoma	I
Ependymoma	II
Anaplastic ependymoma	III

Table 7.
WHO pathological grades of ependymoma.

The current treatment of choice for pediatric patients with cranial ependymoma is resection, if possible, followed by radiation therapy alone [80].

21. Craniopharyngioma

They are low histological grade (WHO I) tumours which arise from epithelial remnants of rathke's pouch. They are usually located in sellar or parasellar location with an overall incidence of 0.5–2.0 new cases per million of the population per year, and constitute 1.2–4.0% of all childhood intracranial tumors.

Symptoms depend upon the location of the tumour:

Craniopharyngimas can present with nonspecific symptoms like headache and nausea due to increased intracranial pressure.

Intrasellar lesions can compress the pituitary gland and hypothalamus involving the hypothalamic-pituitary axes in 52–87% cases, leading to endocrine defects, particularly deficits in the secretion of growth hormone (75% of cases), gonadotropins (40%), adrenocorticotropic hormone (25%) and TSH (25%) [81].

Prechiasmal lesions may compress the optic pathway, leading to visual field cuts, decreased central visual acuity or vision impairment (62–84% of cases in children).

Retrochiasmal lesions may grow into the third ventricle and cause hydrocephalus or compress the optic tracts.

Craniopharyngiomas can cause direct impingement of brain parenchyma and produce neurological deficit.

In case of localized tumours the preferred choice of treatment is complete resection with preservation of visual, pituitary and hypothalamic function [82]. In case of incomplete resection, there are chances of residual tumour progression in 71–90% of patients, whereas the rate of progression after incomplete resection followed by radiotherapy is 21%. Therefore radiotherapy is recommended after surgical resection [83].

22. Conclusion

Since brain tumours are a leading cause of morbidity and mortality among children, the focus lies on how effectively they can be treated. Surgery plays a major role and can be curative in a number of tumours including pilocytic astrocytoma. Radiotherapy is curative in cases of PNET and ependymoma.

The survival and long-term outcome of patients with brain tumors will continue to enhance with future advances in nonsurgical methods, molecular and translational oncology research. For longer survival and reduced morbidity, new molecular diagnostics and new therapies such as immunotherapy, gene therapy and stem cell therapy may be promising.

Author details

Neha Sharma[1] and Deepti Sharma[2]*

1 Department of Radiation Oncology, MAMC and Lok Nayak Hospital, New Delhi, India

2 Department of Radiation Oncology, Max Super Speciality Hospital, New Delhi, India

*Address all correspondence to: drdeeptisharma16@gmail.com

IntechOpen

© 2020 The Author(s). Licensee IntechOpen. This chapter is distributed under the terms of the Creative Commons Attribution License (http://creativecommons.org/licenses/by/3.0), which permits unrestricted use, distribution, and reproduction in any medium, provided the original work is properly cited.

References

[1] Raizer J. Faculty of 1000 evaluation for CBTRUS Statistical Report: Primary brain and other central nervous system tumors diagnosed in the United States in 2010-2014. F1000. 2018. Post-publication peer review of the biomedical literature

[2] Johnson KJ, Cullen J, Barnholtz-Sloan JS, Ostrom QT, Langer CE, Turner MC, et al. Childhood brain tumor epidemiology: A brain tumor epidemiology consortium review. Cancer Epidemiology, Biomarkers & Prevention. 2014;**23**:2716-2736

[3] Ostrom QT, Gittleman H, Xu J, Kromer C, Wolinsky Y, Kruchko C, et al. CBTRUS statistical report: Primary brain and other central nervous system tumors diagnosed in the United States in 2009-2013. Neuro-Oncology. 2016;**18**:v1-v75

[4] Mckinney PA. Central nervous system tumours in children: Epidemiology and risk factors. Bioelectromagnetics. 2005;**26**(S7)

[5] Heuer GG, Jackson EM, Magge SN, Storm PB. Surgical management of pediatric brain tumors. Expert Review of Anticancer Therapy. 2007;**7**(sup1)

[6] Santos MM, Faria CC, Miguéns J. Pediatric central nervous system tumors: Review of a single Portuguese institution. Child's Nervous System. 2016;**32**:1227-1236

[7] Kaatsch P, Rickert CH, Kuhl J, Schuz J, Michaelis J. Population-based epidemiologic data on brain tumors in German children. Cancer. 2001;**92**:3155-3164

[8] Alomar SA. Clinical manifestation of central nervous system tumor. Seminars in Diagnostic Pathology. 2010;**27**:97-104

[9] Borja MJ, Plaza MJ, Altman N, Saigal G. Conventional and advanced MRI features of pediatric intracranial tumors: Supratentorial tumors. American Journal of Roentgenology. 2013;**200**(5)

[10] Ahn ES, Goumnerova L. Endoscopic biopsy of brain tumors in children: Diagnostic success and utility in guiding treatment strategies. Journal of Neurosurgery: Pediatrics. 2010;**5**:255-262. DOI: 10.3171/2009.10.peds09172

[11] Cha S, Knopp EA, Johnson G, Wetzel SG, Litt AW, Zagzag D. Intracranial mass lesions: Dynamic contrast-enhanced susceptibility-weighted echo-planar perfusion MR imaging. Radiology. 2002;**223**:11-29

[12] Wengenroth M, Blatow M, Guenther J, Akbar M, Tronnier VM, Stippich C. Diagnostic benefits of presurgical fMRI in patients with brain tumours in the primary sensorimotor cortex. European Radiology. 2011;**21**:1517-1525

[13] Poussaint TY, Rodriguez D. Advanced neuroimaging of pediatric brain tumors: MR diffusion, MR perfusion, and MR spectroscopy. Neuroimaging Clinics of North America. 2006;**16**:169-192

[14] Sundaram P, Padma S, Tewari APET. CT in paediatric malignancies: An update. Indian Journal of Medical and Paediatric Oncology. 2016;**37**:131

[15] Olivero WC, Dulebohn SC, Lister JR. The use of PET in evaluating patients with primary brain tumours: Is it useful? Journal of Neurology, Neurosurgery & Psychiatry. 1995;**58**:250-252

[16] Naghavi-Behzad M, Meshkini A, Shahzadi S, Alikhah H. Role of stereotactic biopsy in histological

diagnosis of multiple brain lesions. Asian Journal of Neurosurgery. 2013;**8**:69

[17] Chernov MF, Muragaki Y, Kesari S, IE MC, editors. Intracranial Gliomas. Part I: Surgery. Vol. 30. Prog Neurol Surg. Switzerland: Basel, Karger; 2018. pp. 232-243. DOI: 10.1159/000464439

[18] Olivi A, Weingart JD, Liauw J, Raza SM. Frame and frameless stereotactic brain biopsy. In: Youmans Neurological Surgery. Elsevier. 2011. pp. 1254-1260. DOI: 10.1016/b978-1-4160-5316-3.00117-9

[19] Albright L. Diffuse brainstem tumors: When is a biopsy necessary? Pediatric Neurosurgery. 1996;**24**(5):252-255. DOI: 10.1159/000121047

[20] Crawford J. Childhood brain tumors. Pediatrics in Review. 2013;**34**:63-78

[21] Sandri A, Sardi N, Genitori L, Giordano F, Peretta P, Basso ME, et al. Diffuse and focal brain stem tumors in childhood: Prognostic factors and surgical outcome. Child's Nervous System. 2006;**22**:1127-1135

[22] Knab B, Connell PP. Radiotherapy for pediatric brain tumors: When and how. Expert Review of Anticancer Therapy. 2007;**7**(sup1)

[23] Spiegler BJ, Bouffet E, Greenberg ML, Rutka JT, Mabbott DJ. Change in neurocognitive functioning after treatment with cranial radiation in childhood. Journal of Clinical Oncology. 2004;**22**:706-713

[24] Kirsch DG, Tarbell NJ. New technologies in radiation therapy for pediatric brain tumors: The rationale for proton radiation therapy. Pediatric Blood & Cancer. 2004;**42**:461-464

[25] Panosyan EH, Ikeda AK, Chang VY, Laks DR, Reeb CL, Bowles LV, et al. High-dose chemotherapy with autologous hematopoietic stem-cell rescue for pediatric brain tumor patients: A single institution experience from UCLA. Journal of Transplantation. 2011;**2011**:1-11

[26] Nakamura M, Shimada K, Ishida E, Higuchi T, Nakase H, Sakaki T, et al. Molecular pathogenesis of pediatric astrocytic tumors. Neuro-Oncology. 2007;**9**:113-123

[27] Cohen KJ, Broniscer A, Glod J. Pediatric glial tumors. Current Treatment Options in Oncology. 2001;**2**:529-536

[28] Louis DN, Ohgaki H, Wiestler OD, Cavenee WK, Burger PC, Jouvet A, et al. The 2007 WHO classification of tumours of the central nervous system. Acta Neuropathologica. 2007;**114**:97-109

[29] Bar EE, Lin A, Tihan T, Burger PC, Eberhart CG. Frequent gains at chromosome 7q34 involving BRAF in pilocytic astrocytoma. Journal of Neuropathology & Experimental Neurology. 2008;**67**:878-887

[30] Forshew T, Tatevossian RG, Lawson AR, Ma J, Neale G, Ogunkolade BW, et al. Activation of the ERK/MAPK pathway: A signature genetic defect in posterior fossa pilocytic astrocytomas. The Journal of Pathology. 2009;**218**:172-181

[31] Hawkins C, Walker E, Mohamed N, Zhang C, Jacob K, Shirinian M, et al. BRAF-KIAA1549 fusion predicts better clinical outcome in pediatric low-grade astrocytoma. Clinical Cancer Research. 2011;**17**:4790-4798

[32] Lin A, Rodriguez FJ, Karajannis MA, Williams SC, Legault G, Zagzag D, et al. BRAF alterations in primary glial and glioneuronal neoplasms of the central nervous system with identification of 2 novel KIAA1549. Journal of

Neuropathology & Experimental Neurology. 2012;**71**:66-72

[33] Ramkissoon LA, Horowitz PM, Craig JM, Ramkissoon SH, Rich BE, Schumacher SE, et al. Genomic analysis of diffuse pediatric low-grade gliomas identifies recurrent oncogenic truncating rearrangements in the transcription factor MYBL1. Proceedings of the National Academy of Sciences. 2013;**110**:8188-8193

[34] Franz DN, Belousova E, Sparagana S, Bebin EM, Frost M, Kuperman R, et al. Efficacy and safety of everolimus for subependymal giant cell astrocytomas associated with tuberous sclerosis complex (EXIST-1): A multicentre, randomised, placebo-controlled phase 3 trial. The Lancet. 2013;**381**:125-132

[35] Mackay A, Burford A, Carvalho D, Izquierdo E, Fazal-Salom J, Taylor KR, et al. Integrated molecular meta-analysis of 1,000 pediatric high-grade and diffuse intrinsic pontine glioma. Cancer Cell. 2017;**32**(4)

[36] Weiss W. Faculty of 1000 evaluation for hotspot mutations in H3F3A and IDH1 define distinct epigenetic and biological subgroups of glioblastoma. F1000. 2012. Post-publication peer review of the biomedical literature

[37] Korshunov A, Ryzhova M, Hovestadt V, Bender S, Sturm D, Capper D, et al. Integrated analysis of pediatric glioblastoma reveals a subset of biologically favorable tumors with associated molecular prognostic markers. Acta Neuropathologica. 2015;**129**:669-678

[38] Pfister S, Witt O. Pediatric gliomas. Recent Results in Cancer Research Gliomas. 2009;**171**:67-81

[39] Stokland T, Liu J-F, Ironside JW, Ellison DW, Taylor R, Robinson KJ, et al. A multivariate analysis of factors determining tumor progression in childhood low-grade glioma: A population-based cohort study (CCLG CNS9702). Neuro-Oncology. 2010;**12**(12):1257-1268

[40] Finlay JL, Boyett JM, Yates AJ, Wisoff JH, Milstein JM, Geyer JR, et al. Randomized phase III trial in childhood high-grade astrocytoma comparing vincristine, lomustine, and prednisone with the eight-drugs-in-1-day regimen. Childrens cancer group. Journal of Clinical Oncology. 1995;**13**:112-123

[41] Dodge HW. Gliomas of the optic nerves. Archives of Neurology and Psychiatry. 1958;**79**:607

[42] Aihara Y, Chiba K, Eguchi S, Amano K, Kawamata T. Pediatric optic pathway/hypothalamic glioma. Neurologia Medico-Chirurgica. 2018;**58**:1-9

[43] Walker DA, Liu J, Kieran M, Jabado N, Picton S, Packer R, et al. A multi-disciplinary consensus statement concerning surgical approaches to low-grade, high-grade astrocytomas and diffuse intrinsic pontine gliomas in childhood (CPN Paris 2011) using the Delphi method. Neuro-Oncology. 2013;**15**:462-468

[44] Packer RJ, Ater J, Allen J, Phillips P, Geyer R, Nicholson HS, et al. Carboplatin and vincristine chemotherapy for children with newly diagnosed progressive low-grade gliomas. Journal of Neurosurgery. 1997;**86**:747-754

[45] Merchant TE, Conklin HM, Wu S, Lustig RH, Xiong X. Late effects of conformal radiation therapy for pediatric patients with low-grade glioma: Prospective evaluation of cognitive, endocrine, and hearing deficits. Journal of Clinical Oncology. 2009;**27**:3691-3697

[46] Green AL, Kieran MW. Pediatric brainstem gliomas: New understanding leads to potential new treatments for two very different tumors. Current Oncology Reports. 2015;**17**(3)

[47] Fisher PG, Breiter SN, Carson BS, Wharam MD, Williams JA, Weingart JD, et al. A clinicopathologic reappraisal of brain stem tumor classification. Cancer. 2000;**89**:1569-1576

[48] Robertson PL, Allen JC, Abbott IR, Miller DC, Fidel J, Epstein FJ. Cervicomedullary tumors in children: A distinct subset of brainstem gliomas. Neurology. 1994;**44**:1798

[49] Barkovich A, Krischer J, Kun L, Packer R, Zimmerman R, Freeman C, et al. Brain stem gliomas: A classification system based on magnetic resonance imaging. Pediatric Neurosurgery. 1990;**16**:73-83

[50] Wisoff JH, Sanford RA, Heier LA, Sposto R, Burger PC, Yates AJ, et al. Primary neurosurgery for pediatric low-grade gliomas: A prospective multi-institutional study from the children's oncology group. Neurosurgery. 2011;**68**:1548-1555

[51] Ronghe M, Hargrave D, Bartels U, Tabori U, Vaidya S, Chandler C, et al. Vincristineandcarboplatinchemotherapy for unresectable and/or recurrent low-grade astrocytoma of the brainstem. Pediatric Blood & Cancer. 2010;**55**:471-477

[52] Bouffet E, Jakacki R, Goldman S, Hargrave D, Hawkins C, Shroff M, et al. Phase II study of weekly vinblastine in recurrent or refractory pediatric low-grade glioma. Journal of Clinical Oncology. 2012;**30**:1358-1363

[53] Hwang EI, Jakacki RI, Fisher MJ, Kilburn LB, Horn M, Vezina G, et al. Long-term efficacy and toxicity of bevacizumab-based therapy in children with recurrent low-grade gliomas. Pediatric Blood & Cancer. 2012;**60**:776-782

[54] Kieran MW, Yao X, Macy M, Leary S, Cohen K, Macdonald T, et al. Final results of a prospective multi-institutional phase ii study of everolimus (Rad001), an Mtor inhibitor, In pediatric patients with recurrent or progressive low-grade glioma. A poetic consortium trial. Neuro-Oncology. 2014;**16**:iii27

[55] Robison NJ, Campigotto F, Chi SN, Manley PE, Turner CD, Zimmerman MA, et al. A phase II trial of a multi-agent oral antiangiogenic (metronomic) regimen in children with recurrent or progressive cancer. Pediatric Blood & Cancer. 2013;**61**:636-642

[56] Yoshimura J, Onda K, Tanaka R, Takahashi H. Clinicopathological study of diffuse type brainstem gliomas: Analysis of 40 autopsy cases. Neurologia Medico-Chirurgica. 2003;**43**:375-382

[57] Chen H, Panigrahy A, Dhall G, Finlay J, Nelson M, Blüml S. Apparent diffusion and fractional anisotropy of diffuse intrinsic brain stem gliomas. American Journal of Neuroradiology. 2010;**31**:1879-1885

[58] Massimino M, Spreafico F, Biassoni V, Simonetti F, Riva D, Trecate G, et al. Diffuse pontine gliomas in children: Changing strategies, changing results? A mono-institutional 20-year experience. Journal of Neuro-Oncology. 2008;**87**:355-361

[59] Sethi R, Allen J, Donahue B, Karajannis M, Gardner S, Wisoff J, et al. Prospective neuraxis MRI surveillance reveals a high risk of leptomeningeal dissemination in diffuse intrinsic pontine glioma. Journal of Neuro-Oncology. 2010;**102**:121-127

[60] Hoff KV, Rutkowski S. Medulloblastoma. Current Treatment Options in Neurology. 2012;**14**:416-426

[61] Villani A, Malkin D, Tabori U. Syndromes predisposing to pediatric central nervous system tumors: Lessons learned and new promises. Current Neurology and Neuroscience Reports. 2011;**12**:153-164

[62] Wang J, Garancher A, Ramaswamy V, Wechsler-Reya RJ. Medulloblastoma: From molecular subgroups to molecular targeted therapies. Annual Review of Neuroscience. 2018;**41**:207-232

[63] Taylor MD, Northcott PA, Korshunov A, Remke M, Cho Y-J, Clifford SC, et al. Molecular subgroups of medulloblastoma: The current consensus. Acta Neuropathologica. 2011;**123**:465-472

[64] Koeller KK, Rushing EJ. From the archives of the AFIP. Radiographics. 2003;**23**:1613-1637

[65] Millard NE, KCD B. Medulloblastoma. Journal of Child Neurology. 2016;**31**:1341-1353

[66] Merchant TE, Kun LE, Krasin MJ, Wallace D, Chintagumpala MM, Woo SY, et al. Multi-institution prospective trial of reduced-dose craniospinal irradiation (23.4 Gy) followed by conformal posterior fossa (36 Gy) and primary site irradiation (55.8 Gy) and dose-intensive chemotherapy for average-risk medulloblastoma. International Journal of Radiation Oncology Biology Physics. 2008;**70**:782-787

[67] Gajjar A, Chintagumpala M, Ashley D, Kellie S, Kun LE, Merchant TE, et al. Risk-adapted craniospinal radiotherapy followed by high-dose chemotherapy and stem-cell rescue in children with newly diagnosed medulloblastoma (St Jude Medulloblastoma-96): Long-term results from a prospective, multicentre trial. The Lancet Oncology. 2006;**7**:813-820

[68] Bowers DC, Gargan L, Weprin BE, Mulne AF, Elterman RD, Munoz L, et al. Impact of site of tumor recurrence upon survival for children with recurrent or progressive medulloblastoma. Journal of Neurosurgery: Pediatrics. 2007;**107**:5-10

[69] Frühwald MC, Biegel JA, Bourdeaut F, Roberts CW, Chi SN. Atypical teratoid/rhabdoid tumors—Current concepts, advances in biology, and potential future therapies. Neuro-Oncology. 2016;**18**:764-778

[70] Richardson EA, Ho B, Huang A. Atypical teratoid rhabdoid tumour: From tumours to therapies. Journal of Korean Neurosurgical Society. 2018;**61**:302-311

[71] Bambakidis NC, Robinson S, Cohen M, Cohen AR. Atypical teratoid/rhabdoid tumors of the central nervous system: Clinical, radiographic and pathologic features. Pediatric Neurosurgery. 2002;**37**:64-70

[72] Nicolaides T, Tihan T, Horn B, Biegel J, Prados M, Banerjee A. High-dose chemotherapy and autologous stem cell rescue for atypical teratoid/rhabdoid tumor of the central nervous system. Journal of Neuro-Oncology. 2009;**98**:117-123

[73] Zimmerman MA, Goumnerova LC, Proctor M, Scott RM, Marcus K, Pomeroy SL, et al. Continuous remission of newly diagnosed and relapsed central nervous system atypical teratoid/rhabdoid tumor. Journal of Neuro-Oncology. 2005;**72**:77-84

[74] Hoffman HJ, Yoshida M, Becker LE, Hendrick B, Humphreys RP. Pineal region tumors in childhood. Pediatric Neurosurgery. 1994;**21**:91-104

[75] Matsutani M. Pineal germ cell tumors. Progress in Neurological Surgery Pineal Region Tumors. 2009;**23**:76-85

[76] Sato K, Kubota T. Pathology of pineal parenchymal tumors. Progress in Neurological Surgery Pineal Region Tumors. 2009;**23**:12-25

[77] Dhall G, Khatua S, Finlay JL. Pineal region tumors in children. Current Opinion in Neurology. 2010;**23**:576-582

[78] Grill J, Pascal C, Chantal K. Childhood ependymoma. Pediatric Drugs. 2003;**5**:533-543

[79] Foreman NK, Love S, Thorne R. Intracranial ependymomas: Analysis of prognostic factors in a population-based series. Pediatric Neurosurgery. 1996;**24**:119-125

[80] Cage TA, Clark AJ, Aranda D, Gupta N, Sun PP, Parsa AT, et al. A systematic review of treatment outcomes in pediatric patients with intracranial ependymomas. Journal of Neurosurgery: Pediatrics. 2013;**11**:673-681

[81] Müller HL. Childhood craniopharyngioma—Current concepts in diagnosis, therapy and follow-up. Nature Reviews Endocrinology. 2010;**6**:609-618

[82] Fahlbusch R, Honegger J, Paulus W, Huk W, Buchfelder M. Surgical treatment of craniopharyngiomas: Experience with 168 patients. Journal of Neurosurgery. 1999;**90**:237-250

[83] Becker G, Kortmann R, Skalej M, Bamberg M. The role of radiotherapy in the treatment of craniopharyngeoma: Indications, results, side effects. Controversies in neuro-oncology. Frontiers of Radiation Therapy and Oncology. 1999;**33**:100-113

Chapter 7

Role of Sentinel Node Biopsy in Endometrial Cancer

Begoña Díaz de la Noval

Abstract

Lymphadenectomy, for early stages of endometrial cancer (EC), provides a low detection rate of lymphatic metastasis, without having demonstrated a therapeutic effect; so that the collection and histological analysis of the sentinel lymph node (SLN) might be an alternative to lymphadenectomy. The contribution of SLN to surgical staging represents a change in the paradigm of lymphadenectomy in EC, being an intermediate approach between not assessing the condition of the lymph nodes and complete pelvic and paraaortic dissection. Accurate identification of the main uterine drainage pathway increases the likelihood of detecting metastases during lymphatic mapping. In addition, pathological assessment by the ultrastaging of the SLN is the most important advance in the SLN biopsy (SLNB) technique. The application of the SLNB presumes a decrease in surgical and long-term morbidity, with an increase in the detection of lymphatic metastasis, mainly at the expense of detecting low tumour volume, selecting the group of patients that would benefit from a modification in adjuvant therapy. The SLNB can be established as an oncologically safe and effective method in the surgical staging of early-stage EC. Prospective studies are required to determine optimal behaviour and prognosis in the detection of low-volume metastases.

Keywords: endometrial cancer, lymphatic mapping, predictive value of tests, sentinel lymph node biopsy, ultrastaging

1. History and concept

The origins of lymphatic mapping date back more than 100 years, when Sappey injected mercury into the skin of cadavers to delineate the skin's lymphatic pathways [1, 2]. Lymphoscintigraphy was described by Shearman and Ter-Pogossian in 1953, both of whom confirmed Sappey's hypothesis that lymphatic drainage occurs in an orderly and predictable manner [2].

The origin of lymphatic drainage of tumours and its implications for surgical staging are traced back to 1850 with the studies of Virchow and Haldsted on radical axillary lymphadenectomy for breast cancer.

The contribution of SLN to surgical staging represents a change in the paradigm of lymphadenectomy in EC. SLN represented an intermediate approach between not assessing the condition of the lymph nodes and complete pelvic and paraaortic dissection [3, 4]. The accurate identification of the main uterine drainage pathway increases the likelihood of detecting metastases during lymphatic mapping [5].

This information, provided by SLN, will change the therapeutic approach, with a potential benefit in the prognosis, both in survival and quality of life [6].

2. Detection method

Theoretically, the ideal method for studying SLN in EC should meet the following requirements:

1. Cause the least amount of patient discomfort possible, be easy to perform and be reproducible.

2. Be a preoperative procedure that enables planning of the surgical approach according to the anatomical location of the SLN.

3. Enable a laparoscopic approach according to the concept of minimally invasive surgery.

4. Enable the detection of SLN without complete dissection of the retroperitoneal space.

5. Obtain a lymphatic map representative of the tumour drainage or, at least, of the uterine body drainage [7].

2.1 Lymphatic drainage of the uterus

Unlike superficial tumours, such as melanoma, the physiology of lymphatic drainage in deeper/visceral tumours is not well established [8]. Uterine drainage, as well as being bilateral, is therefore complex [9]. Anatomically, three segments of uterine lymphatic drainage have been established:

1. The *lower uterine segment* drains from the paracervix to the parametrium and to the broad ligament, passing by the obturator, internal iliac and interiliac lymph node chains.

2. The *middle third* of the uterus drains the round ligament and the external iliac lymph node chain.

3. The *upper uterine segment* drains through the infundibular pelvic ligament, uterine-ovarian plexus and gonadal vessels towards the common iliac lymph node chain, presacral lymph nodes and paraaortic lymph nodes [10].

Physiologically, there are two main lymphatic pathways and a third accessory for uterine drainage [5]:

1. The main pathway or *upper paracervical*, located in the lymph trunks of the parametrium. The lymphatic vessels of the uterine body often cross the obliterated umbilical artery, which is the most common location of the pelvic SLN, rising over the upper part of the obturator region, medial to the external iliac vessels and ventral to the hypogastric vessels [5].

2. A less common pathway, the *lower paracervical*, is generally observed when the lymphatic vessels do not cross the obliterated umbilical artery and move

cranially over the course of the mesoureter. In these cases, SLN is usually observed in the internal iliac, common iliac or presacral region.

3. A third pathway has been described, the *infundibular pelvic*, but it is very rare except with fundal injections. This pathway has mainly fundal drainage towards the broad ligament and paraaortic chain [11].

2.2 Injection techniques

Three main areas of injection on the uterus have been described: (1) corporal, (2) endometrial and (3) cervical. Each area has been assessed with various approaches: hysteroscopic, laparoscopic and ultrasound-guided transvaginal and even with combined techniques.

1. **Corporal**: The injection can be subserosal or transmyometrial, in the anterior wall, posterior wall or uterine fundus. Corporal injection by laparotomy, using blue dye, was the first technique described. Subserosal injections have the drawback of multiple injections [12] and anatomical distortion when dealing with fibroids [13]. These injections might not be representative of the lesion if the tumour does not infiltrate the uterine fundus. Due to the lack of parametrial drainage, subserosal injections have a detection rate of 75–91% and bilaterality of 80%, which is lower than that of cervical injections ($p = 0.005$) [11], although the former has superior paraaortic drainage (31–40%) [14].

2. **Endometrial**: Intratumoural and peritumoural infiltration have superior validity due to the proximity to the tumour lesion [10, 15]. The disadvantages of this injection pathway are lower rates of bilaterality and paraaortic drainage, which are determined by the location and size of the lesion [16]. Hysteroscopic injections achieve detection rates of 69–80% [17, 18], with greater paraaortic drainage (up to 60%) [15], without having shown superiority against other injection pathways [19]. The hysteroscopic injection procedure is a more complex and uncomfortable technique for the patient. Recent studies have concluded that hysteroscopic injections do not have a correlation between the location of the SLN and the location of the tumour in the uterine cavity [20]. The risk of tumour dissemination to the abdominal cavity has been shown to be irrelevant [21]. Clamping the tubes before or after the injection of the dye interferes with the detection rate by decreasing it [22].

In 2013, the group from the Hospital Clinic of Barcelona published their results with the transvaginal ultrasound-guided myometrial injection of radiotracer (TUMIR) technique, injecting 148 MBq of ^{99m}Tc-albumin nanocolloid (in a volume of 8 mL) in the anterior and posterior peritumoural uterine wall, with migration of 90.5% and laparoscopic identification of 74.3%. The drainage was pelvic in 87.2%, pelvic and paraaortic in 45.4% and exclusively paraaortic in 12.8% of cases. Metastatic involvement of SLN in high-risk histology appeared in 24 patients, with paraaortic extension in 30% of cases. The authors concluded that the TUMIR technique is representative of tumour drainage and can be a promising detection method in high-risk histology, although further studies on the technique are needed [7]. The TUMIR technique has shown no differences compared with hysteroscopic injections ($p = 0.2$) [7].

3. **Cervical**: The cervical injection is the modality most often reported in studies [23]. The technique is reproducible, because the uterine cervix is accessible and

rarely distorted in patients with EC [24]. The meta-analyses by Kang et al. [25] and Bodurtha-Smith et al. [26] showed that hysteroscopic or subserosal injections were associated with lower performance ($p < 0.05$), while cervical administration was correlated with higher detection rates (92%; range, 62–100% [27]; $p = 0.031$) [4] and bilaterality (56 vs. 33%; $p = 0.003$) (bilaterality is defined as the detection of sentinel node on both sides of the pelvis). The disadvantage was lower detection of paraaortic drainage (95% CI 3.4–10.1%) compared with other techniques (7% cervical vs. 27% corporal; $p = 0.001$) [28–31].

In terms of the number of injections, there have been no differences between the injection in two or four quadrants (with detection rates of 92 vs. 88%; $p = 0.38$), but there is less dye dissemination if the injection is limited to two quadrants [31]. Geppert et al. [11] performed pericervical injections at 2, 4, 8 and 10 o'clock thereby obtaining 5% paraaortic drainage. The MSKCC group recommended that cervical injections in EC be bilateral (at 3 and 9 o'clock), both superficial (in the submucosa) to 1–3 mm and deep (in the stroma) to 1–2 cm. In this way, the deep injection would therefore arrive at the isthmus, ensuring parametrial drainage. Applying this technique, a threefold greater detection of lymphatic metastases is achieved ($p = 0.045$), without assuming an increase in the overall detection rates (86%) [32]. The systematic review by Cormier et al. [27] determined that paraaortic detection has been significantly greater with deep cervical infiltration (17 vs. 2%).

Taking into account the critical review of Frumovitz and Levenback [33] and knowing the uterine drainage pathways, the location of the tumour will determine the dissemination of the disease, and the injection technique might reflect the pattern of lymphatic mapping. However, the study by Geppert et al. [11] concluded that the cervical pathway (with submucosal and stromal injection) should be considered the standard pathway, not only due to being a safer injection technique but also because the two main pathways of lymphatic drainage of the uterus were identified regardless of the injection technique employed.

In terms of the lower cervical paraaortic drainage, numerous studies have verified that the incidence rate of paraaortic metastases isolated for EC in initial stages is 5%, with approximately 50% of metastatic pelvic and paraaortic lymph nodes [34]. Ninety percent of detected SLNs are located in the pelvic area; the rest are presacral or paraaortic. The other techniques likely obtain greater paraaortic drainage, at the expense of underestimating the main pathway of pelvic drainage [29, 30].

There is no known technique that detects with absolute bilaterality, and we still do not know why a central organ, such as the uterus, has cases in which bilateral drainage is not observed [20]. Ideally, the technique is considered valid if at least one SLN is identified in each hemipelvis [11].

There is no one ideal or superior technique; all have shown good results, with advantages and disadvantages [25]. Cervical injection is effective and reproduces pelvic drainage. Corporal injection better reproduces paraaortic drainage and the hysteroscopic pathway is representative of tumour drainage, although both are less reproducible than the cervical pathway [4]. A number of authors have advocated combined methods that provide better results. Studies such as the one by Holub et al. [35] have combined cervical and subserosal injections, achieving detection rates of 80%, without observing superiority over the two methods applied individually. In other studies with cervical and fundal injection, detection rates of 72.5% were achieved, comparable results without superior paraaortic drainage (4.9 vs. 9.8%; $p = 0.18$) [6].

Table 1 shows a comparison of the main characteristics of the abovementioned injection techniques.

Characteristic	Corporal	Endometrial	Cervical
Surgical approach for injection:	Subserosal or transmyometrial by laparoscopy or laparotomy	Hysteroscopy Transvaginal Ultrasound-guided	Transvaginal
Multiple injections	++	+	–
Influence on anatomical distortion or tumour size	++	+	–
Increase in economic cost	+/–	+	–
Technical complexity	+/–	+	–
Reproducibility	+	–	++
Detection rate/bilaterality	+	++	++
Paraaortic drainage	+	++	–
Comfort for the patient	+/–	–	+/–

The score was assigned according to the following gradation: (–) = absence of the characteristic or negative evaluation, (+) = meets the characteristic or positive evaluation, (++) = complies being better; (+++) = it fulfils being superior.

Table 1.
Characteristics of injection techniques.

2.3 Sentinel node identification

Various tracers have been shown to be useful. The most commonly used tracers in the lymphatic mapping of EC include ^{99m}Tc-nanocolloid, blue dyes and indocyanine green (ICG), alone or in combination [36].

One inherent and necessary advantage of tracers is their high capacity for penetration and fixation in lymphatic tissues [30]. The objective of lymphatic mapping and preoperative marking with tracer is the ability to analyse at least one lymph node per lymph node chain, two in the case of bilaterality [37].

SLNB was initially performed by the colorimetric method with methylene blue (MB) or synthetic variants of blue dye. SLNB was later combined with the isotopic detection of radiocolloids, thanks to the development of endoscopic gamma-ray detection probes, becoming the standard for use. In recent years, the application of lymphatic mapping by fluorescence in the near-infrared (NIR) electromagnetic spectrum with ICG obviated the need for a nuclear medicine unit and avoiding the adverse effects of blue dye, providing excellent results.

2.3.1 Preoperative marking: radiocolloid

The approach to studying the lymphatic pathways using nuclear medicine techniques has gained considerable momentum in recent years with the development of SLNB.

A radiopharmaceutical is a radioactive compound used for the diagnosis and treatment of diseases. Radiopharmaceuticals's property of transmitting radioisotopes for remote detection is employed to diagnostic purposes [38].

Radiopharmaceuticals can be classified, according to their chemical structure, into primary radionuclides and labelled compounds, the latter of which are essentially a combination of two components: a radionuclide and a particle. The particles are small molecules, colloids, proteins and cells; the most widely used are colloidal sulphur (USA) and albumin (Europe). The particle serves as a vehicle that selectively directs the radiopharmaceutical to a specific tissue in response to physiological conditions or specific patterns of gene expression [38]. The size of the particles is important (range, 2–1500 nm) because it affects the drainage speed and retention of particles in the lymph node [34].

The most widely used diagnostic radiopharmaceutical in nuclear medicine is isomerised metastable ^{99m}Tc [38], which is nontoxic and has almost ideal physical properties: a physical half-life to ^{99}Tc (transition metal) of 6 h, a detectable emission and monochromatic gamma ray of 140 keV, complete disintegration within 24 h and low ionising radiation with negligible exposure [36, 39]. The greatest contribution of radiopharmaceuticals is the ability to use it as a marker of distinct pharmaceutical preparations, known as *cold kits*. The most used cold kit is the Nanocoll® 500 μg/vial (GE Healthcare Bio-Sciences, S.A.U., Madrid), a compound of colloidal particles of human serum albumin measuring ≤80 nm in diameter. The compound therefore has avidity for absorption through the lymphatic capillaries, and the size of its particles does not permit displacement of the lymph node.

To perform the SLNB, low doses of radioactivity are employed (40–185 MBq/ 0.2–4 mCi) because the distribution space is highly reduced. Only the drainage to the first or second lymph nodes needs to be assessed [38]. Furthermore, the injected dose of radiocolloid is calculated based on the estimated time to surgery; the longer the interval, the larger the dose to ensure an adequate signal. The ^{99m}Tc-albumin nanocolloid is injected the day of the surgery (the radiocolloid injection is performed 6 h before the operation with preoperative imaging 30 min after the injection; the dose should be 0.2–1.0 mCi), a method known as the short protocol. If the nanocolloid is injected the day before the surgery (at a dose of 2.0–4.0 mCi), the method is known as the long protocol [40]. Therefore, the radioisotope compound deposited in the interstitial space near the tumour will migrate to the lymphatic capillaries until it reaches the first lymph node encountered by the capillaries. Due to the size of the compound, the capillaries will be trapped, indicating the first sentinel node into which the administered site drains. Moreover, both the short half-life and the low injected dose leave relatively little space for flexibility in surgical scheduling, given that hours-long delays and postponing the operation to the following day due to logistics will compromise the efficacy of the lymphatic mapping [36].

The compound is contraindicated when faced with hypersensitivity to the active ingredient or any of the excipients and during pregnancy. As the radiocolloid is primarily cleared by the kidneys but also by the hepatobiliary system, dose adjustment is required for patients with renal and/or hepatic failure [39]. There have been no reported adverse effects related to the radiopharmaceutical ^{99m}Tc-nanocolloid, except the standard risks of the technical procedure: bleeding, vasovagal syncope and local infection [6].

2.3.1.1 Lymphoscintigraphy and single-photon emission computed tomography

The disadvantages of radiocolloid are the lack of visual assessment and the need for nuclear medicine procedures [30]. Lymphoscintigraphy and single-photon emission computed tomography (SPECT) can obtain preoperative images of the lymphatic drainage [38].

Lymphoscintigraphy obtains a flat static image with morphological information of the lymphatic drainage of the injected radiocolloid [8, 41]. Lymphoscintigraphy in EC offers varying results, depending on the injection method, with poorer detection rates than the overall rates and poor correlation between the preoperative findings and intraoperative detection [42, 43]. In the meta-analysis by Bodurtha-Smith and Tanner [26] of 55 articles and 4915 included patients, preoperative lymphoscintigraphy and the combined use of radiotracer with dye improved the overall SLN detection rates (86 vs. 76%; $p = 0.016$ and 87 vs. 78%; $p = 0.008$, respectively); however, preoperative lymphoscintigraphy showed no benefit. An explanation for the low resolution and correlation could be the proximity of the injection site to the drainage, which can mask the SLN in flat images, and the anatomical complexity of the pelvic area, which can cause confusion in the correct anatomical description.

SPECT obtained a three-dimensional image with the fusion of the scintigraphic image with that of the traditional scanner. SPECT provides image information on the intensity of the scintigraphy and the precise anatomical location of the SLN(s) by scanner [44]. In the study by Naaman et al. [45], SPECT achieved a topographical accuracy of 91%, detecting a higher number of SLNs (1.4 vs. 2.13 SLNs/patient). Buda et al. achieved a detection rate of 50% and bilaterality of 39% for lymphoscintigraphy. For SPECT, the authors achieved a detection rate of 91%, bilaterality of 53% and sensitivity and a negative predictive value of 100% [46]. Compared with lymphoscintigraphy, the high sensitivity of SPECT seems to offer significant improvement in detecting SLNs and in the anatomical location [47, 48].

2.4 Surgical detection

The surgical SLN detection techniques can be applied to open surgery, laparoscopy and robot-assisted surgery [30], with overall detection rates of 60–100% [27]. Regarding the possibility of laparotomic detection, Mais et al. [49] used methylene blue (MB) as tracer and observed a significant difference between the laparoscopic pathway and laparotomy, with detection rates of 82 and 41%, respectively, although with the same false negative rate (FNR).

The mean number of SLNs detected per patient is 2.9 (95% CI 2.5 ± 3.3; range 1–8) [26]. In terms of location, Abu-Rustum et al. [50] reported 89% of SLNs in the territory between the external iliac, obturator and internal iliac areas, with 4% of SLNs in the paraaortic area and 6% in the common iliac areas.

2.4.1 Radiocolloid

The gamma emissions of the radiocolloid can be tracked intraoperatively by a portable gamma probe adapted to open surgery or laparoscopy [42]. The use of laparoscopic gamma probe increases SLN identification guided anatomically by the previous images of SPECT and lymphoscintigraphy [51]. The gamma probe emits a signal proportional to the radioactivity uptake (analogue [counts per second] and auditory), enabling the accurate localisation of the radiocolloid in the lymph node station [38]. The activity will mark this lymph node regardless of whether is it normal or pathological [38].

The radiocolloid is often used along with dye to optimise the detection rate and visual assessment [30]. Studies with only radiotracer are therefore few, with a detection rate in the range of 70–96% [6]. In the Detection Rate and Diagnostic Accuracy of Sentinel node Biopsy in Early Stage Endometrial Cancer (SENTI-ENDO) multicentre study, the long protocol with an injection of radiocolloid increased the detection rate of lymphoscintigraphy versus the short protocol (80.3 vs. 68.2%; $p = 0.02$). The paraaortic detection was more frequent in the long protocol, with no intraoperative differences [40]. There was a weak correlation between preoperative and intraoperative detection ($k = 0.3$) [40]. Other published data indicate good detection rates of 82% [6] and bilaterality with both protocols. While some authors use to perform another lymphoscintigraphy on the morning of the surgery [43, 52], with similarly poor improvement and weak correlation [22]. Other authors have proposed injecting the radiocolloid intraoperatively after the induction of anaesthesia, omitting the preoperative imaging and identifying the SLN directly with the gamma probe 30 min after the injection [36].

The disadvantages of this procedure include the high financial and staff costs, the risk of radioactive exposure and patient discomfort during the preoperative preparation. The advantages include the longer duration of the marking and fixation in the lymph node [15]. The technical limitations are related to the massive and diffuse uptake by the tissue, the interference caused in the gamma probe (which hinders the proper differentiation of the lymphatic tissue, especially in the parametrium and obturator area) and the uptake by the reticuloendothelial system (liver, spleen and bone marrow) [6, 27].

2.5 Dyes

2.5.1 Blue dye

The dye enables the visual identification of the SLN marked or not with the radioisotope. Several dyes have been used: 1% isosulfan blue, 1% MB and 2.5% patent blue. Isosulfan blue is a blue-green hygroscopic powder that is prepared by diluting it in sterile water. MB was created in 1876 and is the first fully synthetic drug used in medicine. Patent blue is a dark blue synthetic dye used as food colouring, and its intensity fades quickly when exposed to sunlight [36].

The detection rates with only blue dye are lower (57–62%), with a bilaterality of 56.1% (50–60%) [17, 53]. MB has lower diffusion but acceptable detection rates (57.5%, range 45–92%) and bilaterality (42.4%, range 50–60%) [54]. Nevertheless, when SLNB is applied to other cancers, such as breast cancer, the various dyes have shown accuracy and equivalence in SLN marking [36]. MB is preferred due to the extensive experience with this dye and its better toxicity profile. Due to the lower detection and given that the combination with ^{99m}Tc or ICG results in higher detection rates, MB is not recommended for use in isolation [21, 27].

After the blue dye is injected interstitially, it binds to the serum proteins and is filtered to the lymphatic vessels passing to the SLN, which will be stained in blue in approximately 5–10 min. This simple method requires no specific logistics, but the SLN must be identified at the start of the procedure before the dye vanishes or is displaced further along the lymphatic system and identifies a second nonsentinel step [36].

MB is more economical and safer than isosulfan blue. The half-life is 5–6 h, with mainly urinary and, to a lesser extent, biliary excretion. The recommendation is to use 2–4 ml of a 1% solution and to not take more than 10–20 min detecting the SLN due to the diffusion of the dye through the lymphatic tissue. A number of authors have estimated the mean procedure time, with an interval of 13.4 ± 6.2 min between the injection and visualisation and a SLN excision time of 17.4 ± 11.2 min [31].

Adverse effects related to the blue dye occur in 2% of cases [36]. The following effects have been reported: severe allergic reactions and anaphylactic crises (0.7–1.9%), thrombophlebitis at the injection site, tissue necrosis, haemolysis or paradoxical methemoglobinemia and serotonin syndrome in patients undergoing treatment with serotonin reuptake inhibitors [30, 55]. Patients and health professionals should be advised of transient colouring of the urine and the possibility of interference with pulse oximetry readings [36]. The use of the dye is contraindicated in cases of hypersensitivity (MD induced allergic reaction and methemoglobinemia), severe renal failure (dosage adjustments may be necessary as serum concentrations are increased in patients with impaired renal function) and glucose-6-phosphate-dehydrogenase deficiency (due to haemolytic anaemia when red blood cells are exposed to the chemical). The dye is not recommended for use during pregnancy or breastfeeding because the dye's safety has not been established.

2.5.2 Indocyanine green

Since the inclusion of fluorescence, the authors such as Holloway et al. [31] have replaced the radiocolloid and achieved equally good results. ICG is a tricarbocyanine dye with a short half-life of 3–4 min and hepatic excretion. ICG was developed by Kodak in the 1950s for use in photography and was approved by the US Food and Drug Administration in 1956 for IV administration [36]. The dye emits an intense blue colour detectable in real time when excited by laser in the near-infrared wavelength (range 750–900 nm, with an absorption peak at 800 nm) [6]. The high avidity by lymphatic tissue enables a high detection rate and accuracy compared with common tracers [4, 56, 57].

ICG has been used for years in laparoscopic and open surgery and in numerous other specialties (cardiology, general surgery, ophthalmology, vascular surgery, urology, etc.). The dye has recently been included in gynaecology. Lymph node mapping by fluorescence with ICG was first described by Furukawa et al. in 2010 in patients with cervical cancer. In 2012, Rossi et al. [58] applied ICG to 20 patients with cervical cancer or EC who underwent robot-assisted laparoscopic detection, achieving a detection rate of 85% and bilaterality of 60%.

The supposed benefits of this technology include high tissue penetration with low autofluorescence [59]. ICG has been shown to be superior to blue dyes, particularly in patients with obesity [30]. Following an interstitial injection, ICG is absorbed to the lymphatic system and travels quickly to the lymph nodes. ICG binds to plasma proteins and is excreted by the liver [36]. The dye lacks significant adverse effects. A single case of a severe allergic reaction after IV injection has been reported (incidence rate of 0.05%) [60]. However, the dye is contraindicated for use in patients with allergies to iodine [23, 56]. Nevertheless, given that iodine is a chemical element and an essential component of the human body, a number of authors have suggested the safety of using ICG in patients with iodine allergies, given that a type I allergic reaction (antibody-mediated and responsible for anaphylactic shock) will not occur [36]. The use of ICG in pregnant patients has been reported as safe [61].

To date, there has been no standard in the concentration and volume to be injected. Rossi et al. [58], Jewell et al. [62] and Holloway et al. [63] established the optimal ICG dose for detecting SLN at 1, 1.25 or 2.5 mg/mL in 4 mL [23]. Unlike ^{99m}Tc, ICG does not remain confined to a lymph node but rather diffuses rapidly through the lymphatic tissue towards the second step lymph nodes without losing intensity. It is therefore crucial to quickly start the search for the SLNs after the administration of ICG, without delaying the start of detection by more than 10 min [23], thereby reducing the risk of sampling too many lymph nodes [36], which limits the technique beyond 25–30 min of the injection [64].

Erikson et al. [65] compared the isolated use of ICG and MB in 472 patients, obtaining a higher detection rate (95 vs. 81%; $p < 0.001$) and bilaterality (85 vs. 54%; $p < 0.001$) with ICG. In 2015, How et al. [66] compared ICG, MB and ^{99m}Tc-nanocolloid, obtaining a higher detection rate (86 vs. 71%; $p = 0.005$) and bilaterality (65 vs. 43%; $p = 0.002$) with ICG than with MB and a similar rate (87 vs. 88%; $p = 0.83$) and bilaterality (65 vs. 71%; $p = 0.36$) to ^{99m}Tc. In 2016, Papadia et al. [67] published the results of a retrospective, multicentre comparative study between detection with the combined technique using radiocolloid and blue dye versus radiocolloid and ICG. The overall detection rate was 97.3% for ^{99m}Tc-blue and 96.9% for ICG ($p = 0.547$). The bilaterality was 84.1% with ICG and 73.5% with the blue dye; ICG was significantly superior ($p = 0.007$). In a series by Martinelli et al. [19] of 202 cases using ICG plus ^{99m}Tc as tracer, there were no differences in the detection rate (93.2%), and the bilateral detection was superior with ICG (72.8 vs. 53.3%; $p = 0.0012$). All of the authors (and many not mentioned here) agree that ICG offers the highest detection rates comparable to those of the standard ^{99m}Tc-blue technique but with superior bilaterality [11, 26].

ICG achieves greater diffusion; better visualisation; greater bilateral detection, which translates into a lower risk of lymphadenectomy (61% with MB vs. 39% with ICG; $p < 0.001$ [63]); a shorter surgical time and long-term financial savings and can obviate the need for an injection of radiotracer [68]. It was initially stated that ICG represented an increase in the number of resected SLNs, a finding that became standard with experience in the technique [69]. Therefore, considering its good toxicity profile, its ease of use and high effectiveness, ICG is the current tracer of choice [70]. The main disadvantage of ICG is that the NIR detection equipment is expensive, because it requires specific optical systems [71].

Advances in the fluorescence technique are ongoing. New NIR detection systems, such as the PINPOINT® Endoscopic Fluorescence Imaging System, specifically identify the uptake intensity with colour codes, such that the primary lymph node is differentiated from the secondary nodes, preventing the excision of nonlymphatic or canalicular tissue [72].

2.6 Combined method

The objective of the double injection method is to optimise the detection rate and bilaterality, given that single dyes (mainly blue dyes) have lower detection rates and bilaterality [27]. The recent systematic review by Cormier et al. [27] achieved superior results with a combination of two tracers. Various combinations have been applied.

2.6.1 Radiocolloid and blue dye

Results vary significantly; however, the conclusion is that a better detection rate (81 vs. 57%; $p = 0.01$) and bilaterality (54 vs. 28%; $p = 0.009$) are achieved with the combination than with the isolated application of each tracer [45]. The multicentre prospective study by the AGO group with 590 patients obtained a better detection rate applying the combined method of radiocolloid and patent blue dye (88.6 vs. 93.5%; $p < 0.001$). Other authors have achieved similarly improved surgical detection results by applying this double method, which has become established as the most appropriate combination of tracers. The review by Ruscito et al. [70] compared the detection by the combined technique (of ^{99m}Tc and MB) with ICG and achieved superior bilaterality with ICG and a tendency to a higher overall detection rate, without differences compared with the combined method.

2.6.2 Radiocolloid and ICG

How et al. [66] compared ICG and isosulfan blue with radiocolloid in a cervical injection in 100 patients with EC. The detection rate (87 vs. 88%; $p = 0.83$) and bilaterality (71 vs. 65%; $p = 0.36$) achieved with ICG and the radiocolloid were comparable to the data obtained with only an injection of ICG. In the meta-analysis by Lin et al. [73], the combined technique with ^{99m}Tc and ICG achieved a detection rate of 92% and bilaterality of 86%, results comparable to those using only ICG (91% and 78%, respectively).

2.6.3 Blue dye and ICG

The prospective cohort study by Holloway et al. [31] combining blue dye with ICG achieved a significant increase in the detection rate (87.8% with blue-ICG vs. 76% for blue alone), bilaterality (83.9% with blue-ICG vs. 40% for blue alone; $p < 0.001$) and detection of lymphatic metastases (21.1% with blue-ICG vs. 13.5% for blue alone; $p = 0.056$) versus the isolated injection of blue dye. In the study by Jewell et al. [62], lymphatic mapping with ICG detected the SLN in 95% of cases, with bilaterality of 79% and no statistically significant differences versus the combined use with isosulfan blue (detection rate of 93%, $p = 0.64$; bilaterality of 77%, $p = 0.8$). Other authors have reached the same conclusion as Jewell: the high effectiveness in the identification with fluorescence is not increased by blue dye. The combination therefore appears unnecessary, which would avoid an increased risk of adverse effects [54].

2.7 Triple tracer

There are few published studies on this subject. How et al. [66] concluded that the triple injection (blue dye, ^{99m}Tc and ICG) in the cervix (submucosa and stroma) provided a detailed mapping of the lymphatic canals, from the parametrium and presacral areas to the hypogastric vessels.

2.8 Paramagnetic tracer

New tracers are being applied. Recently, the Central-European SentiMAG multicentre clinical trial compared the use of the standard tracer (^{99m}Tc-nanocolloid and MB) with superparamagnetic iron oxide (SPIO) labelled nanoparticles, marketed under the name Sienna^{+}®. The preliminary results indicated comparable detection rates of 97.3 versus 98% with the same number of SLNs

Characteristics	^{99m}Tc	Blue	ICG
Economic cost	+	–	+
Technical complexity	+	–	–
Detection rate/ bilaterality	++	+	+++
Comfort for the patient	–	+	+
Need for specific equipment	++ (Radiopharmaceutical/ lymphogammagraphy/SPECT-CT)	–	+ (NIR detection hardware)
Adverse Reactions	– (1–6/100.000)	++ (2%)	– (<0.05%)
Lymphotropism	++	+	+++
Duration marking	24 h/+++	10–20 min/+	20–30 min/++

The score was assigned according to the following gradation: (–) = absence of the characteristic or negative evaluation, (+) = meets the characteristic or positive evaluation, (++) = complies being better; (+++) = it fulfils being superior. ^{99m}Tc = ^{99m}Tc-nanocolloid albumin; ICG = indocyanine green; NIR = near-infrared electromagnetic spectrum. Reference source: Papadia et al. [36].

Table 2.
Characteristics of tracers.

per patient and a tendency for the SPIO tracer to identify more metastatic SLNs, although further research is needed [34].

Table 2 shows a comparison of the main characteristics of the most widely used tracers.

3. Histological analysis

One of the main advantages that the SLN technique offers pathologists is the ability to select and minimise the number of lymph nodes to study, which enables a more exhaustive analysis and search for microscopic metastatic involvement.

3.1 Intraoperative value

Classically, the most widely used method for analysing SLNs has been the intraoperative assessment with haematoxylin-eosin (H&E) of imprint cytology performed in fresh samples and in frozen sections with rapid Diff-Quik staining. Intraoperative examination is questionable due to its limitations, both in the processing and in the results. Its success depends greatly on the collaboration between the surgeon and pathologist [74]. An intraoperative assessment can only examine a small portion of the SLN, has low sensitivity (56–67%) for the intraoperative detection of metastases and has an FNR of 20–30%, which makes the procedure inadequate and unsafe for the patient [75]. The results of Kim et al. [76] indicate an intraoperative understaging of 24%. For Ballester et al. [77], the rate was 43.7%, with little assessment of low-volume metastases. Additionally, the frozen sections distort the lymph node tissue, thereby precluding lymph node ultrastaging [30] and precluding the detection of micrometastatic involvement in the case of initially negative lymph nodes [75]. Currently, the guidelines of the National Comprehensive Cancer Network (NCCN) do not recommend the routine intraoperative assessment of SLNs, except when there is high suspicion and a nonsentinel lymph node [5]. However, other authors have emphasised the importance of intraoperative study to avoid reoperations, especially in high-risk tumours [78].

3.2 Ultrastaging

Conventional histological examination of a nonsentinel lymph node involves a single section along the lymph node's major longitudinal axis and H&E staining, with deeper levels or application of immunohistochemistry (IHC) at the pathologist's discretion [30].

Occasionally, the only evidence of extrauterine disease is the presence of metastases in the SLN. Considering the poorer prognosis associated with the detection of lymphatic metastases, a much more exhaustive analysis is justified [74, 79]. Therefore, pathological assessment by the ultrastaging of the SLN is the most important advance in the SLNB technique [80].

3.2.1 Histological ultrastaging and immunohistochemistry

The histological ultrastaging procedure includes a protocol for the series of microscopic examinations of the SLN block fixed and imbedded in paraffin, with the addition of the immunohistochemical analysis with cytokeratin measurement (pan-cytokeratin kits AE1/AE2 or anti-CK19), thereby increasing the sensitivity [80]. There are no formal evidence-based regimens for the pathology assessment of SLNs in EC, which entails considerable variability among institutions and, therefore, debatable results [30]. The study by Euscher et al. [81] compared two methods of ultrastaging by histological microsection, achieving increased detection of metastatic SLN in 32% of patients, with a mean metastasis size of 0.24–0.38 mm, with no differences in the detection rate by ultrastaging method. The algorithm proposed by the MSKCC consists of an initial assessment by H&E and, if negative, performing two adjacent 5-μm slices at two levels separated by 50 μm in the paraffin block, applying H&E staining and pan-cytokeratins AE1/AE3 in each slice [82]. Holloway et al. [48] performed three slices per level, two of which were then stained with H&E and one with AE1/AE3. Other authors have performed four levels with six slices at 40 μm intervals (levels 1 and 2 with H&E and levels 3 and 4 with AE1/AE3) or five levels (levels 1, 3 and 5 with H&E and 2 and 4 with AE1/AE3) [30] (**Figure 1**).

Cytokeratin-19 (CK-19) is a protein of the intermediate filament responsible for the structural integrity of epidermal epithelial cells, which in normal conditions is not expressed in the lymphatic tissue and is expressed abnormally in more than 90% of cells by EC [83, 84]. CK-19 is a biomarker directly related to the capacity for tumour dissemination in EC, with high sensitivity and a capacity for discriminating between metastatic and nonmetastatic lymph nodes or areas of lymphovascular invasion [84, 85].

Ultrastaging is a more complex procedure, requiring significant dedication, and has the added risk of high intraobserver and interobserver variability. The diagnostic categories of the American Joint Committee on Cancer (AJCC) are applied for breast cancer, with the following classifications for SLN: negative (<200 individual tumour cells or tumour cell aggregates <0.2 mm in size, including the presence of isolated cytokeratin-positive tumour cells [ITC]), micrometastatic (size ≥0.2 and <2 mm) (μM) or macrometastatic (>2 mm) (MM) [86]. The term low tumour volume includes the ITC and μM categories.

The ultrastaging of SLN has improved the validity of the technique and detects an additional 5–15%, with a high rate of low-volume lymph node disease (approximately 50% of patients with metastatic SLN), which would not be identified with the conventional technique. Ultrastaging represents an overall mean increase of 25% (range, 10–60%) in detecting metastatic lymph nodes [80, 84].

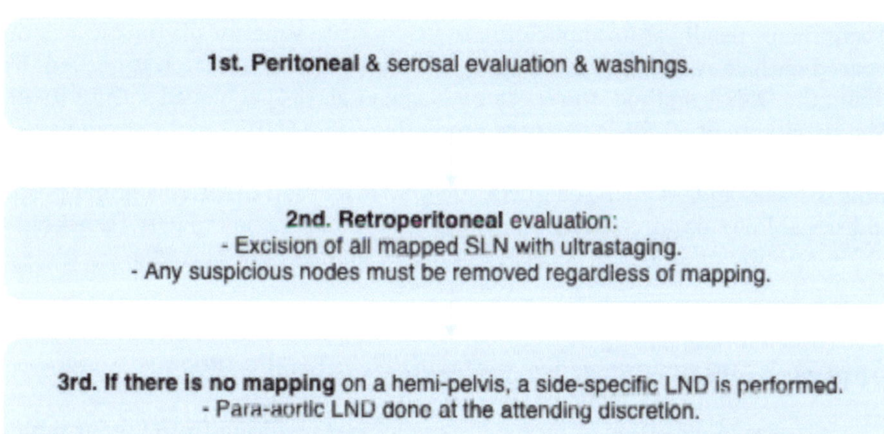

Figure 1.
The SLN algorithm for surgical staging of endometrial cancer. Obtained from NCCN Guideline in Endometrial Carcinoma, Version 4.2019: 'Principles of evaluation and surgical staging when SLN mapping is used, Figure 4: The SLN algorithm for surgical staging of endometrial cancer'. SLN = sentinel lymph node; LND = lymph node dissection.

Analysis by histological microsection and H&E detects 6.9% more patients with metastatic SLN, while the inclusion of IHC provides an additional 4.5% (82.6% with low tumour volume), which represents 12.6% of patients with metastatic SLN [82]. In the multicentre retrospective study by Raimond et al. [87] with 136 low-intermediate risk cases, the detection of SLN and the ultrastaging analysis increased the detection of metastatic lymph nodes threefold over lymphadenectomy (16.2 vs. 5.1%; $p = 0.03$); 11% of the cases were μM and 5.1% were MM, with an FNR of 0 (95% CI 0–1.6%). In the study, 6.1% of the metastatic SLN were detected by histological microsection, and 10.1% were detected by IHC. All MM cases were diagnosed by histological microsection, and 73.3% of the μM cases were diagnosed by IHC readings. Thus, by applying ultrastaging, the SLNB restaged 50% of the patients included in the study to an European Society of Medical Oncology (ESMO) high risk (14.7% of the sample), thereby changing the adjuvant therapy compared with women with negative or unassessed lymph nodes ($p < 0.001$). In the study by Hagen et al. [88], 75% of patients with metastatic SLN were detected with histological microsection and an additional 25% with IHC. For Desai et al. [89], 50% of the metastatic SLNs were detected by IHC.

3.2.2 Molecular ultrastaging

The one-step nucleic acid amplification method (OSNA) is a validated technique for breast cancer and enables a quantitative, systematic, automated, nonobserver-dependent analysis for detecting lymph node metastases [74, 84]. The application of this method always requires prior confirmation of CK-19 expression in the tumour tissue [90, 91]. The application of radiocolloid or dye does not interfere with the process. The number of mRNA copies of CK-19 corresponds to the size of the metastatic foci present in the SLN [92], such that the results are visualised in four separate categories: negative ($<10^2$ copies of mRNA/μL), ITC (10^2 to $<2.5 \times 10^2$ copies of mRNA/μL), μM ($\geq 2.5 \times 10^2$ to $<5 \times 10^3$ copies mRNA/μL) and MM ($>5 \times 10^3$ copies mRNA/μL) [93].

The results of the Breast Complete Lymphadenectomy OSNA Study for Enhanced Review-I (B-CLOSER-I) [94] indicate that histopathology (compared with molecular detection) significantly underestimates the rate of metastases of axillary lymph nodes.

Preliminary results of its application in EC indicate superior diagnostic accuracy compared with conventional ultrastaging, although further research is needed. By applying the OSNA method, the study by Nagai et al. [84] achieved sensitivity of 93.3%, specificity of 99.5%, a negative predictive value (NPV) of 99.5% and a correlation of 99.1%. In the study by López-Ruiz et al. [85] of 34 patients with chronic diseases and 94 analysed SLNs, the OSNA method detected a larger portion of additional low tumour volume metastases, with diagnostic capacity (sensitivity of 100%, specificity of 87.5%, accuracy of 88.3% and an FNR of 2.8%).

4. Approach and prognosis for metastatic sentinel nodes

The increase in detection of lymphatic metastases resulting from the introduction of ultrastaging is mainly at the expense of the detection of low tumour volume. The NCCN guidelines [5] and the consensus of The Society of Gynecologic Oncology (SGO) [30] recommend the study of SLNs by ultrastaging, indicating that the significance of low-volume lymph node involvement is still uncertain and have not established an optimal treatment approach [56, 95, 96].

A number of authors have debated and hypothesised a different tumour biology and therefore a different behaviour between tumours with MM and μM. For other authors, μM metastases appear early and are reflections of isolated metastases in type 2 histology but would be metastases of late evolution in tumours with low oncologic aggressiveness [97]. It has also been suggested that μM metastases could represent an *intermediate state* between negative lymph nodes and positive lymph nodes for MM [98].

One of the aforementioned advantages of the SLNB technique in early stages is avoiding the implementation of lymphadenectomy [87]. However, the therapeutic benefit of completing the lymphadenectomy when faced with the finding of metastatic SLN with low tumour volume remains unknown, and its systematic implementation is not justified [83, 98, 99]. The FIRES trial performed postoperative radiological studies (with scanner or positron emission tomography-computed tomography [PET-CT]). When the findings showed voluminous residual metastases, the proposed treatment was surgical cytoreduction or a change in the adjuvant radiation therapy (RT) to include the paraaortic area [75].

In recent years, research has been conducted on the possible influence of adjuvant therapy and the prognosis for patients with low-volume lymphatic metastases [100]. There is still no evidence from prospective randomised studies on cases with detected low-volume metastatic tumours, resulting in heterogeneity among the published studies [57]. Moreover, it is important to determine the benefit provided to these patients by combining CT and/or adjuvant RT, considering the scarce survival benefit obtained. The study by Plante et al. [101] analysed the impact of adjuvant therapy on survival. Thirty-five percent of the patients with ITC in the SLN underwent CT and external beam RT, 32% only underwent external beam RT or vaginal brachytherapy and 32% underwent follow-up. The overall survival at 3 years in the group with ITC was 95.5%, with no differences compared with the patients without metastatic lymph nodes or with μM in the SLN (87.6 and 85.5%, respectively). However, the low tumour volume SLN was superior to the SLN with MM (58.5%; $p < 0.001$).

Significant differences have not been observed between the prognosis of patients with only SLN excision versus those with lymphadenectomy (disease-free survival [DFS] at 3 years of 94.9 vs. 96.8%; $p = 0.35$). However, it has been observed that the patient group with metastatic SLN increases the portion of adjuvant therapy received (27.1 vs. 10.8%; $p < 0.001$) [102]. In the retrospective series by Raimond et al. [87], neither the absence of metastases in SLN, the detection of metastatic SLN nor the presence of μM in the SLN represented an improvement in DFS ([hazard ratio (HR), 0.89; 95% CI 0.42–1.90; $p = 0.77$], [HR, 0.82; 95% CI 0.18–3.64; $p = 0.8$] and [HR, 0.46; 95% CI 0.03–7.42; $p = 0.59$], respectively). When comparing negative lymphadenectomy with the detection of lymphatic metastases, there were no differences in DFS (HR, 1.13; 95% CI 0.34–3.76; $p = 0.84$) or overall survival (HR, 1.29; 95% CI 0.30–5.59; $p = 0.73$).

Yabushita et al. [92] showed that the detection of μM and SLN was an independent factor for recurrence in early stages of EC. Kim et al. [76] measured a tendency to late distant metastasis when the SLN was metastatic for μM. For Todo et al. [97], ITCs in the paraaortic area were not associated with a greater risk of nonlymphogenic or extrapelvic recurrence. For Kim et al. [76], these ITCs did not represent increased relapses. In the study by Erkanli et al. [103], DFS and overall survival were significantly lower in patients with μM ($p < 0.05$), while the presence of ITCs appeared to have no effect on survival. In another study by Todo et al. [104], the presence of low tumour volume was an independent factor for extrapelvic relapse (RR, 17.9), with 20% lower survival (overall survival of 71.4 vs. 91.9% and DFS of 55.6 vs. 84%; $p = 0.074$) and a tendency towards late relapse

Authors/trial	Journal, year	Injection	Tracer	N	SLN/case	DR	BL	Se	NPN	FNR	FN localization	DR PAO
						(%)						
Ballester et al. (SENTIENDO) [105]	Lancet Oncol. 2011	Cervical	^{99m}Tc + Blue	125	2	89	69	84	97	15	PAO[1]	5
Khoury-Collado et al. [79]	Gynecol Oncol. 2011	Cervical[7]	^{99m}Tc w/o Blue	266	3	84	67	78	93			
Barlin et al.[2] [3]	Gynecol Oncol. 2012	Cervical	Blue	498	3	81	51	98	99.8	1.9	PAO	
How et al. [106]	Gynecol Oncol. 2012	Cervical	^{99m}Tc + Blue	100	2	92	72	89	99	1	PAO	16.3
Raimond et al. [87]	Gynecol Oncol. 2014	Cervical	^{99m}Tc + Blue	304	2.5	87.2	65.4			0[3]		
Touhami et al. [78]	Gynecol Oncol. 2015	Cervical	^{99m}Tc + Blue	268	2	94	73.5	97.2	99.4	0.6[4]		
Hagen et al. [88]	Gynecol Oncol. 2016	Cervical	ICG	108	4	96	78			5.8		
Ehrisman et al. [107]	Gynecol Oncol Reports. 2016	Cervical	ICG or MB	36	2	83	56		92.3	7.7[5]		3
Holloway et al. [48]	Gynecol Oncol. 2016	Cervical	ICG + blue	780	3	98.3	80.7			2.8		9
Rossi et al. (FIRES) [75]	Lancet Oncol. 2017	Cervical	ICG	385		86		97.2	99.6	2.7		1
Plante et al. [101]	Gynecol Oncol. 2017	Cervical	^{99m}Tc + Blue or ICG	519	2.2			98.4	99.7			
Soliman et al. [108]	Gynecol Oncol. 2017	Cervical	^{99m}Tc + Blue or Blue or ICG	101	2	89	58	95	98.6	5[6]		2
	$\sum (\mu \pm \sigma)$			3490	2.3 ± 0.9	89 ± 5.5	67 ± 9.6	92 ± 7.6	97 ± 2.9	4.2 ± 4.5		6 ± 5.7
Bodurtha-Smith et al. Meta-analysis [26]	Am. J Obstet & Gynecol. 2016	Cervical or uterine corpus	Dye (MB or ICG) w/o ^{99m}Tc	4915	2.9	81	50	96	99.7			17
Lin et al. Meta-analysis[7] [73]	Oncotarget. 2017	Various	Various	2236	—	83	56	91				

The results of 13 methodologically comparable studies are cited; studies include more than a hundred of cases, except for the one of Ehrisman et al. [107] because it is one of the recently published studies that includes patients with high-risk endometrial cancer. The studies include cases with all histological type and two papers only high-risk cases, the one mentioned by Ehrisman et al. [107] and Soliman et al. [108] The average of the collected variables is estimated. Results of two meta-analyses, which have not been added in the estimation, are attached to the possibility that the previously mentioned studies were already included in their data. The word "Various" indicates that various injection methods or tracer combinations were collected. The blank box indicates that this information has not been mentioned in the article.

N = patients included; SLN = sentinel lymph node; DR = detection rate; BL = bilaterality; Se = sensibility; NPV = negative predictive value; FNR = false negative rate; FN = false negative; (+) = metastasis; w/o = with or without; (%) = proportion; Σ = summation; (μ ± σ) = mean ± standard deviation; ^{99m}Tc = ^{99m}Tc-nanocolloid albumin; MB = methylene blue; ICG = indocyanine green; PAO = paraaortic.

[1]All three FNR cases had nonendometrioid histology, one with paraaortic positive drainage. There were no cases of isolated paraaortic drainage.

[2]The data are reflected after application of the MSKCC proposed surgical algorithm. Without applying the algorithm: Se of 85.1%, VPN of 98.1% and FNR of 14.9%. One FNR case with isolated paraaortic metastasis.

[3]The estimation of the FNR is performed from the total of negative lymphadenectomies; it does not include negative SLN and positive lymphadenectomy, in which case it would be a FNR of 9.1%.

[4]The predictive capacity is estimated only based on cases with SLN detected bilaterally.

[5]Null FNR with Se and NPV of 100% after the retrospective application of the MSKCC algorithm.

[6]The FNR would be 4.3% after adjusting by MSKCC algorithm.

[7]Surgical detection with dual technique: radiotracer and dye. ICG increases the overall detection rate to 93% and bilaterality of 78%. Cervical injection increases Se to 93% and detection rate to 86%.

Table 3.
Analysis of recent studies: Detection rate, predictive capacity, false negative rate and paraaortic drainage of the sentinel node.

Authors/trial	Journal year	Injection	Tracer	N	SLN+	Single SLN+	LTV	ITC	μM	MM
					(%)					
Ballester et al. (SENTIENDO) [105]	Lancet Oncol. 2011	Cervical	^{99m}Tc + Blue	125	17		8.5	1	7.5	8.5
Khoury-Collado et al. [79]	Gynecol Oncol. 2011	Cervical (7)	^{99m}Tc w/o Blue	266	12		3			9
Barlin et al. [3]	Gynecol Oncol. 2012	Cervical	Blue	498	10					
How et al. [106]	Gynecol Oncol. 2012	Cervical	^{99m}Tc + Blue	100	11	44				
Raimond et al. [87]	Gynecol Oncol. 2014	Cervical	^{99m}Tc + Blue	304	16.2		11		11	5.1
St. Clair et al. [109]	Annals of Surg Oncol. 2015	Cervical	ICG o Blue	844	10.8		5.3	2.7	2.6	5.6
Touhami et al. [78]	Gynecol Oncol. 2015	Cervical	^{99m}Tc + Blue	268	16			4.5	2.6	8.9
Hagen et al. [88]	Gynecol Oncol. 2016	Cervical	ICG	108	16					
Holloway et al. [48]	Gynecol Oncol. 2016	Cervical	ICG + Blue	780	15.8	51.4	5.4	2.2	3.2	10.4
Ehrisman et al. [107]	Gynecol Oncol Reports. 2016	Cervical	ICG o MB	36	15					
Rossi et al. (FIRES) [75]	The Lancet Oncol. 2017	Cervical	ICG	385	12					
Plante et al. [101]	Gynecol Oncol. 2017	Cervical	^{99m}Tc + Blue o ICG	519	16.4		8.1	6	2.1	8.3
Soliman et al. [108]	Gynecol Oncol. 2017	Cervical	^{99m}TC + Azul or Blue or ICG	101	23	40	9.9	2.5	7.4	13.1
	$\sum (\mu \pm \sigma)$			4334	14.7 ± 3.5	45.1 ± 5.8	7.3 ± 2.8	3.1 ± 1.8	5.2 ± 3.4	8.6 ± 2.5

The results of 13 methodologically comparable studies are cited; studies include more than a hundred of cases, except for the one of Ehrisman et al. [107] because it is one of the recently published studies that includes patients with high-risk endometrial cancer. The studies include cases with all histological type and two papers only high-risk cases, the one mentioned by Ehrisman et al. [107] and Soliman et al. [108]. The average of the collected variables is estimated. The blank box indicates that this information has not been mentioned in the article.
N = patients included; SLN = sentinel lymph node; DR = detection rate; (+) = metastasis; LTV = low tumour volume (includes ITC and μM); ITC = isolated tumour cells; μM = micrometastasis; MM = macrometastasis; w/o = with or without; (%) = proportion; Σ = summation; (μ ± σ) = mean ± standard deviation; ^{99m}Tc = ^{99m}Tc-nanocolloid albumin; MB = methylene blue; ICG = indocyanine green.

Table 4.
Analysis of recent studies: proportion of patients with metastatic sentinel node, proportion of single metastatic sentinel node and distribution by type of metastases detected.

(49 vs. 16.5 months; p = 0.066) compared with the patient group without lymphatic metastasis. The conclusion of these studies is that the presence of μM can represent a prognostic biomarker in terms of survival, but whether the presence of ITCs should be used as such, regardless of other clinical-pathological risk factors, is still unknown [30] (**Tables 3** and **4**).

5. Recommendations for the clinical application of selective sentinel node biopsy

The published results of SLNB in EC have shown good diagnostic performance. SNLB is a promising and safe technique from the oncological point of view [10]. Given the mixed results, which have failed to show a therapeutic benefit [9], and the lack of long-term results [5], an appropriate interpretation is recommended [4, 29], considering SNLB a technique under study [79].

As with lymphadenectomy and adjuvant therapy, SNLB can be safely omitted for low-risk patients (endometrioid histology: IA G1, IA G2) [9, 56]. For intermediate-risk (endometrioid histology: IA G3, IB G1, IB G2) patients, SNLB has not shown a clear benefit in survival when performing systematic lymphadenectomy. This group does, however, have a greater risk of lymphatic involvement and typically undergo adjuvant therapy. SLNB in both patient groups has been shown to detect 2–3 times more cases of metastatic EC than lymphadenectomy, without changing the disease prognosis [87, 110]. These results justify extending the technique to low to intermediate risk, with the recommendation of including it in an algorithm or surgical protocol that includes the implementation when faced with failure of the technique. The potential benefit of detecting metastatic SLN in low-risk patients is however diluted by the low incidence of cases and the high proportion of low tumour volume. It appears we need to clarify the role of SLNB and the effect of low tumour volume, which is more frequently detected in this group [87, 110].

Two randomised clinical trials did not show that lymphadenectomy changed overall survival or relapse rates in high-risk patients [111–113], although retrospective series did show this change [114, 115]. The implementation of pelvic and paraaortic lymphadenectomy has been systematised due to the higher rate of lymphatic metastases and poorer prognosis associated with their detection. In contrast, sceptics of lymphadenectomy state that routine nodal assessment of high-risk patients rarely changes the recommendations for adjuvant therapy. EC (especially in high-risk cases) is not just a disease confined to the pelvis [51]. Patients with high-risk EC have a higher probability of recurrence and recidivism with or without detection of lymphatic metastases and should undergo systemic therapy regardless of the nodal state [116]. Nevertheless, published results on high-risk patients have shown no differences compared with those expected from studies that also include low- to intermediate-risk cases, with the same incidence of paraaortic metastasis estimated by lymphadenectomy. Survival data have shown no differences [30], which would assume that the benefit of SNLB in high-risk patients would be equivalent to lymphadenectomy alone [107, 108].

In terms of applying SLNB to high-risk patients, the greatest debate concerns paraaortic drainage, with a greater proportion of undetected metastatic paraaortic nonsentinel lymph nodes. A study by Naoura et al. [117] analysed 180 patients and achieved a much higher FNR in the high-risk group (2.3 vs. 20%; p < 0.001). In this study, it was much more likely that the high-risk subtype (7 vs. 28%; p = 0.03) and the nonendometrioid type (8 vs. 29%; p = 0.02) were poorly assessed.

The FIRES study [75] on 385 patients represents the largest prospective series to date and included low and high-risk patients, achieving a sensitivity of 97.2% and an NPV of 99.6%. Fifty percent of detected metastatic SLNs were in patients with low-risk EC, the most incidental group. Only 1% were isolated paraaortic metastases, with an FNR of 2.7%. Barlin et al. [3] and the FIRES study concluded that a pelvically located SLN could be sufficient for directing the treatment [75].

In light of these results and lacking a therapeutic benefit for lymphadenectomy, the current guidelines recommend that only pelvic SLNs should be determined (and with caution) in this high-risk patient group [5, 30]. Until there is better evidence, the recommendation is to perform systematic lymphadenectomy adding SLNB, which a number of authors have labelled as 'high-precision lymphadenectomy'.

To decrease the number of faults in the technique and the risk of underdiagnosis in high-risk cases, several research groups have performed PET-CT, excluding cases with peritoneal or lymphatic uptake [118]. Other authors have included postoperative scans or PET in cases in which the paraaortic lymphadenectomy was not completed [30]. Another option for managing high-risk patients includes implementing a combined injection pathway, ensuring both pelvic and paraaortic drainage.

The Selective Targeting of Adjuvant Therapy in Endometrial Cancer (STATEC) in the United Kingdom [30] and the Evaluation of Sentinel Node Policy in Early Stage Endometrial Carcinomas at Intermediate and High Risk of Recurrence (SENTIRAD) in France are two studies currently underway on high-risk patients, comparing the effect of SLNB versus systematic lymphadenectomy (bilateral pelvic and paraaortic) in high-risk EC in initial clinical stages. The STATEC study compares SLNB versus lymphadenectomy with the patient as the same control. The SENTIRAD study randomised patients to SLNB or lymphadenectomy, following an algorithm that performs bilateral pelvic and paraaortic lymphadenectomy when faced with a failure in detection or unilateral detection.

In 2014, the NCCN clinical guidelines assessed the technique as an acceptable alternative to systematic lymphadenectomy in selected cases [36]. In the latest edition, NCCN [5] (v.3.2019) accepted the technique as category 2A (based on lower level evidence with uniform consensus by the expert panel that the procedure was appropriate) and established a number of recommendations:

- SLN mapping may be considered
- The application of SLN mapping is appropriate for low intermediate-risk patients or those who do not tolerate standard lymphadenectomy.
- Recent evidence indicates that sentinel node mapping may also be used in high-risk histologies (serous carcinoma, clear cell carcinoma, carcinosarcoma).
- Cervical injection (superficial and optional deep) is a useful and valid option.
- The use of a radiocolloid with blue dye is recommended. The usefulness of ICG is admitted if NIR detection equipment is available.
- The key point in the normalisation of the technique is adherence to a surgical protocol.
- SLNB should be performed in institutions with experience in this procedure. The technique requires proper methodology and demands good anatomical knowledge and surgical ability. The MSKCC group recommends performing SLNB in centres with experience in endoscopic surgery and with an experience of at least 30 supervised cases during the learning process, with a specialised team that enables close collaboration between the surgeon and pathologist [32].

In the study by Papadia et al. [119], the implementation of at least 20 procedures decreased the number of SLNs obtained without compromising the FNR, improving the accuracy of the technique.

- The histological analysis should be performed by ultrastaging. Although the implication and proper management of low tumour volume are not known, its detection has a potential effect on staging.

- Lymphatic mapping implementation is contraindicated in uterine sarcoma.

Recently, the SGO published a first consensus on the application of SLNB in EC [30], which concluded with the following recommendations:

- Lymphatic mapping with cervical injection accurately predicts the detection of lymphatic metastasis, with an FNR <5%. In institutions with higher FNRs, the implementation of lymphadenectomy should be maintained (if it was previously indicated) until an FNR <5% has been ensured. Similarly, the SGO suggests adopting the indications of the American Society of Clinical Oncology applied to SLNB in breast cancer, such that lymphadenectomy is completed after SLNB in the first 20–30 cases. For low-risk patients, the recommendation is to increase the number of supervised cases during the learning process, given the lower risk of detecting lymphatic metastases [36, 120].

- The injection of radiocolloid and dye is acceptable. If ICG is available, it should be used instead.

- For patients with low- to intermediate-grade type I EC and tumour confinement to the uterus, lymphadenectomy can be skipped, performing only the SLNB.

- Although SLNB has been shown to increase the detection of lymphatic metastases, patients should be informed of the potential risk of undetected occult disease.

- The main demonstrated usefulness of SLNB is in detecting pelvic metastasis. The decision to perform paraaortic lymphadenectomy is at the surgical team's discretion, considering the patient's clinicopathological characteristics.

- Ultrastaging is recommended in the analysis of the SLN, although its involvement in detecting ITC requires more research.

- The application of SLNB to high-risk patients (type 1 G3 and type 2 histology) following the NCCN algorithm is feasible and has had good published results [30]. The combination of pelvic and paraaortic lymphadenectomy is reasonable until more safety and efficacy data for SLNB are available.

Abbreviations

CT	chemotherapy
CK19	cytokeratin 19
EBRT	external boost radiotherapy
EC	endometrial cancer

DR	detection rate
FNR	false negative rate
H&E	haematoxylin and eosin
HR	hazard ratio
ICG	indocyanine green
IHQ	Immunohistochemistry
ITC	isolated tumour cells
MB	methylene blue
MM	macrometastases
NPV	negative predictive value
OSNA	one-step nuclear acid amplification
PET-CT	positron emission tomography-computed tomography
RR	relative risk
RT	radiotherapy (includes EBRT y vaginal-cuff brachytherapy)
Se	sensibility
SLN	sentinel lymph node
SLNB	sentinel lymph node biopsy
Sp	specificity
SPECT	single photon emission computed tomography
vs.	versus
95%CI	confidence interval of 95%
^{99m}Tc	^{99m}Tc-albumin nanocolloid
μM	micrometastases
μ	mean
$\sum$	summation or total
σ	standard deviation

Author details

Begoña Díaz de la Noval
Consultant at Gynaecology and Obstetrics, Hospital Universitario Central de Asturias, Spain

*Address all correspondence to: begodelanoval@gmail.com

IntechOpen

© 2019 The Author(s). Licensee IntechOpen. This chapter is distributed under the terms of the Creative Commons Attribution License (http://creativecommons.org/licenses/by/3.0), which permits unrestricted use, distribution, and reproduction in any medium, provided the original work is properly cited.

References

[1] Tanis PJ, Nieweg OE, Valdés Olmos RA, Th Rutgers EJ, Kroon BB. History of sentinel node and validation of the technique [Review]. Breast Cancer Research. 2001;**3**(2):109-112

[2] Nieweg OE, Uren RF, Thompson JF. The history of sentinel lymph node biopsy. Cancer Journal. 2015;**21**(1):3-6

[3] Barlin JN, Khoury-Collado F, Kim CH, Leitao MM, Chi DS, Sonoda Y, et al. The importance of applying a sentinel lymph node mapping algorithm in endometrial cancer staging: Beyond removal of blue nodes. Gynecologic Oncology. 2012;**125**(3):531-535

[4] Bogani G, Ditto A, Martinelli F, Signorelli M, Perotto S, Lorusso D, et al. A critical assessment on the role of sentinel node mapping in endometrial cancer. Journal of Gynecologic Oncology. 2015;**26**(4):252-254

[5] NCCN Clinical Practice Guidelines in Oncology. Uterine Neoplasms. v4.2019 [Internet]. National Comprehensive Cancer Network (NCCN). Available from: https://www.nccn.org/professionals/physician_gls/pdf/uterine.pdf [Accessed: 24 September 2019]

[6] Smith B, Backes F. The role of sentinel lymph nodes in endometrial and cervical cancer. Journal of Surgical Oncology. 2015;**112**(7):753-760

[7] Torné A, Pahisa J, Vidal-Sicart S, Martínez-Roman S, Paredes P, Puerto B, et al. Transvaginal ultrasound-guided myometrial injection of radiotracer (TUMIR): A new method for sentinel lymph node detection in endometrial cancer. Gynecologic Oncology. 2013;**128**(1):88-94

[8] Pelosi E, Arena V, Baudino B, Bellò M, Giusti M, Gargiulo T, et al. Pre-operative lymphatic mapping and intra-operative sentinel lymph node detection in early stage endometrial cancer. Nuclear Medicine Communications. 2003;**24**(9):971-975

[9] Touboul C, Bentivegna E, Uzan C, Gouy S, Pautier P, Lhommé C, et al. Sentinel lymph node in endometrial cancer: A review. Current Oncology Reports. 2013;**15**(6):559-565

[10] Abu-Rustum NR. Sentinel lymph node mapping for endometrial cancer: A modern approach to surgical staging. Journal of the National Comprehensive Cancer Network. 2014;**12**(2):288-297

[11] Geppert B, Lönnerfors C, Bollino M, Arechvo A, Persson J. A study on uterine lymphatic anatomy for standardization of pelvic sentinel lymph node detection in endometrial cancer. Gynecologic Oncology. 2017;**145**(2):256-261

[12] Burke TW, Levenback C, Tornos C, Morris M, Wharton JT, Gershenson DM. Intraabdominal lymphatic mapping to direct selective pelvic and paraaortic lymphadenectomy in women with high-risk endometrial cancer: Results of a pilot study. Gynecologic Oncology. 1996;**62**(2):169-173

[13] Biliatis I, Thomakos N, Koutroumpa I, Haidopoulos D, Sotiropoulou M, Antsaklis A, et al. Subserosal uterine injection of blue dye for the identification of the sentinel node in patients with endometrial cancer: A feasibility study. Archives of Gynecology and Obstetrics. 2017;**296**(3):565-570

[14] Abu-Rustum NR. The increasing credibility of sentinel lymph node mapping in endometrial cancer. Annals of Surgical Oncology. 2013;**20**(2):353-354

[15] Sahbai S, Taran F-A, Fiz F, Staebler A, Becker S, Solomayer E, et al.

Pericervical injection of ^{99m}Tc-nanocolloid is superior to peritumoral injection for sentinel lymph node detection of endometrial cancer in SPECT/CT. Clinical Nuclear Medicine. 2016;**41**(12):927-932

[16] Niikura H, Kaiho-Sakuma M, Tokunaga H, Toyoshima M, Utsunomiya H, Nagase S, et al. Tracer injection sites and combinations for sentinel lymph node detection in patients with endometrial cancer. Gynecologic Oncology. 2013;**131**(2): 299-303

[17] Levinson KL, Escobar PF. Is sentinel lymph node dissection an appropriate standard of care for low-stage endometrial cancers? A review of the literature. Gynecologic and Obstetric Investigation. 2013;**76**(3):139-150

[18] Kataoka F, Susumu N, Yamagami W, Kuwahata M, Takigawa A, Nomura H, et al. The importance of para-aortic lymph nodes in sentinel lymph node mapping for endometrial cancer by using hysteroscopic radio-isotope tracer injection combined with subserosal dye injection: Prospective study. Gynecologic Oncology. 2016;**140**(3): 400-404

[19] Martinelli F, Ditto A, Signorelli M, Bogani G, Chiappa V, Lorusso D, et al. Sentinel node mapping in endometrial cancer following hysteroscopic injection of tracers: A single center evaluation over 200 cases. Gynecologic Oncology. 2017;**146**(3):525-530

[20] Perrone AM, Casadio P, Formelli G, Levorato M, Ghi T, Costa S, et al. Cervical and hysteroscopic injection for identification of sentinel lymph node in endometrial cancer. Gynecologic Oncology. 2008;**111**(1):62-67

[21] Zivanovic O, Khoury-Collado F, Abu-Rustum NR, Gemignani ML. Sentinel lymph node biopsy in the management of vulvar carcinoma, cervical cancer, and endometrial cancer. Oncologia. 2009;**14**(7):695-705

[22] Mais V, Cirronis MG, Piras B, Silvetti E, Cossu E, Melis GB. Intraoperative lymphatic mapping techniques for endometrial cancer. Expert Review of Anticancer Therapy. 2011;**11**(1):83-93

[23] Rocha A, Domínguez AM, Lécuru F, Bourdel N. Indocyanine green and infrared fluorescence in detection of sentinel lymph nodes in endometrial and cervical cancer staging—A systematic review. European Journal of Obstetrics, Gynecology, and Reproductive Biology. 2016;**206**:213-219

[24] Abu-Rustum NR. Update on sentinel node mapping in uterine cancer: 10-year experience at Memorial Sloan-Kettering Cancer Center. The Journal of Obstetrics and Gynaecology Research. 2014;**40**(2):327-334

[25] Kang S, Yoo HJ, Hwang JH, Lim M-C, Seo S-S, Park S-Y. Sentinel lymph node biopsy in endometrial cancer: Meta-analysis of 26 studies. Gynecologic Oncology. 2011;**123**(3):522-527

[26] Bodurtha-Smith AJ, Tanner EJ. Sentinel lymph node assessment in endometrial cancer: A systematic review and meta-analysis. American Journal of Obstetrics and Gynecology. 2016; **216**(5):459.e10-476.e10

[27] Cormier B, Rozenholc AT, Gotlieb W, Plante M, Giede C, Communities of Practice (CoP), et al. Sentinel lymph node procedure in endometrial cancer: A systematic review and proposal for standardization of future research. Gynecologic Oncology. 2015;**138**(2):478-485

[28] Mariani A, Dowdy SC, Cliby WA, Gostout BS, Jones MB, Wilson TO, et al. Prospective assessment of lymphatic dissemination in endometrial cancer:

A paradigm shift in surgical staging. Gynecologic Oncology. 2008;**109**(1): 11-18

[29] Khoury-Collado F, Abu-Rustum NR. Lymphatic mapping in endometrial cancer: A literature review of current techniques and results. International Journal of Gynecological Cancer. 2008; **18**(6):1163-1168

[30] Holloway RW, Abu-Rustum NR, Backes FJ, Boggess JF, Gotlieb WH, Lowery WJ, et al. Sentinel lymph node mapping and staging in endometrial cancer: A Society of Gynecologic Oncology literature review with consensus recommendations. Gynecologic Oncology. 2017;**146**(2): 405-415

[31] Holloway RW, Ahmad S, Kendrick JE, Bigsby GE, Brudie LA, Ghurani GB, et al. A prospective cohort study comparing colorimetric and fluorescent imaging for sentinel lymph node mapping in endometrial cancer. Annals of Surgical Oncology. 2017; **24**(7):1972-1979

[32] Khoury-Collado F, Glaser GE, Zivanovic O, Sonoda Y, Levine DA, Chi DS, et al. Improving sentinel lymph node detection rates in endometrial cancer: How many cases are needed? Gynecologic Oncology. 2009;**115**(3): 453-455

[33] Frumovitz M, Levenback CF. Is lymphatic mapping in uterine cancer feasible? Annals of Surgical Oncology. 2008;**15**(7):1815-1817

[34] Maccauro M, Lorenzoni A, Crippa F, Manca G, Chondrogiannis S, Giammarile F, et al. Sentinel lymph node biopsy in pelvic tumors: Clinical indications and protocols under investigation. Clinical Nuclear Medicine. 2016;**41**(6):e288-e293

[35] Holub Z, Jabor A, Lukac J, Kliment L. Laparoscopic detection of sentinel lymph nodes using blue dye in women with cervical and endometrial cancer. Medical Science Monitor. 2004; **10**(10):CR587-CR591

[36] Papadia A, Gasparri ML, Buda A, Mueller MD. Sentinel lymph node mapping in endometrial cancer: Comparison of fluorescence dye with traditional radiocolloid and blue. Journal of Cancer Research and Clinical Oncology [Internet]. 2017;**143**(10): 2039-2048

[37] Fishman A, Klein A, Zemer R, Zimlichman S, Bernheim J, Cohen I, et al. Detection of micrometastasis by cytokeratin-20 (reverse transcription polymerase chain reaction) in lymph nodes of patients with endometrial cancer. Gynecologic Oncology. 2000; **77**(3):399-404

[38] Chain Y, Illanes L. Radiofármacos en medicina nuclear. In: Fundamentos y Aplicación Clínica. 1st ed. Buenos Aires, Argentina: Universidad Nacional de la Plata, Libros de Cátedra; 2015. 188p

[39] Nanocoll Ficha Técnica y Resúmen de las Características del Producto [Internet]. Ministerio de Sanidad, Política Social e Igualdad - Agencia Española de Medicamentos y Productos Sanitarios. Available from: https://www.aemps.gob.es/cima/pdfs/es/ft/71080/71080_ft.pdf [Accessed: August 13, 2017]

[40] Frati A, Ballester M, Dubernard G, Bats AS, Heitz D, Mathevet P, et al. Contribution of lymphoscintigraphy for sentinel lymph node biopsy in women with early stage endometrial cancer: Results of the SENTI-ENDO study. Annals of Surgical Oncology. 2015; **22**(6):1980-1986

[41] Resino MC, Sánchez Hermosa C, Lapeña G, Pardo C, Ruibal A, Medina C, et al. Linfogammagrafía prequirúrgica para la identificación del ganglio centinela en el cáncer de mama. Revista

Española de Medicina Nuclear. 2016; **22**(6):410-417

[42] Frumovitz M, Levenback CF. Lymphatic mapping and sentinel node biopsy in vulvar, vaginal and cervical cancers. Oncology. 2008;**22**(5):529-536

[43] Niikura H, Okamura C, Utsunomiya H, Yoshinaga K, Akahira J, Ito K, et al. Sentinel lymph node detection in patients with endometrial cancer. Gynecologic Oncology. 2004; **92**(2):669-674

[44] Mucientes Rasilla J, Farge Balbín L, Cardona Arboniés J, Moreno Elola-Olaso A, Delgado-Bolton R, Izarduy Pereyra L, et al. SPECT-TAC: Una nueva herramienta para la localización del ganglio centinela en pacientes con cáncer de mama. Revista Española de Medicina Nuclear. 2008;**27**(3):183-190

[45] Naaman Y, Pinkas L, Roitman S, Ikher S, Oustinov N, Vaisbuch E, et al. The added value of SPECT/CT in sentinel lymph nodes mapping for endometrial carcinoma. Annals of Surgical Oncology. 2016;**23**(2):450-455

[46] Buda A, Elisei F, Arosio M, Dolci C, Signorelli M, Perego P, et al. Integration of hybrid single-photon emission computed tomography/computed tomography in the preoperative assessment of sentinel node in patients with cervical and endometrial cancer: Our experience and literature review. International Journal of Gynecological Cancer. 2012;**22**(5):830-835

[47] Perissinotti A, Paredes P, Vidal-Sicart S, Torné A, Albela S, Navales I, et al. Use of SPECT/CT for improved sentinel lymph node localization in endometrial cancer. Gynecologic Oncology. 2013;**129**(1):42-48

[48] Holloway RW, Gupta S, Stavitzski NM, Zhu X, Takimoto EL, Gubbi A, et al. Sentinel lymph node mapping with staging lymphadenectomy for patients with endometrial cancer increases the detection of metastasis. Gynecologic Oncology. 2016;**141**(2):206-210

[49] López-De la Manzanara Cano C, Cordero García JM, Martín-Francisco C, Sánchez Hidalgo L, Delgado Portela M, Haya Palazuelos J. Eficacia del Estadiaje Quirúrgico con Ganglio Centinela en el Carcinoma de Endometrio [Internet]. Comunicación Oral 31 Congreso Nacional de la Sociedad Española de Ginecología y Obstetricia, Sevilla-2011. Available from: http://www.sego.es/Content/pdf/CONGRESO_SEVILLA_2011/COMUNICACIONES/ONCOLOGIA/Files04/4.pdf [Accessed: 13 August 2017]

[50] Abu-Rustum NR, Khoury-Collado F, Pandit-Taskar N, Soslow RA, Dao F, Sonoda Y, et al. Sentinel lymph node mapping for grade 1 endometrial cancer: Is it the answer to the surgical staging dilemma? Gynecologic Oncology. 2009; **113**(2):163-169

[51] Bogani G, Martinelli F, Ditto A, Signorelli M, Chiappa V, Recalcati D, et al. Sentinel lymph node detection in endometrial cancer: Does injection site make a difference? Journal of Gynecologic Oncology. 2016;**27**(2):e23

[52] Farzaneh F, Moridi A, Azizmohammadi Z, J MA, Hosseini MS, Arab M, et al. Value of sentinel lymph node (SLN) mapping and biopsy using combined intracervical radiotracers and blue dye injections for endometrial cancer. Asian Pacific Journal of Cancer Prevention. 2017;**18**(2):431-435

[53] Vidal F, Leguevaque P, Motton S, Delotte J, Ferron G, Querleu D, et al. Evaluation of the sentinel lymph node algorithm with blue dye labeling for early-stage endometrial cancer in a multicentric setting. International Journal of Gynecological Cancer. 2013; **23**(7):1237-1243

[54] Sinno AK, Fader AN, Roche KL, Giuntoli RL, Tanner EJ. A comparison of

colorimetric versus fluorometric sentinel lymph node mapping during robotic surgery for endometrial cancer. Gynecologic Oncology. 2014;**134**(2): 281-286

[55] Methylene Blue 1% Aqueous, Safety Data Sheet [Internet]. LabChem—EE. UU. Available from: http://www.labchem.com/tools/msds/msds/LC16940.pdf [Accessed: 13 August 2017]

[56] Darin MC, Gómez-Hidalgo NR, Westin SN, Soliman PT, Escobar PF, Frumovitz M, et al. Role of indocyanine green in sentinel node mapping in gynecologic cancer: Is fluorescence imaging the new standard? Journal of Minimally Invasive Gynecology. 2016; **23**(2):186-193

[57] Cibula D, Oonk MHM, Abu Rustum NR. Sentinel lymph node biopsy in the management of gynecologic cancer. Current Opinion in Obstetrics & Gynecology. 2015;**27**(1):66-72

[58] Rossi EC, Ivanova A, Boggess JF. Robotically assisted fluorescence-guided lymph node mapping with ICG for gynecologic malignancies: A feasibility study. Gynecologic Oncology. 2012; **124**(1):78-82

[59] Frangioni JV. In vivo near-infrared fluorescence imaging. Current Opinion in Chemical Biology. 2003;7(5):626-634

[60] Hope-Ross M, Yannuzzi L, Gragoudas E, Guyer D, Slakter J, Sorenson J, et al. Adverse reactions due to indocyanine green: A case report and a review of the literature. Ophthalmology. 1994;**101**(3):529 533

[61] Papadia A, Mohr S, Imboden S, Lanz S, Bolla D, Mueller MD. Laparoscopic Indocyanine green sentinel lymph node mapping in pregnant cervical cancer patients. Journal of Minimally Invasive Gynecology. 2016;**23**(2):270-273

[62] Jewell EL, Huang JJ, Abu-Rustum NR, Gardner GJ, Brown CL, Sonoda Y, et al. Detection of sentinel lymph nodes in minimally invasive surgery using indocyanine green and near-infrared fluorescence imaging for uterine and cervical malignancies. Gynecologic Oncology. 2014;**133**(2):274-277

[63] Holloway RW, Bravo RAM, Rakowski JA, James JA, Jeppson CN, Ingersoll SB, et al. Detection of sentinel lymph nodes in patients with endometrial cancer undergoing robotic-assisted staging: A comparison of colorimetric and fluorescence imaging. Gynecologic Oncology. 2012;**126**(1): 25-29

[64] Surynt E, Reinholz-Jaskolska M, Bidzinski M. Laparoscopic sentinel lymph node mapping after cervical injection of indocyanine green for endometrial cancer—Preliminary report. Videosurgery and Other Miniinvasive Techniques. 2015;**10**(3):406-412

[65] Eriksson AG, Beavis A, Soslow RA, Zhou Q, Abu-Rustum NR, Gardner GJ, et al. A comparison of the detection of sentinel lymph nodes using indocyanine green and near-infrared fluorescence imaging versus blue dye during robotic surgery in uterine cancer. International Journal of Gynecological Cancer. 2017; **27**(4):743-747

[66] How J, Gotlieb WH, Press JZ, Abitbol J, Pelmus M, Ferenczy A, et al. Comparing indocyanine green, technetium, and blue dye for sentinel lymph node mapping in endometrial cancer. Gynecologic Oncology. 2015; **137**(3):436-442

[67] Papadia A, Zapardiel I, Bussi B, Ghezzi F, Ceccaroni M, De Ponti E, et al. Sentinel lymph node mapping in patients with stage I endometrial carcinoma: A focus on bilateral mapping identification by comparing radiotracer Tc99m with blue dye versus indocyanine green fluorescent dye.

Journal of Cancer Research and Clinical Oncology. 2016;**143**(3):475-480

[68] Laios A, Volpi D, Tullis IDC, Woodward M, Kennedy S, Pathiraja PNJ, et al. A prospective pilot study of detection of sentinel lymph nodes in gynaecological cancers using a novel near infrared fluorescence imaging system. BMC Research Notes. 2015;**8**:608

[69] Buda A, Passoni P, Corrado G, Bussi B, Cutillo G, Magni S, et al. Near-infrared fluorescence-guided sentinel node mapping of the ovary with Indocyanine green in a minimally invasive setting: A feasible study. Journal of Minimally Invasive Gynecology. 2017;**24**(1):165-170

[70] Ruscito I, Gasparri ML, Braicu EI, Bellati F, Raio L, Sehouli J, et al. Sentinel node mapping in cervical and endometrial cancer: Indocyanine green versus other conventional dyes—A meta-analysis. Annals of Surgical Oncology. 2016;**23**(11):3749-3756

[71] Buda A, Crivellaro C, Elisei F, Di Martino G, Guerra L, De Ponti E, et al. Impact of indocyanine green for sentinel lymph node mapping in early stage endometrial and cervical cancer: Comparison with conventional radiotracer (99m) Tc and/or blue dye. Annals of Surgical Oncology. 2015; **23**(7):2183-2191

[72] Lopez Labrousse MI, Frumovitz M, Guadalupe Patrono M, Ramirez PT. Sentinel lymph node mapping in minimally invasive surgery: Role of imaging with color-segmented fluorescence (CSF). Gynecologic Oncology. 2017;**146**(3):676-677

[73] Lin H, Ding Z, Kota VG, Zhang X, Zhou J. Sentinel lymph node mapping in endometrial cancer: A systematic review and meta-analysis. Oncotarget. 2017; **8**(28):46601-46610

[74] Guillén-Paredes MP, Carrasco-González L, Chávez-Benito A, Aguayo-Albasini JL. Aplicación de la técnica OSNA en el análisis intraoperatorio del ganglio centinela en el cáncer de mama. Cirugía Española. 2011;**89**(4):261-262

[75] Rossi EC, Kowalski LD, Scalici J, Cantrell L, Schuler K, Hanna RK, et al. A comparison of sentinel lymph node biopsy to lymphadenectomy for endometrial cancer staging (FIRES trial): A multicentre, prospective, cohort study. The Lancet Oncology. 2017;**2045**(17):1-9

[76] Kim CH, Khoury-Collado F, Barber EL, Soslow RA, Makker V, Leitao MM, et al. Sentinel lymph node mapping with pathologic ultrastaging: A valuable tool for assessing nodal metastasis in low-grade endometrial cancer with superficial myoinvasion. Gynecologic Oncology. 2013;**131**(3): 714-719

[77] Ballester M, Dubernard G, Bats A-S, Heitz D, Mathevet P, Marret H, et al. Comparison of diagnostic accuracy of frozen section with imprint cytology for intraoperative examination of sentinel lymph node in early-stage endometrial cancer: Results of senti-endo study. Annals of Surgical Oncology. 2012; **19**(11):3515-3521

[78] Touhami O, Trinh X-B, Gregoire J, Sebastianelli A, Renaud M-C, Grondin K, et al. Predictors of non-sentinel lymph node (non-SLN) metastasis in patients with sentinel lymph node (SLN) metastasis in endometrial cancer. Gynecologic Oncology. 2015;**138**(1):41-45

[79] Khoury-Collado F, Murray MP, Hensley ML, Sonoda Y, Alektiar KM, Levine DA, et al. Sentinel lymph node mapping for endometrial cancer improves the detection of metastatic disease to regional lymph nodes. Gynecologic Oncology. 2011;**122**(2): 251-254

[80] Altgassen C, Müller N, Hornemann A, Kavallaris A, Hornung D, Diedrich K, et al. Immunohistochemical workup of sentinel nodes in endometrial cancer improves diagnostic accuracy. Gynecologic Oncology. 2009;**114**(2): 284-287

[81] Euscher E, Sui D, Soliman P, Westin S, Ramalingam P, Bassett R, et al. Ultrastaging of sentinel lymph nodes in endometrial carcinoma according to use of 2 different methods. International Journal of Gynecological Pathology. 2017;**2**:1-10

[82] Kim CH, Soslow RA, Park KJ, Barber EL, Khoury-Collado F, Barlin JN, et al. Pathologic ultrastaging improves micrometastasis detection in sentinel lymph nodes during endometrial cancer staging. International Journal of Gynecological Cancer. 2013;**23**(5): 964-970

[83] Stewart CJR, Crook ML, Lacey J, Louwen K. Cytokeratin 19 expression in normal endometrium and in low-grade endometrioid adenocarcinoma of the endometrium. International Journal of Gynecological Pathology. 2011;**30**: 484-491

[84] Nagai T, Niikura H, Okamoto S, Nakabayashi K, Matoda M, Utsunomiya H, et al. A new diagnostic method for rapid detection of lymph node metastases using a one-step nucleic acid amplification (OSNA) assay in endometrial cancer. Annals of Surgical Oncology. 2015;**22**(3):980-986

[85] López-Ruiz ME, Diestro MD, Yébenes L, Berjón A, Díaz de la Noval B, Mendiola M, et al. One-step nucleic acid amplification (OSNA) for the detection of sentinel lymph node metastasis in endometrial cancer. Gynecologic Oncology. 2016;**143**(1):54-59

[86] Amoroso V, Generali D, Buchholz T, Cristofanilli M, Pedersini R, Curigliano G, et al. International expert consensus on primary systemic therapy in the management of early breast cancer: Highlights of the Fifth Symposium on Primary Systemic Therapy in the Management of Operable Breast Cancer, Cremona, Italy (2013). Journal of the National Cancer Institute. Monographs. 2015;**2015**(51): 90-96

[87] Raimond E, Ballester M, Hudry D, Bendifallah S, Daraï E, Graesslin O, et al. Impact of sentinel lymph node biopsy on the therapeutic management of early-stage endometrial cancer: Results of a retrospective multicenter study. Gynecologic Oncology. 2014;**133**(3): 506-511

[88] Hagen B, Valla M, Aune G, Ravlo M, Abusland AB, Araya E, et al. Indocyanine green fluorescence imaging of lymph nodes during robotic-assisted laparoscopic operation for endometrial cancer. A prospective validation study using a sentinel lymph node surgical algorithm. Gynecologic Oncology. 2016; **143**(3):479-483

[89] Desai P, Hughes P, Graebe K, Tchabo N, Heller P, Tobias D, Slomovitz B. Robotic Sentinel Lymph Node Detection (RSLD) for Patients with Endometrial Cancer (EC) [Internet]. ESGO eAcademy. 2013. p. 38305. Available from: https://eacademy.esgo.org/esgo/2013/18th/38305/brian.slomovitz.robotic.sentinel.lymph.node.detection.28rsld29.for.patients.html?f=m2 [Accessed: 13 August 2017]

[90] Ojima T, Kinami S, Nakamura K, Oyama K, Inokuchi M, Fujita H, et al. Advantages of the rapid double-staining method for intraoperative detection of micrometastasis in sentinel lymph nodes. Oncology Reports. 2013;**30**(3): 1067-1072

[91] Bernet L, Piñero A, Vidal-Sicart S, Peg V, Giménez J, Algara M, et al. Consenso sobre la biopsia selectiva del

ganglio centinela en el cáncer de mama. Revisión 2013 de la Sociedad Española de Senología y Patología Mamaria. Revista de Senología y Patología Mamaria. 2014;**27**(1):43-53

[92] Yabushita H, Shimazu M, Yamada H, Sawaguchi K, Noguchi M, Nakanishi M, et al. Occult lymph node metastases detected by cytokeratin immunohistochemistry predict recurrence in node-negative endometrial cancer. Gynecologic Oncology. 2001;**80**(2):139-144

[93] RD-100 OSNA, Folleto Informativo [Internet]. Sysmex España S.L. Available at: https://www.sysmex.es/fileadmin/media/f117/OSNA/OSNA_RD-100i_6p_ES.pdf [Accessed: 13 August 2017]

[94] Vegué LB, Rojo F, Hardisson D, Iturriagagoitia AC, Panadés MJ, Velasco A, et al. Comparison of molecular analysis and histopathology for axillary lymph node staging in primary breast cancer: Results of the B-CLOSER-I study. Diagnostic Molecular Pathology. 2012;**21**(2):69-76

[95] Colombo N, Creutzberg C, Amant F, Bosse T, González-Martín A, Ledermann J, et al. ESMO-ESGO-ESTRO consensus conference on endometrial cancer: Diagnosis, treatment and follow-up. International Journal of Gynecological Cancer. 2016;**26**(1):2-30

[96] Weaver DL, Krag DN, Manna EA, Ashikaga T, Harlow SP, Bauer KD. Comparison of pathologist-detected and automated computer-assisted image analysis detected sentinel lymph node micrometastases in breast cancer. Modern Pathology. 2003;**16**(11):1159-1163

[97] Todo Y, Suzuki Y, Azuma M, Hatanaka Y, Konno Y, Watari H, et al. Ultrastaging of para-aortic lymph nodes in stage IIIC1 endometrial cancer: A preliminary report. Gynecologic Oncology. 2012;**127**(3):532-537

[98] Morice P, Leary A, Creutzberg C, Abu-Rustum N, Darai E. Endometrial cancer. Lancet. 2016;**387**(10023):1094-1108

[99] Buda A, Guerra L, Signorelli M. Regarding: Pathologic ultrastaging improves micrometastasis detection in sentinel lymph nodes during endometrial cancer staging. International Journal of Gynecological Cancer. 2014;**24**(6):964-965

[100] Bats A, Clément D, Larousserie F, Le Frère-Belda M, Pierquet-Ghazzar N, Hignette C, et al. Does sentinel node biopsy improve the management of endometrial cancer? Data from 43 patients. Journal of Surgical Oncology. 2008;**97**(2):141-145

[101] Plante M, Stanleigh J, Renaud M-C, Sebastianelli A, Grondin K, Grégoire J. Isolated tumor cells identified by sentinel lymph node mapping in endometrial cancer: Does adjuvant treatment matter? Gynecologic Oncology. 2017;**146**(2):240-246

[102] Eriksson AGZ, Ducie J, Ali N, McGree ME, Weaver AL, Bogani G, et al. Comparison of a sentinel lymph node and a selective lymphadenectomy algorithm in patients with endometrioid endometrial carcinoma and limited myometrial invasion. Gynecologic Oncology. 2016;**140**(3):394-399

[103] Erkanli S, Bolat F, Seydaoglu G. Detection and importance of micrometastases in histologically negative lymph nodes in endometrial carcinoma. European Journal of Gynaecological Oncology. 2011;**32**(6):619-625

[104] Todo Y, Kato H, Okamoto K, Minobe S, Yamashiro K, Sakuragi N. Isolated tumor cells and micrometastases in regional lymph

nodes in FIGO stage I to II endometrial cancer. Journal of Gynecologic Oncology. 2016;**27**(1):e1

[105] Ballester M, Dubernard G, Lécuru F, Heitz D, Mathevet P, Marret H, et al. Detection rate and diagnostic accuracy of sentinel-node biopsy in early stage endometrial cancer: A prospective multicentre study (SENTI-ENDO). The Lancet Oncology. 2011;**12**(5):469-476

[106] How J, Lau S, Press J, Ferenczy A, Pelmus M, Stern J, et al. Accuracy of sentinel lymph node detection following intra-operative cervical injection for endometrial cancer: A prospective study. Gynecologic Oncology. 2012; **127**(2):332-337

[107] Ehrisman J, Secord AA, Berchuck A, Lee PS, Di Santo N, Lopez-Acevedo M, et al. Performance of sentinel lymph node biopsy in high-risk endometrial cancer. Gynecologic Oncology Reports. 2016;**17**:69-71

[108] Soliman PT, Westin SN, Dioun S, Sun CC, Euscher E, Munsell MF, et al. A prospective validation study of sentinel lymph node mapping for high-risk endometrial cancer. Gynecologic Oncology. 2017;**146**(2):234-239

[109] St Clair CM, Eriksson AGZ, Ducie JA, Jewell EL, Alektiar KM, Hensley ML, et al. Low-volume lymph node metastasis discovered during sentinel lymph node mapping for endometrial carcinoma. Annals of Surgical Oncology. 2015;**23**(5):1653-1659

[110] Jewell E. Chapter 76: Lymphadenectomy for endometrial cancer: Pro. In: ESGO Textbook of Gynaecological Oncology. Ankara, Turquía: Güneş, Publishing; 2016. pp. 660-664

[111] Panici PB, Basile S, Maneschi F, Lissoni AA, Signorelli M, Scambia G, et al. Systematic pelvic lymphadenectomy vs no lymphadenectomy in early-stage endometrial carcinoma: Randomized clinical trial. Journal of the National Cancer Institute. 2008;**100**(23):1707-1716

[112] Uccella S, Podratz KC, Aletti GD, Mariani A. Re: Systematic pelvic lymphadenectomy vs no lymphadenectomy in early-stage endometrial carcinoma: Randomized clinical trial. JNCI: Journal of the National Cancer Institute. 2009;**101**(12): 897-898

[113] ASTEC Study Group, Kitchener H, Swart A, Qian Q, Amos C, Parmar M. Efficacy of systematic pelvic lymphadenectomy in endometrial cancer (MRC ASTEC trial): A randomised study. Lancet. 2010; **373**(9658):125-136

[114] Todo Y, Kato H, Kaneuchi M, Watari H, Takeda M, Sakuragi N. Survival effect of Para-aortic lymphadenectomy in endometrial cancer (SEPAL study): A retrospective cohort analysis. Lancet. 2010;**375**(9721): 1165-1172

[115] Kim HS, Suh DH, Kim M-K, Chung HH, Park NH, Song YS. Systematic lymphadenectomy for survival in patients with endometrial cancer: A meta-analysis. Japanese Journal of Clinical Oncology. 2012; **42**(5):405-412

[116] Bendifallah S, Genin AS, Naoura I, Chabbert Buffet N, Clavel Chapelon F, Haddad B, et al. A nomogram for predicting lymph node metastasis of presumed stage I and II endometrial cancer. American Journal of Obstetrics and Gynecology. 2012;**207**(3):197. e1-197.e8

[117] Naoura I, Canlorbe G, Bendifallah S, Ballester M, Daraï E. Relevance of sentinel lymph node procedure for patients with high-risk endometrial cancer. Gynecologic Oncology. 2015;**136**(1):60-64

[118] Mayoral M, Paredes P, Domènech B, Fusté P, Vidal-Sicart S, Tapias A, et al. 18F-FDG PET/CT and sentinel lymph node biopsy in the staging of patients with cervical and endometrial cancer. Role of dual-time-point imaging. Revista Española de Medicina Nuclear e Imagen Molecular. 2016;**36**(1):20-26

[119] Papadia A, Imboden S, Gasparri ML, Siegenthaler F, Fink A, Mueller MD. Endometrial and cervical cancer patients with multiple sentinel lymph nodes at laparoscopic ICG mapping: How many are enough? Journal of Cancer Research and Clinical Oncology. 2016;**142**(8):1831-1836

[120] Lyman GH, Giuliano AE, Somerfield MR, Benson AB, Bodurka DC, Burstein HJ, et al. American Society of Clinical Oncology Guideline recommendations for sentinel lymph node biopsy in early-stage breast cancer. Journal of Clinical Oncology. 2005;**23**(30):7703-7720